KU-274-271

Contents

Contributors

Sally Anne Argyle MVB PhD CertSAC MRCVS
Royal (Dick) School of Veterinary Studies, University of Edinburgh, Hospital for Small Animals, Easter Bush Veterinary Centre, Roslin, Midlothian EH25 9RG

Sue Dallas CertEd VN
Walford and North Shropshire College, Baschurch, Shrewsbury, Shropshire

Paula Hotston Moore CertEd VN
University of Bristol, Langford House, Langford, Bristol BS40 5DU

Joy Howell DipAVN (Surg) VN
Bayer Animal Health, Strawberry Hill, Newbury, Berkshire RG14 1JA

Alan Hughes BVSc MRCVS
The Roebuck Veterinary Group. Roebuck Gate, Stevenage, Hertfordshire SG2 8HP

Jo Masters CertEd VN
Langport Veterinary Centre, Langport, Somerset TA10 9PS

Anna Meredith MA VetMB CertLAS DZooMed MRCVS
Royal (Dick) School of Veterinary Studies, University of Edinburgh, Hospital for Small Animals, Easter Bush Veterinary Centre, Roslin, Midlothian EH25 9RG

Elizabeth Mullineaux BVM&S CertSHP MRCVS
Quantock Veterinary Hospital, The Drove, Bridgwater, Somerset TA6 4BA

Dawn Platten VN
Cerberus Training and Consultancy, Yewgate Cottage, Remenham Hill, Henley-on-Thames, Oxfordshire RG9 3ES

Sharon Redrobe BSc (Hons) BVetMed CertLAS DZooMed MRCVS
Head of Veterinary Services, Bristol Zoo Gardens, Bristol BS8 3HA

Heather Roberts BSc (Hons) VN
Mypetshop Pet Resort and Care Centre, Topcliffe Close, Capitol Park, Tingley, West Yorkshire WF3 1BU

Freda Scott-Park BVM&S PhD MRCVS
Portnellan, Gartocharn, Alexandria, Dunbartonshire G83 8NL

Maggie Shilcock BSc CMS DipLib
Anmer, Norfolk

Jennifer Soloman-Kretay VN
Stevenage, Hertfordshire

Kim Willoughby BVMS PhD MRCVS
Virus Surveillance Unit, Moredun Research Institute, Penicuik, Midlothian EH26 0PZ

Foreword

This, the second edition of the *BSAVA Manual of Practical Animal Care*, provides an important introduction to those wishing to pursue a career in, and gain information about, the general care and management of those species seen in veterinary practice.

The first key chapter within the book gives an insight into the development of the veterinary profession and the qualification structure available to those who embark on a career within it.

The book provides a logical progression through the various aspects of the practical application of basic nursing care of patients within a veterinary practice, including first aid, preventive health care, nutrition, development and behaviour. This knowledge is vital for those working in a nursing capacity within the veterinary field.

Another key role within practice is that of client communication. The chapter written by Maggie Shilcock explores this fully from basic reception work through to dealing with euthanasia, ensuring the reader will have a sound understanding of this important role.

The book has been written by authors respected in their field and provides an excellent introduction to practical animal care. It is a valuable book presented in an easy to read format.

Andrea Jeffery MSc CertEd DipAVN (Surg) VN
Division of Companion Animals, University of Bristol,
Langford House, Langford, Bristol BS40 5DU

Preface

The first edition of this manual (the *BSAVA Manual of Veterinary Care*) was aimed at those with an interest in basic animal care and anyone wishing to work with animals in their career. In this second edition, we have deliberately focussed more on those working specifically in veterinary practice. The *BSAVA Manual of Practical Animal Care* has been written with the syllabuses of the Animal Nursing Assistant and the Veterinary Care Assistant qualifications uppermost in our minds, but also as an introduction to animal care for all those contemplating careers as veterinary nurses. The manual will also be useful for those members of the veterinary team, such as receptionists, administrators and kennel assistants who would like to learn more about the care of the patients in their practice.

As the first volume in a series of three, this manual is designed to complement the *BSAVA Manual of Practical Veterinary Nursing* and the *BSAVA Manual of Advanced Veterinary Nursing*, and to provide the ideal first step on a road which for many will hopefully lead to becoming a Registered Veterinary Nurse and even holder of the Diploma of Advanced Veterinary Nursing.

Eight of the chapters from the first edition have been extensively re-written, and the authors have worked hard to ensure that all the information provided is of real practical use and is presented in an accessible, stimulating and attractive manner. These, we believe, will prove to be an invaluable source of underpinning knowledge, essential for anyone beginning a career involving the care and nursing of animals. As such, they include the latest information on legislation and regulations governing health and safety in the veterinary practice and the dispensing of veterinary drugs. There are also two completely new chapters – one describing the increasingly complex veterinary world and the opportunities for caring and nursing careers within it, and another that discusses the vital skills and knowledge required when interacting with the owners of our patients.

A significant proportion of the authors of this manual are veterinary nurses. This is a reflection and recognition of the skill and expert knowledge now available in the veterinary nursing profession, and this is something that we, as editors, are very proud to acknowledge.

Without the help of a dedicated team at BSAVA the publication of this book would not have been possible. Our combined thanks are extended to Nicola Lloyd, Marion Jowett and their team at BSAVA – thank you all for your help in the presentation and editing of this book. We would both like to thank all the authors for their expertly written contributions.

Paula would like to thank Alasdair, Esme and Alice for their continued support. Alan would like to thank Janet, Daniel, Natalie and Alice, and all his colleagues at the Roebuck Veterinary Group for their patience and support.

Paula Hotston Moore
Alan Hughes

June 2007

An introduction to veterinary practice

Freda Scott-Park

This chapter is designed to give information on:

- The historical relationships between humans and animals
- The role of animals in modern society
- The organization of the veterinary profession
- The history of veterinary nursing
- A career in veterinary nursing

Relationship between humans and animals

Domestication of animals

Pets

Between 20,000 and 10,000 years ago, two species hunted the huge mammals that roamed on the sub-arctic tundra of Europe and Asia. The hunters were wolves and humans; both were much smaller and weaker than the species on which they preyed but the hunters were able to organize themselves into social structures that permitted hunting in packs. Over time it came about that the two species teamed up: for the wolf, human ingenuity and the use of weapons meant a share in a greater number of kills; for humans, the wolf's speed and ferocity were equivalent to a new weapon. It is suggested that the relationship solidified when humans nurtured and raised young wolf cubs and they adapted well to the rules of the hierarchical human society. It is thought that the majority of domesticated dogs are descended from wolves.

The earliest known evidence of a domesticated dog is a jawbone found in a cave in Iraq dated ca. 12,000 years ago. This evidence indicated a species of dog with a smaller jaw and teeth than a wolf. Images in Egyptian paintings, Assyrian sculptures and Roman mosaics showed that these civilizations nurtured many different types of dog. How closely they relate to modern breeds is unknown, but a dog recognizable as a Pekingese existed in China in the 1st century AD. Roman ladies around the same time had 'lap dogs', their warmth believed to be a cure for stomach ache. A Roman writer gave a fascinating insight into coat colour selection, with shepherd's dogs selected to have white tails to distinguish them in the dark from predator wolves, and farmyard dogs having black coats to frighten thieves.

Apart from the dog, the cat was the only domesticated species to dwell indoors with humans. It is not known exactly when cats became domesticated but the Egyptians considered them to be sacred animals and so they were probably adapting to live with humans from 3000 BC. Cats are solitary in the wild and as a result have remained closer to their wild cousins while accepting the comforts (food, shelter, warmth) that humans can provide. When human support is withdrawn they are generally well able to fend for themselves, whatever their environment – urban or rural.

Food-producing animals

The first animals to be domesticated as a source of food were sheep and goats and evidence for this comes again from the Middle East. At the time (9000–7000 BC) humans were nomadic pastoralists who moved in tribes with their flocks, driven by the need to find fresh grazing for their animals. These pastoralists no longer relied on hunting as a source of food; hunting was dangerous, the kill was not guaranteed and, if too much meat was produced by the hunt, it soon turned rotten in the absence of storage facilities. By keeping sheep, goats, cows and pigs, early humans provided a source of food-on-the-hoof, which could be killed when necessary to ensure a ready supply of fresh meat. Cattle and pigs were kept by more settled communities, probably from around 7000 BC. The relationship between people and their animals evolved as early humans found a use for almost every by-product of the food-producing animals: the dung provided fertilizer for crops, the wool and leather were used for garments, horn and bone were used to make tools (needles and arrows), the hooves made glue and the fat provided candles.

Working beasts

From ca. 4000 BC, cattle were not always slaughtered to provide food but they were milked and also put to work in harness. By pulling wagons they enabled people to start moving equipment and crops over greater distances. By dragging a plough they allowed the cultivation of much larger tracts of land, with increases in the yields of wheat and rice. Mechanization is now worldwide but there remain countries where the terrain is unsuitable for tractors or where the economy cannot support the purchase of expensive machines and so horses and oxen are still used to work the land.

Transport

When the horse was domesticated in approximately 3000 BC it provided yet another food source but, more importantly, allowed humans to move great distances very quickly. The first horses (those that would now be called ponies) were tamed on the steppes of central Asia some 5000 years ago. Small horses of this kind were discovered in Mongolia in the 1870s and named Przewalski's horse; they now only survive in zoos. The entire range of horses from the carthorse to the tiny Shetland pony have arisen from human breeding programmes. Donkeys were tamed where they roamed wild in northern Africa and ridden or used as beasts of burden in Egypt. Both the horse from the north and the donkey from the south became available to the earliest civilizations in Mesopotamia and Egypt.

Other beasts of burden and transport are camels, llamas and alpacas. Llamas and alpacas were domesticated around 3000 BC in South America; however, neither was strong enough to pull a plough or drag a cart and this was a disadvantage to the South Americans. Camels were probably domesticated sometime around 1500 BC and both species (the single-humped Arabian and the double-humped Bactrian) became important transport animals, with an ability to resist dehydration by absorbing water from the fat stored in their humps.

Other food sources

It is probable that all poultry are descended from the red jungle fowl, which was kept for eggs and meat in Thailand and Indonesia some 8000 years ago. Pigeons were kept as a food source by the Egyptians in 2000 BC and it was not until 3000 years later that their other talent was discovered – they could be trained to fly home. From the 1st century AD rabbits were considered to be a good food source and were kept when they could be in domestication, but rabbits were able to burrow and then often destroyed crops. Many rabbits were placed on islands as a food source for passing ships. Now rabbits are the third most popular pet after cats and dogs.

A child's pet

In 1930 a female hamster with twelve young was captured in Syria and taken to a laboratory, where the animals were bred for experiments. Each female had several litters per year and the numbers grew. It was not long before someone noticed that this tiny creature with its puffed-out cheeks would make a wonderful children's pet. All golden hamsters are descended from this single Syrian hamster.

The role of animals in modern society

Rural communities

The British countryside is a patchwork of fields, woodland, rivers and hills and moorland. The reason that the countryside looks as it does is mainly because of farming practices; crops and animals are important contributors both to the landscape and to the rural economy.

Rural communities are diverse and are facing substantial change as agriculture has declined in importance and prices for farm produce have been driven down by wider economic forces. The reform of the Common Agricultural Policy and the introduction of the Single Farm Payment in 2005 required farmers to ensure their animals' health and welfare and to keep their farms in good agricultural and environmental condition (GAEC). Farm incomes remain static in real terms and many farmers are opting out of agriculture, choosing instead to claim their Single Farm Payment for maintaining their land in good condition without keeping animals.

This decline in agriculture has meant that farms and estates are less able to employ the numbers of staff that were once considered necessary to run the enterprises and many rural properties are available, allowing people to move out of the towns. Once the exclusive preserve of rural communities wholly employed in land-based occupations, the countryside is now becoming an extension of the city.

Dogs in sport

Traditional mounted foxhunting in England and Wales has a relatively short history. Although King Edward I had a royal pack of foxhounds in the 13th century, it was not until several centuries later that foxhunting was taken up by the rest of the nobility.

One of the biggest changes in the countryside to occur in recent years is the ban on hunting with dogs that was introduced in 2003. Hunting played an important role in the social and cultural life of some rural communities. There were many different types of hunt, depending on the prey pursued – foxes, stags, hares and mink – and they all had dedicated registered and non-registered dog packs. It was generally accepted before the ban that the hunt played a part in population control of the species involved. Since the ban, some hunts have closed or contracted; others have retrained their dogs to diversify into related activities such as drag hunting and bloodhound hunting.

Lurchers and other 'long dogs' have been used for pest control by farmers and gamekeepers for many years. Terrier work (digging out and bolting) was also practised by gangs of terrier men as a sport or in response to requests for help in pest control.

The origins of hare coursing go back to the Egyptian and Greek empires and the sport was probably introduced to Britain by the Romans. It became very popular in the late 19th and early 20th centuries, when there were approximately 300 coursing clubs. There are now some 24 greyhound coursing clubs affiliated to the National Coursing Club, as well as clubs for other breeds such as whippets and salukis. An extension to hare coursing is greyhound racing (Figure 1.1): six greyhounds make up the race and the speed at which they travel is breathtaking. The sport began in 1926 and now attracts attendances of four million viewers per year.

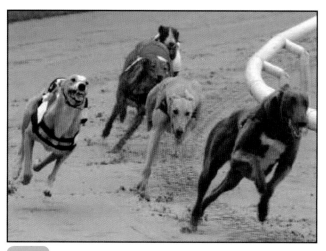

1.1 Greyhound racing.

Companion animals

Many city workers now live in the countryside and commute to work on a daily basis or have country weekend retreats. With this relocation of population, there has been a marked shift in the predominant breeds of dogs in the countryside from mainly working dogs (sheepdogs, terriers, foxhounds, beagles, bassets, harriers and gundogs) to pets of every shape and size.

Concurrently there is a huge increase in the number of farm animals kept as companions: pigs, goats, sheep, poultry, llamas and alpacas (see *BSAVA Manual of Farm Pets*). Horses are kept mainly for personal pleasure and used in competitions. Thus, as farmers leave agriculture a new population is taking up hobby farming and the diversity of animals in the countryside continues to provide work for veterinary practices.

The value of the companion animal is often underestimated by those who do not understand the benefits of owning a pet. A growing body of scientific opinion recognizes that companion animals have an important role to play in human health and wellbeing.

Work in the 1960s showed that human psychiatric patients became less withdrawn and were able to be better rehabilitated when they owned a pet. Cats, dogs and fish introduced into nursing homes have been used to improve the general atmosphere and quality of life of patients and the elderly.

Wildlife and conservation

The British countryside has a wide variety of wild birds, mammals, reptiles, amphibians and fish. Unfortunately many of these species are brought injured, apparently abandoned or diseased to the veterinary practice by the general public. Many wildlife casualties can be cured but the dilemma comes when the veterinary surgeon has to decide whether it is correct to intervene. The *BSAVA Manual of Wildlife Casualties* suggests that veterinary medicine should not be used to prevent or treat diseases in wild animals living in their natural state. However, it is suggested that it is a different matter when the disease or injury is caused by human agency. Provided that the veterinary care does not further compromise the animal's welfare, it seems to be justifiable to treat the problem.

Rehabilitation centres are found throughout the country and vary considerably in their practical and human resources. Many are one-man bands run out of a garden shed but the level of care and expertise often matches that of a large purpose-built centre.

There is an obligation laid on veterinary surgeons to provide care as long as a clinical assessment justifies the stress to the animal while it is in captivity and allows for a return to the wild. If these conditions cannot be met, euthanasia may be the best and kindest option.

Working dogs

An illustration of the mutual benefits of the human–animal bond can be found in the highly developed teamwork required by working dogs and their handlers. Police dogs are trained to detect, for example, drugs and items of forensic importance. Search-and-rescue dogs locate casualties in the mountains and urban disaster environments far more quickly than human searchers alone. Military working dogs (Figures 1.2 and 1.3) are employed in many roles to protect the armed forces, for

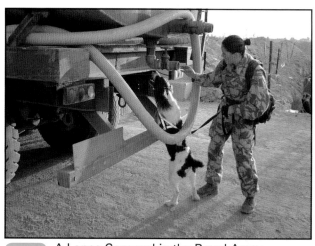

1.2 A Lance Corporal in the Royal Army Veterinary Corps, with her 'Search' dog, checking out a tanker at a permanent vehicle check point.

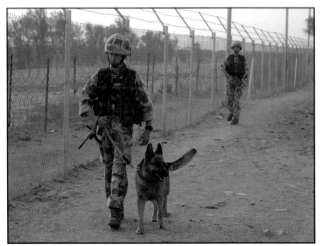

1.3 A Lance Corporal in the Royal Army Veterinary Corps, with his 'Protection' dog, patrolling a perimeter fence.

example by giving warning of ambushes in the jungle or by searching for weapons, ammunition or other terrorist materials. Many such dogs are donated by members of the public because they cannot meet the commitment that dog ownership demands. The quality of the dogs' lives is often transformed by the fulfilment of working for reward and the relationship they develop with their handler. At the same time the results they achieve contribute immeasurably to society.

The veterinary profession

Royal College of Veterinary Surgeons (RCVS)

The RCVS is the regulatory body for veterinary surgeons in the UK. Its roles are:

- To safeguard the health and welfare of animals committed to veterinary care through the regulation of the educational, ethical and clinical standards of the veterinary profession, thereby protecting the interests of those dependent on animals and assuring public health
- To act as an impartial source of informed opinion on animal health and welfare issues and their interaction with human health.

The RCVS is made up of three distinct organizations with different roles: as a statutory regulator; as a Royal College; and as a charitable Trust.

Statutory regulator

The RCVS was established in 1844 by Royal Charter to be the governing body of the veterinary profession. Its statutory duties, currently laid out in the Veterinary Surgeons Act 1966, are:

- To maintain a register of veterinary surgeons eligible to practise in the UK
- To regulate veterinary education
- To regulate professional conduct.

The RCVS safeguards the interests of the public and animals by ensuring that only those registered with the RCVS can carry out acts of veterinary surgery.

In order to carry out its statutory duties, a Council of 40 Members governs the RCVS and meets three times a year. Council is supported by a system of Committees. RCVS policy issues put forward by working parties or the secretariat go first to Committees for recommendation and, if recommended, on to Council for approval or rejection.

The President, Senior Vice-President, Junior Vice-President and Treasurer are elected by Council from its number. Together with the Registrar, they form a team of Officers and have the main responsibility for running the RCVS.

RCVS Veterinary Nurses Council

The RCVS Veterinary Nurses Council was established in 2002 and replaced the Veterinary Nurses Committee. It has overall responsibility for all matters concerning veterinary nurse training, post-qualification awards and the registration (listing) of qualified veterinary nurses. The Veterinary Nurses Council comprises elected veterinary nurses, appointed veterinary surgeons (RCVS Council members and non-Council members), lay members and Industry Group representatives.

Royal College

The RCVS as a 'Royal College' exercises powers under the Royal Charter to award Fellowships, Diplomas and Certificates to veterinary surgeons, veterinary nurses and others, and to act as an informed and impartial source of opinion on veterinary matters.

RCVS Trust

The Trust is a separate charity established to promote and advance the study and practice of the art and science of veterinary surgery and medicine, by providing the RCVS Library and Information Service and a range of grants, largely to support educational and research activities.

British Veterinary Association (BVA)

The BVA is the national representative body for the veterinary profession. Although membership is voluntary there are over 10,000 members and the Association has evolved, over 118 years, into the public relations house for the profession at home and overseas. In promoting the interests of members and the animals under their care, the BVA is committed to developing and maintaining channels of communication with the RCVS, Government, parliamentarians and the media.

It is important to distinguish between the BVA and the Royal College of Veterinary Surgeons. The RCVS is a *statutory* body set up to administer the Veterinary Surgeons Act and as such is responsible for the registration, education and discipline of the profession. The BVA is a *representative* body and must act to support the needs of its members. The BVA also provides a media and parliamentary information service and maintains a list of Honorary Associates, the majority of whom are MPs and peers who can be lobbied on matters that affect the profession.

The business of the BVA is driven through three committees:

- Veterinary Policy Group: drives policy initiatives forward (e.g. guidance on avian influenza, a policy document on bovine tuberculosis)
- Member Services Group: provides services for BVA members (e.g. practice insurance, health insurance, reduced travel rates)
- Ethics Committee: considers the ethical issues relating to society's use of animals. It prioritizes the issues that the profession should address and recommends policy development where necessary. It is not concerned with professional ethics; that is the role of the Royal College of Veterinary Surgeons.

The BVA Council is made up of representatives of the specialist divisions, such as the British Small Animal Veterinary Association, the British Cattle Veterinary Association and the Fish Veterinary Society, as well as the territorial divisions, such as West of Scotland, the Essex Veterinary Society and so on. In total the BVA can call on 52 specialist and territorial divisions for opinion and comment.

BVA Animal Welfare Foundation (BVA AWF)

The BVA also has its own charity, the BVA AWF. The principal aim of the Foundation is to apply the knowledge, skill and compassion of veterinary surgeons in an effective way through a variety of projects and activities. Through veterinary science, education and debate, the BVA AWF is committed to finding practical solutions to the welfare problems of all animals, and then disseminating this information amongst veterinary practitioners, nurses, students, farmers, animal care workers and the general public.

British Small Animal Veterinary Association (BSAVA)

The BSAVA exists to promote high scientific and educational standards of small animal medicine and surgery in practice, teaching and research. The Association encourages veterinary surgeons to develop their professional skills and runs numerous continuing education courses and seminars throughout the UK. It holds the biggest annual small animal conference in the world, attracting over 7000 delegates.

Through its charity Petsavers the BSAVA funds clinical investigations into the diseases of companion animals.

British Equine Veterinary Association (BEVA)

The BEVA promotes veterinary and allied sciences related to horse welfare and provides a forum for discussion and exchange of ideas on the management, health and diseases of the horse.

Private practice

Most veterinary surgeons graduate from university intending to work in general practice, with many new graduates looking for a position in a mixed practice. A mixed practice is one that treats both large animals (farm animals and horses) and small animals (dogs, cats, rabbits and other small pets and birds). By working in a truly mixed practice the new graduate is able to gain experience in a wide range of species and to use all their newly acquired knowledge before deciding whether to specialize in a particular species or in one particular area (e.g. orthopaedics, internal medicine, dermatology). There are many veterinary surgeons who specialize in, say, just horses or just cats.

Historically, large animal practice was the backbone of the profession and it was unusual for a veterinary surgeon to specialize in small animals. With the downturn in farm economics, there has been a complete reversal of this situation and the majority of practices now treat small animals, either exclusively or as the main income generator in a mixed practice. Few large animal practices survive and there are many areas of the country – both in rural areas and on the urban fringes – where veterinary cover for farm animals is lacking.

Government veterinary surgeons

Government veterinary surgeons work in a number of different spheres and in different departments and agencies where the work is varied and often very challenging. The Veterinary Head of Profession within the Civil Service is called the Chief Veterinary Officer (CVO), supported in this role by a Veterinary Professional Unit (VPU), which is located within the Department for Environment, Food & Rural Affairs (Defra). Defra and its agencies employ the largest number of veterinary surgeons within the Civil Service, including those in the following departments:

- Animal Health (formerly State Veterinary Service, SVS)
- Food Standards Agency (FSA)
- Meat Hygiene Service (MHS)
- Ministry of Defence (MOD)
- Home Office
- Centre for Environment, Fisheries and Aquaculture Science (CEFAS)
- Department for International Development (DFID)
- Veterinary Laboratories Agency (VLA)
- Department of Agriculture and Rural Development in Northern Ireland (DARDNI)
- Scottish Executive Environment and Rural Affairs Department (SEERAD)
- Veterinary Medicines Directorate (VMD).

Charities

Many animal charities employ veterinary surgeons to help care for the animals that they work with. Among those charities, the People's Dispensary for Sick Animals (PDSA) employs approximately 200 veterinary surgeons and nearly 250 veterinary nurses across the country, while the Blue Cross has four animal hospitals that provide top-quality veterinary care to pets whose owners cannot afford private animal care.

Armed forces

Army Veterinary Officers (VOs) provide preventive care and treatment wherever military working animals (MWAs) are deployed in support of military operations, often in challenging and hostile environments. The Royal Army Veterinary Corps (RAVC) is a small Corps and its manpower is sufficient only to deliver operational capability and essential military training. In peacetime, the most appropriate and cost-effective source of veterinary support, to those MWAs that are employed far from a military veterinary facility, is often the local civilian veterinary practice.

The horses of the Household Cavalry and The King's Troop Royal Horse Artillery are familiar sights in London. Military horses, once the source of the Army's mobility, are now used only for ceremonial purposes, but for over 200 years the Army Veterinary Service has been responsible for their health and welfare.

These days, the dog has become the species of greatest military importance and the versatility of dogs and their willingness to please make them ideal partners in force protection. Soldiers on patrol at night with a dog know that they can never be taken by surprise, so acute are the dog's senses. In search operations, the dog's sense of smell is capable of rapidly and safely locating small, hidden but potentially lethal quantities of terrorist materials such as arms and explosives. The Veterinary Officers, Veterinary Technicians and Dog Trainers of the RAVC supervise every aspect of the lives of service animals: procurement, training, health and employment (Figure 1.4). When animals eventually retire from the services, their continuing welfare is also carefully arranged.

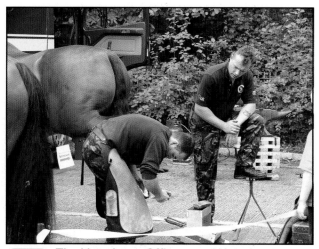

1.4 The Veterinary Officers and Veterinary Technicians of the Royal Army Veterinary Corps supervise every aspect of the lives of service animals and are responsible for their health and welfare.

Veterinary surgeons in industry

There are many different roles for veterinary surgeons within the pharmaceutical and animal food industries. Veterinary surgeons may become company representatives and their communication skills in marketing and sales bring veterinary products to the attention of the profession. Pharmaceutical company employees are engaged in a wide variety of tasks. Veterinary surgeons may be at the forefront of research as veterinary scientists who work at the cutting edge of science and technology, using and developing state-of-the-art techniques to provide the medicines of the future. They may be employed in

pharmaceutical and academic research establishments as Named Veterinary Surgeons, looking after the health and welfare of animals used in research.

Academia

Universities have been instrumental in shaping history for over 400 years and offer opportunities to work in a vibrant, research-led academic community. University veterinary staff teach students, conduct research programmes and contribute to wider continuing professional development of the profession by lecturing at regional, national and international meetings. Veterinary surgeons also teach veterinary nurses in colleges of further or higher education.

Zoos and conservation

Veterinary surgeons often choose to work with more exotic species of animal. They work in conservation of wild animals, contribute to the maintenance of captive stocks of endangered species and provide animal management and wildlife veterinary skills.

Veterinary nursing

History of veterinary nursing

The origins of the 'veterinary nurse' are unclear but animal nurses may have played a key part in the late 1880s when history records the presence of hospitals devoted to the nursing of dogs. In 1908 a Canine Nurses Institute was established, which had a philosophy of using properly trained nurses to look after ill dogs and which wrote rules of conduct that could be equally applied today:

1. The nurse, behaving herself with tact, gentleness and discretion, shall faithfully tend and minister the sick animal. She shall report any symptoms she may observe to the veterinary attendant and she must carry out his directions to the best of her ability. She shall abstain from expressing an opinion on a diagnosis or treatment as beyond the province of a nurse, referring enquiries on such subjects to the veterinary surgeon in charge of the case.
2. She shall not divulge any facts which may come to her knowledge regarding the private affairs of the animal's owners.

It is recorded that qualified nurses were supplied by the Institute but further details of the establishment are not available. One of the next references to a veterinary nurse identified a Mrs Florence Bell of the Royal Veterinary College, described as being in charge of the 'Subscribers' in-patients'.

Canine nurses continued to play a role throughout the middle years of the 20th century but the next leap in their position was probably linked to the formation of the BSAVA in 1956. BSAVA members realized that it would be advantageous to have veterinary nurses trained to a similar standard and, after approaches to the RCVS, a scheme was inaugurated in 1961. Because the term 'nurse' was protected and could only be applied to those involved in human work, the new veterinary nurses were called Registered Animal Nursing Auxiliaries (RANAs). Practices could apply to become Approved Training Centres and in 1963, after two years of training, the very first RANAs appeared in practice. In 1965 the first veterinary nursing association was set up: the British Veterinary Nursing Association (BVNA), the aim of which was 'to foster and promote the standard of veterinary nursing and the interests and status of the RANA'.

A close relationship continued between the BSAVA and the newly formed BVNA and that relationship continues today. The BVNA itself went through some changes, as the term 'veterinary nurse' was not recognized and therefore the name changed at the first AGM in 1966 to the British Animal Nursing Auxiliaries' Association (BANAA).

In the early 1960s there were no textbooks dedicated to RANAs in training; veterinary textbooks were too complex and human nursing books were completely inappropriate. What a contrast today with this, the second edition of a very successful manual, one of many books dedicated to the modern RANA – the veterinary nurse.

In 1984, following a change to human nurses' legislation, RANAs could apply for a new certificate as a veterinary nurse, bearing the date 1 November 1984. Shortly afterwards, the name of the association was changed back to BVNA, since the term 'veterinary nurse' was now acknowledged, though it has no protection in statute (unlike the term 'veterinary surgeon').

A career in veterinary nursing

Qualified veterinary nurses are key members of the veterinary team, providing skilled care for sick animals and support for their owners (Figures 1.5 and 1.6). In order to qualify, most student veterinary nurses undergo a two-year period of vocational training, which is assessed at work and through examination by the RCVS. An increasing number of nurses now train via university entrance, undertaking an academic course of study supported by vocational training in clinical practice. In 2005 approximately 20% of entrants to veterinary nurse training were undergraduates.

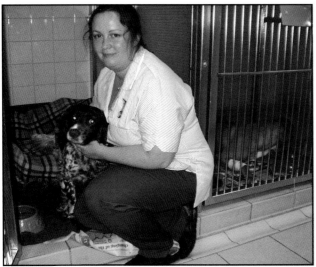

1.5 A student veterinary nurse attending to patients. (Photograph by Freda Scott-Park, courtesy of The Blue Cross.)

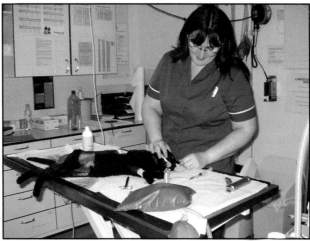

1.6 A veterinary nurse assessing a patient under anaesthesia. (Photograph by Freda Scott-Park, courtesy of The Blue Cross.)

The role of the veterinary nurse

Veterinary nurses:
- **Provide expert supportive care for sick animals by:**
  - **Assessing the nursing needs of patients**
  - **Providing nursing care**
  - **Undertaking medical treatments**
  - **Making diagnostic tests**
  - **Performing minor surgical procedures**
- **Play a significant role in client education on animal health matters**
- **Add value to the services provided by the practice by holding:**
  - **Puppy parties**
  - **Obesity clinics**
  - **Over-8 checks**
  - **Arthritis and lameness clinics**
  - **Worming and vaccination seminars**
  - **Support clinics for chronically sick animals, e.g. diabetics**
- **Supply medicines to clients under the supervision of the veterinary surgeon.**

The RCVS and the veterinary nurse

The RCVS is associated with veterinary nursing through the Veterinary Nurses' Council and its functions include:

- The maintenance of the List of Veterinary Nurses and, from 2007, the Register
- The award of veterinary nursing National Vocational Qualifications (NVQs) and Vocationally Related Qualifications (VRQs)
- The award of veterinary nursing certificates and diplomas (under RCVS Charter powers)
- Non-statutory regulation of veterinary nurses with effect from ca. 2010 if no statutory framework has been introduced by then.

The RCVS is the Awarding Body for veterinary nursing vocational qualifications. The Awarding Body works with the Sector Skills Council and the veterinary industry to ensure that nationally agreed standards for training are met. The National Occupational Standards in Veterinary Nursing must be met by every veterinary nurse seeking to register on the RCVS list of veterinary nurses. The RCVS Awarding Body accredits NVQ centres (known as Veterinary Nurse Approved Centres or VNACs) and course providers and sets the required standard for training practices. It also ensures that both NVQ centres and course providers are quality assured through visits from its external verifiers. The Awarding Body also sets and marks the external written and practical veterinary nursing examinations. This work is controlled by the RCVS Veterinary Nursing Awarding Body Management Board.

Qualified veterinary nurses may enter the RCVS List of Veterinary Nurses. On entering the List they are entitled by law to undertake a range of veterinary treatments and procedures on animals under veterinary direction. There are currently two parts of the RCVS List: one for small animal veterinary nurses and one for equine veterinary nurses (Figure 1.7). Nurses who are already qualified in one of these disciplines may undertake a shortened 'top up' training in order to register on the other part of the List.

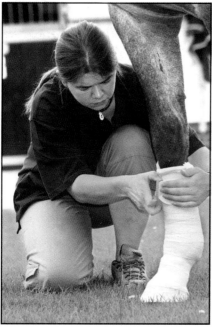

1.7 An equine veterinary nurse attending a horse with an injured fetlock. (Courtesy of Rossdale & Partners.)

The RCVS guide to professional conduct and Schedule 3B

The Veterinary Surgeons Act 1966 (Section 19) states that, subject to a number of exceptions, only registered members of the Royal College of Veterinary Surgeons may practise veterinary surgery. This is to ensure that animals are treated only by people qualified to do so. Veterinary nurses are considered to be one of the exceptions under the Act under the Schedule 3 Amendment, commonly called 'Schedule 3':

The Veterinary Surgeons Act 1966 (Schedule 3 Amendment) Order 2002 extends the exceptions to include qualified veterinary nurses whose names are on the List of Veterinary Nurses maintained by the RCVS and student nurses registered for training with the RCVS.

Under this exemption the privilege of giving medical treatment and carrying out minor surgery, not involving entry into a body cavity, is given to *listed* veterinary nurses under the direction of their veterinary surgeon employer and the animals must be under the care of that veterinary surgeon. The directing veterinary surgeon must be satisfied that the veterinary nurse is qualified to carry out the medical treatment or minor surgery.

Student nurses are also allowed the same privilege under the direction of their veterinary surgeon employer to animals under their employer's care but in addition the medical treatment or minor surgery must be supervised by a veterinary surgeon or listed veterinary nurse and in the case of minor surgery the supervision must be direct, continuous and personal. The medical treatment or minor surgery must be given in the course of the student's training.

A veterinary nurse or student nurse must always work under veterinary direction and is not entitled to undertake either medical treatment or minor surgery independently.

In considering whether to direct an RCVS Listed Veterinary Nurse to carry out 'Schedule 3' procedures, a veterinary surgeon must consider how difficult the procedure is in the light of any associated risks, whether the nurse is qualified to treat the species concerned, understands the associated risks and has the necessary experience and competence to react appropriately if any problem should arise. The veterinary surgeon must also be sure that he/she will be available to answer any call for assistance, and, finally, should be satisfied that the nurse feels capable of carrying out the procedure competently and successfully. When a veterinary nurse is negligent the liability is likely to rest with the directing veterinary surgeon.

Dated: November 2005

The veterinary nurse register

The establishment of the veterinary nurse Register in September 2007 was a major milestone in the development of the veterinary nursing profession, and is designed to reassure employers, colleagues and animal owners that registered veterinary nurses (RVNs) are prepared to be accountable for their professional practice. Currently there is no legislative requirement for veterinary nurses to be registered, unlike their human counterparts, and therefore the registration is non-statutory.

Any veterinary nurses listed on or after 1st January 2003 are automatically entered on to the Register (in either the small animal or equine section). Those listed before that date can choose to transfer on to the Register or remain on the unregulated list. Annual registration cards are issued to all registered veterinary nurses as evidence of their professional status, and they are entitled to the letters 'RVN' after their name.

Accountability will be relevant in three ways in particular:

1. Registered veterinary nurses have to demonstrate that they are committed to maintaining their professional skills through a minimum of 6 days continuing professional development (CPD) over a 3-year period.
2. Veterinary nurses returning to work after a break of 5 or more years will need to undergo a 3-month period of supervised practice, including a programme of updating skills, before they can join or rejoin the Register.
3. Registered veterinary nurses will be required to adhere to *The Guide to Professional Conduct for Veterinary Nurses* published by the RCVS on similar lines to that for veterinary surgeons.

Although the RCVS monitors complaints and the uptake of CPD, there will be no enforcement through disciplinary proceedings until 2010, allowing Registered veterinary nurses to become familiar with the obligations of the new Register without fear of punishment.

Routes to veterinary nursing

There are several routes to becoming a veterinary nurse, but whatever the route of training, all veterinary nurses in the UK must meet the nationally agreed Occupational Standards for veterinary nursing. These are incorporated into all training programmes approved by the RCVS.

Training in a higher education establishment

Universities offer a range of qualifications in veterinary nursing. The most usual are honours and foundation degrees and Higher National Diplomas. These courses take up to four years to complete and include supervised and assessed placements in clinical veterinary practice.

A BSc honours in veterinary nursing degree is available, which consists of four years of full-time study. During the degree programme, students are eligible to take Level 2 (Part 1) and Level 3 (Part 2) of the RCVS veterinary nursing examination leading to the professional qualification for veterinary nursing. It is also possible for qualified veterinary nurses to 'top up' their basic qualification to the BSc (Hons) in veterinary nursing.

Higher National Diplomas in veterinary nursing are also available at a number of colleges.

Training in an approved training practice

Student veterinary nurses undertake a clinically based training that takes at least two years. All student veterinary nurses, whether undertaking vocational NVQ-based training or a degree or HND course, undertake practically based vocational training in practices, supported by theoretical study courses at colleges or universities. Clinical training takes place in practices that have been approved by the RCVS Awarding Body to provide suitable resources and experience to support veterinary nurse training. These practices are known as Training Practices (TPs) and are affiliated to an approved veterinary nurse centre (VNAC) for NVQ or degree/HND provision. VNACs have a close working relationship with their affiliated TPs and ensure that all students in training are well supported and rigorously assessed.

Once students have achieved their NVQ at Level 3, or their qualifying degree or HND, they can enter the RCVS List of Veterinary Nurses and use the letters VN after their name, or from September 2007 enter the Register and use the letters RVN.

Entry requirements

The entry requirements to enrol as a student veterinary nurse are:

- Aged 17 years or over
- A minimum level of qualifications that are:
  - Five GCSEs at Grade C or higher
  - Five Scottish standard grades 1 to 3.

These passes must include English Language, mathematics and a science subject.

Alternative entry qualifications may be acceptable at the discretion of the RCVS. For instance:

- The BVNA Level 2 Certificate for Animal Nursing Assistants
- The Veterinary Care Assistant Level 2 qualification.

Since the entry requirements can alter, it is essential to contact the RCVS for information.

Alternatively, for a BSc honours in veterinary nursing degree, the minimum requirements are as above and usually at least two A-levels, BTEC National Diploma in a science subject or Advanced GNVQs. Equivalent qualifications (including the VN Certificate) will also be considered. Those who are over 21 without formal qualifications may also apply if they can show high levels of ability and experience.

If the entry qualifications are met, the RCVS may be contacted for enrolment as a student veterinary nurse. Once enrolled, the RCVS will provide:

- A syllabus
- A copy of the National Occupational Standards (NOS)
- An assessment document.

National Occupational Standards (NOS)

Continual assessment takes place at work and students must provide evidence that they have been assessed on the National Occupational Standards. These Standards define the level of basic veterinary nursing competence required in order to register on the List. They are divided into **units**, which cover the main areas of training, and **elements**, which contain more detail about what the student veterinary nurse must know and be able to do.

Each element is made up of four parts:

- **Performance criteria**: what the student must be able to do practically
- **Knowledge and understanding**: theoretical knowledge
- **Scope**: ranges to be covered (for example, the species to be dealt with)
- **Notes**: any other requirements, such as the requirement for a simulation.

Competence is determined through a series of work-based assessments. The NVQ assessor is a person who has received special training to be able to evaluate the practical competence of a student veterinary nurse against the NOS. Assessors are experienced (and listed) veterinary nurses or registered veterinary surgeons (MRCVS).

The assessment portfolio

The portfolio helps a student veterinary nurse to provide evidence that they have achieved the competencies detailed in the National Occupational Standards. This evidence may take many forms, such as a written description of a nursing case; a report by the assessor of work they have observed the student undertaking; photographs; and copies of observation sheets. Sometimes the portfolio may simply contain a reference to assessment evidence located in the veterinary practice records (e.g. a radiograph taken by the student). Whatever the type of evidence, it will be referenced against the elements of the NOS in order that the achievement of the required competencies is clear to see. Guidance and forms to use for assessments are provided in the RCVS *Candidate Handbook*.

Level 2 certificate for animal nursing assistants (ANA)

This qualification was designed by the BVNA for candidates seeking a specialized qualification to enhance their existing contribution in the workplace, with the overall aim being to prepare candidates, based within a veterinary practice, for a career in animal care or as an entry to the veterinary nursing qualification.

The course covers a number of units, including biological science, animal husbandry and the welfare and care of a wide range of small animals encountered within a veterinary practice. Candidates enrolled on this course learn skills to play a valuable support role to veterinary surgeons and qualified veterinary nurses. The candidate also learns basic reception skills, handling of finances and retailing of products. The ANA is awarded jointly by the BVNA and ABC and is recognized by the RCVS as a direct entry into the Veterinary Nursing scheme, provided that the student also has Key Skills Level 2 awards in Application of Number and Communication.

This course would suit candidates from the following categories:

- School leavers with no or insufficient GCSEs to register as a student veterinary nurse
- School leavers with enough GCSEs but under 17 years of age
- School leavers unsure of their chosen career
- Non-qualified staff
- Mature candidates with insufficient GCSEs.

There is no minimum academic entry requirement for this course but each candidate must be in either of the following:

- Full-time (35 hours or more per week) employment in a veterinary practice, which does not have to be an approved TP. Candidates must be enrolled for 9 months prior to the date of the examination
- Part-time (20 hours or more per week) employment in a veterinary practice (not necessarily a TP). Candidates must be enrolled for 18 months prior to the date of the examination.

The syllabus may be studied at an approved college. To complete this work-based course there is ongoing evaluation by the staff and candidates in the following ways:

- Candidate self-evaluation
- Regular review of learning outcomes against agreed criteria
- Validation by the student's supervisor
- Eight case logs to be completed throughout the year in the workplace and assessed by a suitably competent professional in the workplace.

The qualification is awarded when the student has completed:

- Their time working in practice
- Multiple-choice examinations
- The case logs, which are examined by external examiners.

National certificate for veterinary care assistants

This qualification has been created for those involved in providing basic veterinary care to animals under the direction or supervision of a veterinary surgeon. It is designed to provide practical skills and underpin knowledge relevant to the job of a veterinary carer in a modern veterinary practice. This course would suit candidates from the following categories:

■ Career progression within the veterinary care sector

■ Mature adults seeking a career change

■ Existing employees (either full-time or part-time) seeking to achieve a recognized qualification that reflects the role that they play in the successful provision of quality veterinary care

■ Those wishing to achieve RCVS listed Veterinary Nurse status.

The programme was developed in response to demands by veterinary employers for a nationally recognized qualification for the veterinary care staff. The programme consists of three separate modules, all of which must be achieved to gain the whole award. Assessment is via multiple-choice questions set by City and Guilds and a series of assignments, all of which must be passed.

Topics covered include: introduction to common animal species; animal husbandry; health and hygiene; reception duties; record keeping; health and safety; and employment issues. The qualification provides a means by which all veterinary care staff can be trained to a single national standard based on the needs and working practices of the modern veterinary practice.

To enrol on the Veterinary Care Assistants programme, the student does not need to be employed in a training practice but must spend 800 hours working in a veterinary care environment to achieve this award. This may be through full- or part-time employment or by gaining real work experience in a suitable veterinary practice.

The veterinary team

Often veterinary nurses take on other roles within the practice. In small practices, the veterinary nurse may be receptionist, kennel cleaner, theatre nurse and practice manager all rolled into one. However, as practices become more streamlined and with larger staff numbers, these different roles are achieving their own status and in some cases specific qualifications have been developed to ensure competence in a specific field.

Veterinary receptionists

In addition to the veterinary nurse, practice manager and animal nursing assistant, a veterinary receptionist is an essential part of the practice staff team. The receptionist is often the first person a new or existing client talks to on the telephone or sees when they visit their veterinary practice, and they are therefore key to creating a favourable impression of the practice (see Chapter 9). In addition to dealing with clients, veterinary receptionists often deal with financial aspects of the practice, including invoices, payments and client records. Veterinary receptionists are often trained in-house but both the ANA and VCA qualifications have reception modules, which can be taken as a stand-alone qualification.

Veterinary practice managers

The Veterinary Practice Management Association (VPMA) exists to provide individuals who are involved in the management of veterinary practice with an effective means of communication and interaction with others with similar interests, and a forum for promoting, providing and recognizing training and excellence in all aspects of veterinary practice management.

The Certificate in Veterinary Practice Management (CVPM) is a qualification recognizing proficiency in administrative and management tasks. The qualification was established in 1995 and is designed to be relevant to managers and employers in general practice and to indicate that the successful candidate has the appropriate knowledge, experience and expertise to manage a practice.

Access is open to anyone involved in veterinary practice management who self-certifies relevant experience. There is no formal course of training and qualification is via portfolio submission and examination. The CVPM is aimed at those willing to undertake self-study, but there are many courses around the country providing suitable 'modules' in all of the general business areas. A volunteer examination board, appointed from within the VPMA, examines the candidates.

The CVPM syllabus is published in the VPMA document 'Certificate in Veterinary Practice Management', which is available from the secretariat and can be downloaded from the certification section at www.vpma.co.uk. To sit the CVPM, the registrant must be a member of the VPMA.

Members of the VPMA with appropriate levels of knowledge and experience and who are actively involved in veterinary practice management may apply to the VPMA to be registered for the CVPM examination.

Veterinary practice administrators

Administrative assistants use specific skills to complete defined tasks (such as entering data into accounts software or running the payroll). They are answerable to a supervisor or manager who takes overall responsibility for an area or policy or even the whole business.

The Veterinary Practice Administration Course (VPAC) is designed to cover the skills required to carry out administrative tasks efficiently with the minimum of supervision and to be able to present the finished task to the supervisor, manager or employer. A reasonable understanding of the tools being used and the way they work (e.g. accounts software) is necessary to complete the task, but it is not necessary to have an in-depth knowledge or understanding of the impact of that work on the overall business strategy.

To enrol, practice administrators are normally expected to have gained three GCSEs at grade A–C within the last five years, but other relevant experience will be considered and the college offering the course will check individual circumstances. Only members of the VPMA may be awarded the Certificate.

Employment issues for veterinary nurses

Importance of a well presented curriculum vitae (CV)

Most people still train to be a veterinary nurse through employment at a training practice. When applying for a post in the chosen practice, the job seeker is unlikely to have much relevant experience, but a well written CV can make their application stand out from the rest of the letters that the practice receives requesting employment opportunities. Poor presentation may prevent the practice from reading the CV.

Simple tips

- Keep the CV simple and uncluttered in an easy-to-read font on plain white A4 paper.
- Do not put in unnecessary details (e.g. personal anecdotes about hobbies).
- Make sure that the spelling and grammar are perfect – get someone to check them.
- Double-check personal details (e.g. phone number, email address) before sending.
- If the advertisement has described the job specification, try to match your relevant skills against it.
- A CV should be between one and three pages long – concise is better than long.

What a CV should include

- Personal details: title, name, address and contact details, age, marital status, children.
- Education details: state the most recent qualifications and briefly cover older less relevant ones.
- Work experience: put the most recent first and work backwards.
- Key skills (e.g. languages, IT skills, customer care, pharmacy training, dog training).
- Hobbies and interests: keep this section short unless it is relevant to the job application.

It would be ideal to include a mobile telephone number. There is a good chance that a call could be missed when not at home. There should be a professional message on the answer phone.

Photos or references should not be included with an initial application (references will be asked for at a later date as part of the interview process). A common mistake is to detail every academic qualification, which is not necessary.

When emailing a CV, the email address should be taken into consideration. Email addresses such as 'sexylady123@emailaddress.com' will not present a professional image. Consideration should be given to obtaining a free email account and keeping job application emails separate from personal email. If sending a CV by post, a suitable A4 envelope should be used so that the CV does not have to be folded.

Preparing for an interview

Before the interview

Once an interview has been arranged, attempts should be made to find out some information about the practice. This could involve asking local people if they know the practice or looking at the practice's website (if it has one). Any questions about the practice should be written down and asked at the interview. Asking the interviewer questions will actually work to

the interviewee's advantage as it will show that they are interested in the practice and the position being applied for.

One of the easiest things that can be done before an interview is to *practise*. This can be done at home in front of the mirror, however silly it might feel. Practising will reduce the chance of sounding so nervous at the interview and it will also give a general idea as to what needs to be said before even beginning. Some local recruitment agencies allow clients to perform a 'dummy' interview with them.

On the day

Some people underdress (or even overdress) when attending an interview. As with a CV, first impressions are the most important. Here are some tips for any interview:

- Look neat and tidy
- Try to keep make-up, jewellery, aftershave or perfume to a minimum
- Wear sensible shoes (remember that you will almost certainly be shown around the practice and high heels or open toes are often not practical or safe)
- Take a pad and pen to the interview, giving the opportunity to make notes and keep track of any questions that you are planning to ask the interviewer
- Arrive on time for the interview. Turning up late may suggest to the interviewer that the applicant would always be late if given the position. Consider planning the journey before the interview and if possible try to arrive around 15 minutes before the appointment to allow time for preparation. Get detailed directions to the practice online (e.g. Streetmap or Multimap)
- At the start of the interview, try to be aware of body language. When shaking hands, make sure the grip is firm and look at the person to whom you are being introduced; this shows confidence. Everyone gets nervous at some point but if the interviewee appears too nervous, the interviewer might think they are not capable of doing the job
- Listen to the questions and keep answers short
- It is a common mistake to complain about responsibilities in a previous position. Avoid making negative comments about previous jobs or employers. Remember: employers want to hire someone who is positive and enthusiastic
- There will be an opportunity to ask questions. Do not ask about salary or holidays. Before the interview, think up some interesting questions on current issues in the veterinary profession (for example, is the practice part of the RCVS Practice Standards scheme or does the practice support further education for veterinary nurses?). If relevant, ask whether the practice does any horse or large animal work, particularly if you have an interest in working with other species.

After the interview

After the interview, a letter should be sent to the interviewer thanking them for taking time to interview you. The letter gives an opportunity to polish up on any details that may have been overlooked in the interview. It is also polite and professional to say thank you.

Starting the job

A new job is in a strange environment and it will take some time to find your feet. Most practices will hold an induction process where new staff are introduced to their new colleagues and where the practice procedures, including health and safety measures, are explained. Notes should be taken if the practice does not provide a practice manual.

It is important to receive either a contract or Terms and Conditions from the practice. These documents will set out the expectations of the practice, detailing the expected hours of work along with the salary and holiday allowance, continuing professional development (CPD) allowance, insurance, pension (if applicable), grievance procedures, pregnancy clauses, termination of employment and disciplinary procedures. This document is for the employee's benefit as much as that of the practice and its principal or manager, and the new employee should sign it and keep their copy safe.

Appraisals

Practices may require their staff to undergo appraisals. These are (usually) one-to-one sessions with an immediate superior (line manager) in the practice. Appraisals, when done well, provide the perfect opportunity for the employer to give employees feedback, which will motivate them and encourage them to improve their performance. They also give line managers the opportunity to identify training needs, provide career counselling and ensure that staff are reaching their full potential. If there is any question of poor performance, this can be quickly identified and action taken to ensure that work reaches expectations.

The employee will be given adequate notice of an appraisal (at least two weeks) and should prepare any questions or problems that they wish to raise with their line manager, who in turn will take time to find out how well they are working with colleagues. The appraisal is an opportunity for the employee to talk about themselves in the context of the job that they are doing. A good appraiser will know a considerable amount about them, the relationship with their colleagues and their performance before starting the process. The appraiser is there to listen for most of the time (at least 80%) but the communication is a two-way process and they will also ask questions to direct the employee's commentary.

The appraisal should be a positive process with measurable outcomes such as:

- Identifying areas in which the employee has excelled where they could offer training to others less competent
- Setting aims and objectives for them to achieve over the next 6 months
- Identifying training needs either in the practice or at conferences and setting the date of the next appraisal.

Continuing professional development

One of the outcomes of the appraisal process is the requirement for continuing education. Continuing professional development (CPD) is an essential part of life-long learning. The practice should give details of the time allowed off for CPD in the employment contract or terms and conditions or in the practice procedures manual, with details of how much money will be allocated to an individual's CPD. An employee might be expected to work within a budget, so that it is their own choice either to use the whole lot on a trip to the USA for a technician's conference, say, or to attend a number of short weekend courses in the UK. Or an employer might stipulate a course of learning that fits in with the practice plan; for instance, the employer might wish a member of staff to attend courses in small animal nutrition or animal behaviour so that they can run puppy parties or obesity clinics. It is probably wise for student veterinary nurses to attend courses that will augment their college and work-based learning.

Further education for veterinary nurses

- **Diploma in Advanced Veterinary Nursing.**
- **BSc (Hons) in Veterinary Nursing.**
- **BVNA Dentistry course.**
- **Pharmacy training to SQP level.**

Health and safety in the workplace

To comply with the law, the practice must 'manage health and safety'. If a practice has five or more employees, a written health and safety policy statement is needed. It is the responsibility of a practice to do all that is reasonably practicable to ensure the safety, health and welfare of all staff, clients and visitors.

To this end the practice should adopt policies on all matters of health and safety that are compatible with the Health and Safety at Work etc. Act 1974. Therefore **'rules'** (what the practice *must* do) and **'codes of practice'** (what the practice *will* do and how it will be done) form the basis of the practice health and safety management system.

General duties of individual employees include:

- Taking reasonable care for the maintenance of health and safety of oneself and others who may be affected by acts or omissions at work
- Acting in such a way as to allow the practice to comply with its legal obligations under the Health and Safety at Work etc. Act
- Avoiding the misuse of any items in the practice that may be involved in health and safety.

Health and safety covers many aspects of working in a veterinary practice, including lifting of heavy weights, working with anaesthetics, safety of electrical equipment, laboratory procedures and reporting of accidents – to name but a few (see also *BSAVA Manual of Practical Veterinary Nursing*).

2

General care and management of the dog

Alan Hughes and Jennifer Soloman-Kretay

This chapter is designed to give information on:

- The history of the dog and its role in society
- How a client should select a suitable dog
- The different dog breeds
- How to prepare for the arrival of a new dog
- General dog care by the owner
- Routine veterinary care of dogs
- Feeding a dog
- Breeding from a dog
- Dog behaviour and training

History of the dog and its association with humans

The dog (*Canis familiaris*) has been a close companion of humans for thousands of years. The very earliest domestication of dogs, most likely from the wolf, possibly coincided with the evolution of modern humans one million years ago, but selective breeding did not begin until 10,000–20,000 years ago. The earliest fossil records of domestic dogs date from about 12,000 years ago from the Middle East, but more widespread records date back 8000–10,000 years.

A number of theories exist to explain how domestication first occurred:

- Humans exploited the animal's success as a hunter of prey, and the social organization of wolf packs is such that the members of the pack learn to respond to a single leader
- Dogs may originally have been kept as pets or companions, especially for children
- They may have been kept as guards
- Rather than active domestication, dogs and humans may have developed their relationship alongside each other with mutual benefits.

It is likely that several or all of these factors may have been involved, but since early domestication selective breeding has led to a huge variety of breeds to fulfil a large number of uses for humans. Some of these functions have been lost through history as civilization changed (e.g. war dogs, carriage dogs, turnspits, bull- and bear-baiting dogs) but the modern dog is still widely used in many human activities (Figure 2.1).

Selecting a suitable dog

There are many points to consider when choosing a dog and clients will often seek the advice of veterinary staff to help them in making an informed decision. The average life expectancy of a dog is 10–12 years and a prospective owner should be aware of the necessary dedication that would be required over this period of time if they choose to take on such a commitment. A client needs to consider their reasons for wanting a dog and should be discouraged from rushing in and selecting an inappropriate breed for their lifestyle. Some of the factors to be considered are: exercise, training, grooming, puppy *versus* adult, dog *versus* bitch, being at home alone, size, activity and expense.

Area of activity	Examples
Work	Sniffer dogs for detecting drugs, explosives, chemicals, banknotes Police dogs for aiding in crime control Guard dogs for security of people and property Sled dogs in Arctic society Assistance dogs for the blind, deaf or disabled
Sport	Greyhounds and whippets for racing Gundogs for detection, flushing and retrieval of gamebirds
Hobbies	Agility trials and fly-ball competitions Obedience trials Showing
Companion	Pet dogs have been clearly shown to confer many health and social benefits to people of all ages and circumstances. Dogs from the other groups often fulfil this function as well

2.1 Examples of the role of dogs in modern society.

Exercise and training

All dogs, regardless of their size, require daily exercise. Ideally this should be two walks a day, which must be provided in all weathers, in order to give the dog physical exercise and mental stimulation vital for its wellbeing.

It is essential that all dogs receive some basic training in order to stimulate them mentally and to ensure that they are under control in public situations.

Grooming

Each breed has different grooming requirements. For example, the coat of an Afghan Hound or Old English Sheepdog will require thorough daily grooming and this will be very time consuming, compared with caring for the coat of a short-coated breed such as a Boxer.

Age and sex

There are advantages and disadvantages to owning either a new puppy or a new adult dog:

- A puppy will require toilet training, which takes time and patience, whereas an adult will usually be house trained already
- A puppy can be trained from the first day to fit into the life of its new family and to behave to the standard required, whereas adult dogs may have learned bad habits and require some retraining.

Whether to choose a dog or a bitch is often a matter of personal preference, sometimes for ill-defined reasons, but there are some specific pros and cons to be considered, as described in Figure 2.2.

Home alone

Dogs can and often do become bored and destructive if left alone for long periods of time, especially as puppies. If a prospective owner is unable to spend adequate time with a dog during the day, especially at first, it may be possible to arrange for someone to visit and offer the dog company on a regular basis. If it is likely that the new dog will be left alone for long periods of time each day, is the client's lifestyle really suitable for dog ownership?

Size and activity

As a species, dogs show a unique variety of adult size, from the tiny Chihuahua of less than 1 kg, to giant breeds such as the St Bernard of up to 100 kg. The size of the prospective owner's house and garden is obviously an important consideration here, as someone with a small flat would be more suited to a smaller breed requiring less space.

The size of the dog also partly determines their cost, larger breeds necessarily being more expensive in feeding, equipment, veterinary treatment, etc. Lifespan is also partly determined by size, the giant breeds only having an average longevity of approximately 8 years, whereas smaller breeds, such as the terriers, will often live to 16 years of age.

	Advantages	Disadvantages
Bitches	Less aggressive towards other dogs More companionable with people More easily trained, more biddable	Six-monthly seasons unless neutered Risk of unwanted pregnancy
Dogs	No seasons Usually larger Usually bolder, less nervous	May be more aggressive More boisterous, less biddable May roam, territory mark, show sexual behaviour

2.2 Advantages and disadvantages of bitches *versus* dogs as pets.

Some breeds and breed-types are by nature far more active than others and therefore require more exercise, and possibly more space at home. For example, the gundog and hound breeds (e.g. Labrador Retriever, Springer Spaniel, Beagle) often demand longer periods of vigorous exercise, requiring a reasonably fit owner – unlike breeds considered to be 'lapdogs' (e.g. Pekingese, King Charles Spaniel), which may be content with one or two gentle lead-walks each day and are therefore suited to more elderly or infirm owners. Activity levels are not directly related to size, and the giant breeds are often considered quite lazy, only demanding short walks with long periods of relative inactivity in between.

Expense

For most people owning a dog is a luxury, not a necessity, and although very rewarding, dogs are inevitably time consuming. Dog ownership is also associated with significant expense, which needs to be appreciated in advance of choosing a new pet:

- Cost of purchase or adoption (even rescue centres will now usually make a charge for people rehoming a rescued dog)
- Veterinary fees for annual vaccination, preventive treatments (e.g. flea and worm control), one-off expenses for microchipping and neutering
- Health insurance: annual premium and excess charges made for each claim. Without this, dog owners need to appreciate the potential unexpected costs involved with treatment of illnesses and injuries, which can be considerable if serious
- Feeding, especially a large dog
- Training classes
- Grooming: some breeds require professional grooming at regular intervals
- Boarding kennels, house-sitters, or Pet Passports for when owners take holidays
- Essential equipment: collar, lead, harness, food and water bowls, bed, indoor kennel, dog guard or seat belt harness for car travel, toys.

Finding the right dog

Having considered all of these points and decided that they can offer a suitable home for a pet dog, the potential owner now needs to choose the right one for them. If they are interested in a specific breed, they need to be sure that the breed is really suitable for their lifestyle; they should be encouraged to visit breeders, talk to other owners and attend dog shows or one of the Discover Dogs events organized by the Kennel Club.

Ideally puppies should be seen with their litter mates and mother in the breeder's home to see how they all interact with each other, and to allow an assessment of the bitch (and father if he is also present). Well reared puppies should never show aggression and should be bold and inquisitive. The timid puppy, or the one that cries or appears afraid when handled, should always be avoided, no matter how appealing.

Selecting the correct pedigree puppy may involve considerable time, expense, effort and travelling, but this will be amply rewarded if the correct choice is made. Reputable and caring breeders will:

- Spend time ensuring that the prospective owner and the puppy are suited, considering all of the factors discussed above
- Discuss and provide information about grooming, exercise, insurance, feeding and training
- Encourage the new owner to seek veterinary advice regarding vaccination, preventive healthcare, neutering, etc. and will advise that the new puppy is taken to a veterinary surgeon for a general health check soon after purchase
- Encourage the prospective owner to see the litter with the bitch at 3–5 weeks of age and then to return when the puppy is 8–10 weeks old, when it will be ready to go to its new home.

Many breed organizations have their own advisers, and often run rescue organizations that are happy to offer breed-specific advice and may have adult dogs requiring a home. For those who are less interested in a specific breed, or are prepared to take a crossbred dog, there are many excellent rescue shelters (e.g. those run by The Dogs Trust, RSPCA, Wood Green Animal Shelters) where members of the public are welcome to visit and will often be helped by staff to select the most suitable dog for their circumstances. Good rescue centres sometimes also offer behavioural advice for the dogs rehomed through their shelters, and may assist new owners with the initial costs of neutering and vaccination if necessary.

Dog breeds

Dogs may be classified according to their breeding, as follows:

- Purebred: the parents are both of the same breed
- Pedigree: a purebred dog that is registered with the governing body (in the UK this is the Kennel Club) and whose ancestors are recorded
- Crossbred: the parents are of recognized but different breeds
- Mongrel: one or both parents are of mixed breeding.

Nearly 200 different breeds are recognized by the Kennel Club, and each has a Breed Standard, which determines the ideal conformation, size, coat characteristics and colour, movement, behaviour and temperament for the breed. For the purposes of judging shows, each breed is assigned to a group, usually with some common features or functions. The groups include: hounds; working dogs; terriers; gundogs; pastoral dogs; utility dogs; and toys. Figure 2.3 gives some popular examples of breeds within each group.

Examples of many of these breeds, as well as people with particular knowledge and experience, are to be seen at the Kennel Club's Discover Dogs events held at Crufts and in London each year.

Group		Description	Examples
Hounds	 (a)	Breeds originally used for hunting, either by sight or by scent The scent hounds particularly are noted for requiring a lot of exercise	Scent hounds: Bloodhound, Bassett, Beagle, Foxhound Sight hounds: Afghan Hound (Figure 2.3a), Greyhound, Whippet, Saluki, Wolfhound, Deerhound Dachshunds are also included in this group
Working	 (b)	Breeds selectively bred to produce the guarding and search-and-rescue breeds, characterized by their courage and toughness	Bernese Mountain Dog, Boxer, Mastiffs (Figure 2.3b), Dobermann, Great Dane, Newfoundland, Rottweiler, St Bernard and Husky
Terriers	 (c)	Originally bred and used for hunting vermin, both above and below ground; most originate in the UK	Airedale, Bedlington (Figure 2.3c), Staffordshire and English Bull Terriers; Fox Terriers; Norfolk, Norwich, Border, Cairn, Scottish and West Highland White Terriers
Gundogs	 (d)	Trained to find live game and to retrieve game that has been shot. Generally make good family dogs but require plenty of exercise and attention. Probably the most intelligent group and therefore easier to train than others. Divided into four subgroups, according to their main activity (but are often capable of several functions in the field)	Retrievers including Golden, Labrador, Curly-coated and Flat-coated Spaniels including Cocker, Springers and Irish Water Setters including Irish, Gordon and English (Figure 2.3d) Hunters, Pointers and Retrievers (HPR – multipurpose) including English and German Pointers, Vizsla and Weimaraner
Pastoral	 (e)	Traditionally used for herding cattle, sheep and deer	Collies (Figure 2.3e), Shepherd Dogs, Sheepdogs, Samoyed, Pyrenean Mountain Dog, Corgis

2.3 Dog breed groups, with examples of popular breeds. **(a)** Afghan Hound. **(b)** Mastiff. **(c)** Bedlington Terrier. **(d)** English Setter. **(e)** Border Collie. (Photographs © The Kennel Club.) (continues) ▶

Group		Description	Examples
Utility	(f)	Miscellaneous group of non-sporting breeds, bred for a variety of purposes	Boston Terrier, Bulldogs, Chow Chow, Dalmatian (Figure 2.3f), Lhasa Apso, Keeshond, Poodles, Schnauzers, Shar pei, Shih Tzu, Tibetan Spaniel, Tibetan Terrier
Toy	(g)	Small companion or lapdogs, bred deliberately for that purpose or included in this group as a product of their small size	Bichon Frise (Figure 2.3g), Cavalier King Charles Spaniel, Chihuahua, Italian Greyhound, Papillon, Pekingese, Pug, Pomeranian, Yorkshire Terrier

2.3 (continued) Dog breed groups, with examples of popular breeds. **(f)** Dalmatian. **(g)** Bichon Frise. (Photographs © The Kennel Club.)

Preparing for the new arrival

Before bringing a new dog into the home, everything should be prepared to ensure that the dog settles quickly.

Space

All dogs should be provided with an area that they can go to for rest, and this should be considered to be a space of their own.

Ideally all dogs should be trained to use an indoor kennel. These are especially useful for puppies (Figure 2.4) as they can be shut away to ensure adequate periods of rest, to prevent them from damaging property when left alone, and to help with house training (even young puppies will eventually avoid toileting near their bed, and should be taken out into the garden to relieve themselves after every period in their kennel and before they are allowed the freedom of the house).

It is important that both the owner and their new pet do not consider the indoor kennel as a prison or form of punishment. To ensure speedy acceptance:

- The dog should be encouraged to use its kennel as a sleeping area
- Food or food treats should be provided in the kennel
- Initially, the dog should only be confined for short periods.

Older dogs may resent being confined to a cage and a quiet area of the house should be chosen where their bed is placed to allow undisturbed rest.

It is essential to have a securely fenced garden free from potentially toxic plants, other toxic substances (such as rodent poison) and any other source of possible injury.

Collar and lead

An appropriate collar should be worn from the outset, with an identification disc attached (note that this is a legal requirement for all dogs over 6 months of age). As puppies grow rapidly, their collars should be checked regularly to ensure that they are not too tight. For an adult dog, a well fitting nylon or leather collar is best; check or choke chains should be avoided as they may damage the dog's neck.

A suitable lead will be required. Extending leads have their place, as they give more freedom to dogs that are not trained to come when called off lead, but they should not be used when walking near roads.

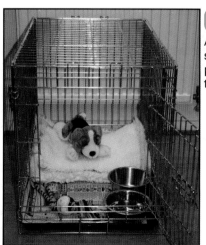

2.4 An indoor cage set up for a new puppy of a small to medium breed.

A number of products are available to prevent dogs from pulling on the lead and to give the owner more control, such as harnesses and head collars, and clients will often seek advice on selecting and fitting these.

Feeding equipment, bedding and grooming equipment

An appropriately sized food bowl should be chosen from the range discussed in the 'Feeding' section (below). A feeding stand (Figure 2.5) is useful for larger and giant breeds; it prevents them from stooping down to eat and it is thought that this may reduce the intake of air with the food, which may otherwise lead to the life-threatening condition commonly known as bloat (which is gastric dilatation and volvulus).

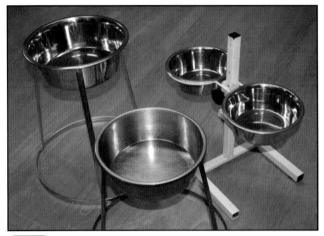

2.5   Some raised dog-feeding bowls.

Appropriate bedding should be selected from the types discussed in the 'General care' section, below.

Grooming equipment should be purchased and this will vary depending on the breed chosen (see 'General care', below, and Chapter 6).

Diet

Initially, in order to minimize the risk of digestive upsets, a dog should be kept on the diet it has previously been fed. Breeders will often provide diet sheets for a new puppy. Although diets can be changed after approximately 2 weeks, the transition must be gradual.

Toys

A variety of good quality dog toys are available (Figure 2.6) but even with these dogs should always be supervised to prevent injury or ingestion of damaged toys. All toys must be large and sturdy enough to withstand chewing and to ensure that they cannot be swallowed or obstruct the throat. They must be checked regularly and discarded when broken or worn. It is never a good idea to give a puppy old shoes or clothing, as they will not be able to differentiate between what is 'theirs' and what is the owner's.

Training classes

Clients should be encouraged to attend a variety of training classes *before* acquiring their new pet, in

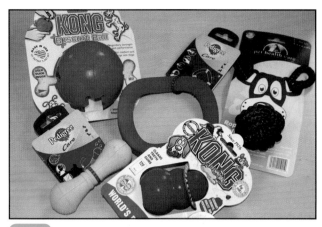

2.6   Some suitable and safe toys for dogs.

order to decide which one they feel more comfortable with and which they feel would provide a stimulating and enjoyable environment for themselves and their dog to learn in.

Behaviour and training

Socialization

Early socialization of puppies is particularly important: the more situations, noises, etc. that they experience in the first few weeks, the more likely it is that they will become confident, calm adults. A new puppy may not have experienced the everyday noises of, say, a washing machine, the television, trees or traffic and will need to be introduced to these in a gentle and reassuring fashion to avoid an excessively nervous reaction. Even before the puppy has completed its vaccination course and is allowed out of the home for exercise, it is beneficial for the owner to carry the puppy outside as this will greatly reduce the fears shown when first walked in the 'big wide world'. Continued supervised contact with other dogs after the puppy has left its litter (provided that the other dogs are healthy and fully vaccinated) is helpful in the puppy's social development and should avoid nervousness or aggression towards other dogs in future. This vital period of early socialization only lasts until 12 weeks of age, after which the opportunities to mould the dog's character are greatly reduced.

Early training

Training should start from the instant a new dog is brought into the home. It should be consistent and fair, with all members of the family knowing what they want to achieve and using the same commands. Results from training a young puppy will only be achieved slowly, and owners must be prepared to adopt a patient and methodical approach and realize that it is far better to have short training sessions repeated several times each day, rather than longer less frequent sessions during which the puppy will become bored and the owner frustrated. Early training should include sitting on command, walking on a lead, coming when called and staying in one place for a time; all of these should be reinforced using lavish praise and food treat rewards.

Puppy classes

The main purpose of puppy classes is to continue the socialization of the puppy with a variety of other dogs and people. If properly organized, this can significantly increase a puppy's confidence and teach it self-control in the face of distractions. Many veterinary practices now run these classes, and they also help to instruct new owners in various aspects of preventive healthcare and give them an opportunity to ask the nursing staff any questions on their puppy's health and development.

Play and exercise

Play and exercise must be part of the daily routine for all dogs. For younger dogs these play sessions must be short but repeated frequently (as with more formal training sessions) to be effective and to avoid boredom. Playing led by family members helps to bond them with their pet, is an important and enjoyable form of exercise for all concerned and is an additional form of training. Encouraging the whole family, especially children, to play games with the dog helps to maintain gentle control over their pet.

Toilet training

Success in early toilet training can only be achieved using a system of rewards. When the puppy urinates or defecates in the appropriate place, be that outside on the grass or yard or indoors on newspaper, it must be rewarded with a food treat or praise – and the latter needs to be lavish in the early stages. The young puppy will need to relieve itself whenever it wakes up or after eating or drinking, so it is essential that, after rest or meals and after a period in the indoor kennel, the puppy should be taken outside or to the newspaper and amply rewarded when it 'performs'. A puppy should never be punished for toileting in the 'wrong' place (and that includes rubbing the puppy's nose in it). Clients should be advised not even to clean up 'accidents' in front of their puppy, as this can create considerable confusion and anxiety in the dog's mind and often all that it achieves is to ensure that the dog never toilets in front of its owner. With patience, this principle of training will usually produce rapid results.

Training classes

A range of different training classes, all of which should be fun and stimulating for both the dog and the owner, is available for young and adult dogs (Figure 2.7):

- Pet dog obedience
- Competitive obedience
- Heelwork to music
- Ringcraft for show dogs
- Agility
- Fly-ball.

Avoiding dominance problems

A dominance hierarchy is thought to play an important role in the social organization of pack animals such as dogs, avoiding unnecessary conflict between pack members. Dogs need to understand their position in the 'pack' that is their family, and

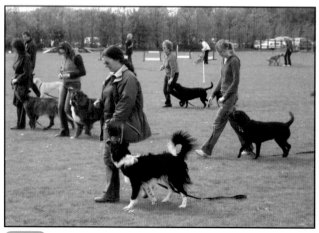

2.7   A pet dog obedience class in action.

the human family members should always be alpha (superior) to any dogs.

Many dogs will go through phases during their development when they will see how much they can challenge their owners, and this should be discouraged. The early signs of dominance may be obvious, such as the dog growling when a family member approaches the dog's resting place, food or toys, or more subtle such as the dog that continually demands attention for food, petting, to be let out and so on. Dogs that are very protective of the home or its family members may, in fact, be demonstrating an expression of dominance. Even young puppies may demonstrate signs of attempted dominance, such as growling or biting when being picked up, groomed or examined by the veterinary surgeon. These signs must be taken very seriously, dealt with firmly by all the family, and never viewed with amusement.

Owners should be strongly advised never to resort to physical chastisement to achieve dominance over a dog. There are a number of methods recommended to achieve this end:

- The humans in the family should eat their meals first, before feeding the dog
- The dog should always be kept physically lower than the humans, and not allowed on to beds or chairs
- Always walk through doors and gateways ahead of a dog
- When a member of the family enters the home, they should effectively ignore the dog at first: it should always be greeted after any other humans
- Always try to be very firm and appear unafraid when confronting a dog that is showing dominance aggression. The dog should be told off sharply and sternly, provided that this does not provoke a worsening aggression
- From when first acquired, puppies should be accustomed to having their food, toys, favourite bedding, etc. removed by any of the family members. If the puppy accepts this, it is praised warmly and the item concerned is returned. If the puppy shows an aggressive reaction, it should be spoken to sternly and excluded from the room ('time out') if necessary until it calms down, at which time the dog should again be warmly

praised (it is important for a puppy to know that its owners love it, even if they do tell it off)

- Try to avoid tugging and pulling games with a dominant dog unless you are confident of winning. These games are used by the dog as a test of physical strength.

Body language

It is important for veterinary staff and the new dog owner to understand a dog's body language so that behaviour can be modified appropriately, and dangerous situations avoided. Facial expressions, tail position and movement, stance, vocalization and elimination all give clues to a dog's behaviour (Figure 2.8). For example:

- Ears held erect may indicate that a dog is alert or preparing to attack
- The eyes are half closed when a dog is greeting someone with pleasure or submissively, but will be wide open if aggressive
- Drawing back the lips to show the teeth in a snarl is a familiar sign of aggression

- Raising the hair on the back or neck (the 'hackles') indicates aggression
- The tail clamped low against the anal region is a sign of fear
- The dog has a number of vocal signals whose meaning may vary with the context. For example, a growl will often indicate aggression and threat, but will also be used in mock dominance when playing, and in some dogs a low varying growl is a form of greeting. There are also barks of different types, howls, whimpers and whining, all of which may signal different attitudes.

Routine veterinary care

Vaccination

Dogs can be protected against a number of serious infectious diseases by regular vaccination (Figure 2.9). Although there has been some controversy in recent years about the need for, and the possible risks of, repeated vaccination, the overwhelming weight of scientific evidence is that all dogs should receive some immunization to avoid potentially fatal diseases.

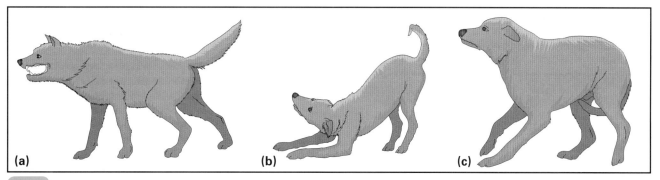

(a)   (b)   (c)

2.8   Body language: **(a)** posture of aggression; **(b)** typical 'play-bow' stance; **(c)** posture of fear.

Disease	Causal organism	Main features of the disease
Distemper ('hardpad')	Canine distemper virus (CDV)	Fever Respiratory and digestive signs Thickened footpads Eventually nervous clinical signs with fitting, coma and death
Infectious hepatitis (Rubarth's disease)	Canine adenovirus I (CAV I)	Blue discoloration of eyes Acute liver failure and haemorrhage
Parvovirus	Canine parvovirus (CPV)	Acute severe gastroenteritis, often haemorrhagic
Leptospirosis	*Leptospira icterohaemorrhagiae* and *L. canicola*	Acute or chronic kidney and/or liver disease May be contracted from contaminated water, as carried by rats and excreted in their urine Can be infectious to humans (i.e. is a zoonosis) (Weil's disease)
Kennel cough	A number of organisms, either together or alone, including: canine parainfluenza virus, canine adenoviruses I and II, *Bordetella bronchiseptica* and mycoplasmas	Acute upper respiratory clinical signs, rarely serious (NB: *Bordetella* vaccine is administered intranasally)
Rabies	Rhabdovirus	Mainly neurological/behavioural clinical signs, including aggression A zoonosis (NB: vaccine is usually only administered to dogs travelling abroad)

2.9   Diseases commonly protected against by vaccination.

Recommended vaccination regimes vary with different vaccine manufacturers, different veterinary practices and the particular circumstances of any individual dog, but most commonly puppies will receive an initial course of two doses of vaccine at 6–8 weeks of age, then at 10–12 weeks of age. Vaccination at earlier than 6 weeks may be rendered ineffective by interference from antibodies derived from the puppy's mother via the placenta and the milk (maternally derived antibodies). As full immunity takes some time to develop, it is usually advised that puppies should not be exposed to risk of infection (i.e. by walking outside and meeting other unprotected dogs) for 1–2 weeks following completion of the vaccination course.

Immunity from vaccination is not necessarily life-long, and it is still common practice to recommend annual revaccination to maintain the best protection. There is some evidence that it may not be necessary to give booster vaccinations against every disease every year, depending on a dog's circumstances; reference should be made to the vaccine manufacturer's recommendations. Annual boosters do have the great advantage of encouraging dog owners to bring their pets to the veterinary practice for regular health checks, when other problems may be identified. Boarding kennels will also often require evidence of regular vaccinations.

Parasite control

There are two main groups of parasites:

- Endoparasites – those living inside the body (e.g. 'worms')
- Ectoparasites – those living on the outside of the body.

Endoparasite control

Potentially, a large number of different worm species may be seen in dogs, but only two groups are common and considered important for *routine* control.

Roundworms (*Toxocara canis*)

Roundworms are particularly prevalent in puppies and nursing bitches, and the eggs are passed out in the dog's faeces. Transmission to humans is possible and roundworm control is therefore an important public health issue, especially in avoiding exposure of children to the worm eggs. Pregnant bitches and new puppies should be wormed at least monthly and all adult dogs should be wormed every three months. A wide range of very effective drugs is available from veterinary practices.

Tapeworms

These include *Taenia* and *Dipylidium* species. They are more common in adult dogs and are passed on either through fleas or from eating raw meat; therefore flea control, feeding only cooked meat and prevention of scavenging are all measures that are helpful in preventing infection. Drug treatment is also advisable on a routine basis every 3–12 months, depending on the dog's lifestyle.

Ectoparasite control

There is a wide range of ectoparasites but routine treatment is only concerned with two: fleas and ticks.

Fleas

The commonest flea seen on dogs is, in fact, the cat flea (*Ctenocephalides felis*) and is therefore most often seen in dogs living alongside cats. To prevent infestations, regular treatment of all affected dogs and cats in the household, as well as the animals' environment (soft furnishings, carpets, bedding), is essential – especially during the warmer months of the year, but central heating and fitted carpets provide ideal breeding conditions for fleas all year round. Clients should seek veterinary advice on the wide range of flea preparations available.

Ticks

Although seen most often in dogs that have walked through long grass (especially rough grazing frequented by deer and sheep), other vectors such as hedgehogs and cats ensure that ticks may also affect dogs with an exclusively urban lifestyle. Ticks are much more difficult than fleas to prevent, as only a small number of antiparasitic agents are effective. These parasites occasionally carry a serious disease (Lyme disease), which is also a zoonosis.

Neutering

If a dog or bitch is not likely to be required for breeding, early neutering around the age of puberty is generally recommended for a number of reasons.

Castration

This surgical procedure involves removal of the testicles and is performed from 6 months of age, depending on factors such as breed and circumstances.

The advantages of castration are that it:

- Reduces unwanted puppies
- Prevents hypersexual behaviour (e.g. mounting people and furniture)
- Prevents scent marking with urine
- Reduces aggressive tendencies towards other (especially male) dogs
- Reduces risk of some hormone-related diseases (e.g. prostatic enlargement and cancer, perineal hernias, tumours of the anal sphincter)
- Prevents testicular cancer.

It is a commonly held misconception that castration is an effective way of curbing a dog's excitable nature. The procedure should not be advised just to 'calm a dog down': it might have a calming effect on a dog's personality, but it is not guaranteed to calm down lively behaviour.

To avoid obesity after castration, it is important to advise owners that a dog's calorie intake should be reduced.

Spaying

This involves the surgical removal of the ovaries and the uterus, or the ovaries alone. It is best performed before the bitch has her second season, and is usually done 2–3 months after her first season.

The advantages of spaying are that it:

- Prevents unwanted puppies
- Prevents the nuisance and mess of seasons
- Prevents false pregnancies
- Reduces the risk of mammary tumours if performed before the second season
- Prevents ovarian cancer
- Prevents the serious infection of the uterus known as pyometra.

Again, it is important to counsel owners to monitor their bitch's weight after spaying, especially in those breeds prone to obesity.

Microchipping

Loss from straying or theft is of genuine concern to responsible pet owners. The law requires that all dogs over the age of 6 months should wear a collar and an identity disc at all times. To improve the chances of a dog that goes missing being reunited with its owners, a microchip can be implanted (Figure 2.10). This device consists of a tiny electrical transponder and battery encased in a glass capsule which is injected under the dog's skin between the shoulder blades. When a special reader (now possessed by most veterinary practices, rescue centres and warden services) is passed over the site of the microchip, an identity number unique to that animal appears on the screen. A telephone call to Petlog, the database company, will then provide the owner's details to allow them to be contacted. An increasing number of puppies are microchipped at the time of vaccination.

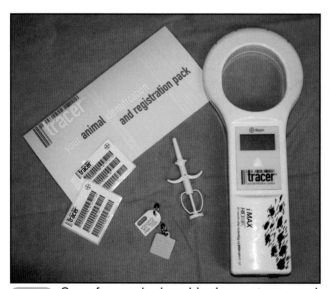

2.10 One of several microchipping systems used for the permanent identification of pets.

Insurance

The small animal veterinary profession in the UK offers an increasingly wide range of effective and sophisticated treatments and other services for pet owners. The elaborate surgical and medical facilities that are now available for dogs are something of which veterinary staff are justifiably proud. However, the full range of veterinary services is only available at a cost, and the successful treatment of chronic illnesses and serious injuries may involve considerable expense – a fact that may be underestimated in a society in which medical costs are largely hidden by a National Health Service.

Pet insurance is now available from a large number of companies, offering cover to help with the costs of veterinary treatment as well as other features such as third party liability, boarding costs if an owner becomes ill, costs involved in recovering a lost pet, or costs of replacing a pet that has died. The level and type of cover vary considerably, as do the premiums, and advice should be sought from a veterinary practice as to which *type* of policy would be suitable for a particular pet owner's needs (note that the Financial Services regulators now control quite strictly precisely what information can be given by a practice). It is important to understand that most pet insurance policies do not cover *routine* costs such as neutering and vaccination.

Illness and injury

Dog owners should be encouraged to be aware of a number of aspects of their pet's day-to-day lives as this may help them to recognize when their dog is ill or injured, and they will play an important role in helping the veterinary surgeon to diagnose the problem.

Activity level

This will obviously vary greatly from one dog to another, depending on factors such as breed, age, lifestyle and ambient temperature. A sudden or unexpected reduction in activity will be a common general presenting sign when a dog is ill.

Appetite

Again, this varies between individuals, but either a reduction or complete loss of appetite, or a significant increase in appetite, from the dog's normal level, may be an indication of disease.

Defecation

Healthy dogs will normally defecate at least once a day and should pass properly formed stools. A change in the nature of the faeces (e.g. softer, diarrhoea, changed colour, presence of mucus or blood) or the frequency of defecation should be noted, as should any apparent difficulty in the passage of faeces.

Drinking

Dogs should always have access to fresh water. Given this, a healthy dog will always drink as much as it needs. As a guide, the average normal maintenance requirement of a dog is 50 ml water/kg bodyweight per day. An increase in thirst that cannot be easily explained by normal circumstances, such as hot weather, increased exercise, change to dried diet or salty snacks, may be significant. It is always useful to ask clients to quantify the increased thirst if possible and it is usually a simple matter for owners to measure a dog's water intake over 24 hours, or, at the very least, make a rough estimation from the number of bowlfuls drunk in one day.

Urination

An increase in the frequency or amount of urination will often accompany increased drinking (the polydipsia/polyuria signs often referred to in veterinary practice). Sometimes a dog will urinate more frequently, but only small amounts, and this may be associated with obvious straining.

The nature of the urine – colour, smell, presence of blood – may be helpful, and it is often necessary to ask owners to collect a urine sample (into a clean container) from any dog exhibiting clinical signs of possible urinary tract disease or polydipsia, to aid in diagnosis.

Itchiness and skin irritation

External inflammation will often produce clinical signs of irritation (pruritus), depending on the part of the body affected:

- Skin disease will often result in scratching and/or biting of the affected areas
- Ear disease may cause head shaking or scratching
- Inflamed feet will often be nibbled and licked repeatedly
- Anal gland over-filling or infection may cause the dog to lick the anal area or rub its bottom along the ground ('scooting').

Some of these disorders will be accompanied by an unpleasant odour.

Lameness

Pain or stiffness in a limb will usually be exhibited as lameness. It is sometimes difficult, but very helpful, if the owner is able to identify (and then remember) which leg is affected, as mild lameness may be difficult to detect in the veterinary surgeon's consulting room.

Breathing

Laboured, rapid or noisy breathing may be an indication of disease and may be accompanied by coughing, sneezing or nasal discharge.

Injuries

Wounds, abscesses, external bleeding and painful swellings should all be checked by a veterinary surgeon, as they may require treatment.

External lumps

Skin tumours are quite common in dogs and some are highly malignant. All abnormal lumps, however innocuous they appear to the owner, should be examined by a veterinary surgeon.

Vomiting

Dogs vomit very easily – their omnivorous and scavenging nature makes this an important protection against the ingestion of unsuitable food. However, if a dog vomits more than once or twice in a day, and especially if this is accompanied by other signs such as lethargy, inappetence or diarrhoea, veterinary advice should be sought. The appearance of the vomit, the frequency and its timing in relation to any feeding or drinking should all be noted.

Temperature, pulse and respiratory rate (TPR)

The more experienced or knowledgeable owner, and certainly all veterinary nurses and surgeons, will measure a dog's body temperature, pulse or heart rate, and respiratory rate (Figure 2.11) as a routine procedure in the examination of an ill or injured animal.

The elderly dog

The age at which a dog is classed as elderly depends on its breed: smaller breeds are considered elderly at 11–12 years of age, whilst a Great Dane is considered elderly at 7 years of age.

The recommendation for regular routine health checks for all dogs, often combined with the annual booster vaccination, has already been mentioned. Once dogs enter old age, these routine examinations by a veterinary surgeon become even more important and could usefully be performed every 6 months, so that age-related disease is identified as early as possible. Blood testing, and other laboratory investigations, may be an integral part of these checks.

Although not a specific disease in its own right, old age in dogs is associated with an increase in the frequency of a number of conditions, as follows.

Arthritis

Degenerative joint disease is often seen as stiffness or lameness in one or more limbs, especially after rest. Large breeds are more commonly affected. Although not curable, a number of treatments are available that will effectively alleviate the clinical signs and may slow the progression of the disease.

Measurement	Method	Normal values
Temperature	A lubricated thermometer is gently inserted into the rectum for the required time	38.3–38.7°C
Pulse	Feel the heart beat through the chest wall, listen to the heart with a stethoscope, or feel for a peripheral arterial pulse such as the metacarpal pulse (distal to the carpal pad on the palmar aspect of the forefoot)	60–140 beats per minute
Respiratory rate	Count the movements of the chest when the dog is at rest	10–30 breaths per minute

2.11 Normal TPR values in the dog.

Tumours (neoplasia)

Dogs are subject to a wide range of tumours, which are usually classified as either benign or malignant:

- Benign tumours may enlarge with time but are not locally destructive and do not spread to elsewhere in the body
- Malignant tumours have the potential to cause significant local destruction of the tissues in which the tumour develops and may spread to other parts of the body. These are commonly described as cancerous.

Both types of tumours require assessment with a view to treatment or removal, if possible, but obviously the malignant type necessitates a more urgent and vigorous approach if fatal disease is to be avoided.

Heart disease

Many older dogs develop a heart murmur, usually caused by wear and distortion of valves within the heart. Only a proportion of these will be clinically significant, producing coughing, breathlessness, reduced exercise tolerance and lethargy. Many different treatment regimes exist to help to alleviate the clinical effects of heart disease.

Kidney and liver failure

Degeneration of the internal organs is an inevitable consequence of ageing. Although a number of signs may result, specific diagnosis is often only possible with further investigation, including blood tests, radiography and ultrasonography.

Hormonal (endocrine) diseases

A number of these are more likely to be seen in older animals. For example:

- Diabetes mellitus, due to inadequate production of insulin
- Cushing's syndrome, due to excessive secretion of cortisone
- Hypothyroidism, due to inadequate production of thyroxine.

Laboratory testing will play a crucial role in diagnosis of these diseases.

Behavioural changes

Senile deterioration, especially in dogs of a great age, is a common cause of concern to owners. Changes in temperament, loss of house-training, confusion, restlessness, vacant episodes, separation anxiety and changed sleep patterns can all result from this, especially as the dog's eyesight and hearing deteriorate.

Dental disease

Tartar accumulates on teeth with age, and this can lead to gum disease and loosening of teeth. These problems can be minimized by regular brushing with a veterinary toothpaste, or by the use of special diets, treats or chew toys, but many older dogs will have dental treatment under anaesthetic to prevent pain, difficulty in eating and halitosis.

Skin disease

Although common at all ages, some skin conditions increase in prevalence in older dogs, particularly some of the chronic oil imbalances (seborrhoeas) seen in the terrier breeds especially. Chronic pressure sores over the bony prominences of the elbows and hocks are frequently seen in larger, heavier dog breeds.

Obesity

This is especially common in older dogs, as activity levels inevitably decline but appetite may not (see 'Feeding', below).

The Pet Passport scheme

To prevent the introduction of rabies into the UK, it used to be the case that all dogs that had travelled abroad were required to be held in quarantine kennels for 6 months following re-entry to this country. In recent years, a Pet Passport scheme has been introduced to allow dogs to travel abroad, often accompanying their owners on holiday or during temporary periods of employment abroad, and to return home without the need for quarantine. The key features of the scheme are as follows:

- The dog must be over 6 months of age
- The dog must be microchipped
- The dog must have been vaccinated against rabies, and this must be boosted within the time intervals recommended by the vaccine manufacturers
- Two to four weeks after the first rabies vaccination, a blood sample is taken and sent to an approved laboratory where immunity to rabies is established. Only those dogs with written evidence to indicate sufficient immunity are entitled to a passport
- The passport to allow the dog to re-enter the UK does not become valid immediately after successful blood tests are obtained; at the time of writing the time interval is 6 months after the blood sample has been taken, but this may be reduced in the future
- Dogs are allowed to return under the passport scheme if they have travelled only to countries on an approved list, which includes most of western Europe, North America and Australasia
- To reduce the risk of introducing other zoonotic canine diseases from abroad, the dog must be treated for ticks and endoparasites at a veterinary practice 24–48 hours before re-entering the UK.

General care of the dog

With the ownership of a dog comes a responsibility to look after the pet to the best of the owner's ability. All veterinary staff play an important role in encouraging owners, especially those new to caring for a dog, to take seriously the health and wellbeing of their canine companion. Veterinary nurses, especially, are a vital source of sound and sensible advice on the general care of a dog.

Regular checks

Owners should be encouraged to examine their dog regularly and systematically (Figure 2.12; see also Chapter 6). This enables health problems to be identified early and often whilst they are still relatively minor. A set routine for examining the dog should be performed at least once a week. While the pet is still a puppy these checks should be carried out daily and by different members of the family, as this quickly accustoms the puppy to being handled and looked at, and makes future visits to the veterinary practice far less upsetting.

Body part	Possible abnormalities
1. Eyes	Pain and resentment on examination Excessive discharge: increased tears will appear as wetting of the fur around the eyelids; a green or yellow discharge may indicate infection Reddening of the 'white' of the eye and the lining of the eyelids Rubbing the eye(s)
2. Ears	Pain and resentment on examination Unpleasant smell Discharge – this may be wax or pus Swelling of the pinna Scratching the ear(s) and/or head shaking
3. Mouth	Halitosis Reddening of the gums, especially around base of teeth (indicates gingivitis) Brown deposit on teeth (tartar) Loose and/or painful teeth Rubbing/pawing the mouth
4. Coat and skin	Unpleasant odour Skin scaling Bald areas/coat thinning Evidence of ectoparasites (e.g. flea dirt) Painful red areas Pustules
5. Anal area	Swelling and pain around and just below anus, including anal gland area Faecal material adhering to anal area
6. Genital opening	Unpleasant smell Excessive discharge Excessive licking of the area
7. Feet and claws	Overgrown or broken nails Sore skin and swellings between toes
8. Nose	Excessive discharge (clear fluid, mucus, blood or pus) NB: A cold wet nose is not a reliable indication that a dog is healthy
9. General body surfaces	Abnormal lumps, sometimes painful
10. Joints and limbs	Pain on palpation or manipulation of limbs

2.12 Parts of the body included in a routine check.

Dental care

From when a puppy is first acquired, owners should be advised to brush their dog's teeth every day. The lips are pulled back on one side of the mouth and the outer surfaces of the teeth and gums are gently brushed, using a veterinary toothpaste and the correctly sized brush (Figure 2.13). There is no need to brush the inner surfaces of the teeth, as the dog's tongue tends to keep these clean. To accustom a dog to tooth brushing, it may be a good idea to use just a fingertip instead of the brush at first, then a damp cloth, before progressing to a soft toothbrush.

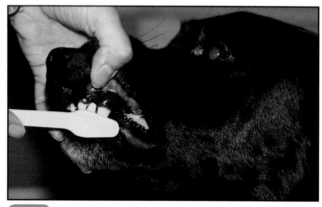

2.13 Brushing a dog's teeth.

For dogs that will not allow daily brushing, there are proprietary dental chews, chewing toys and special diets that are all designed to reduce the accumulation of tartar. Regular and correct brushing, however, will minimize the need for dental treatments in later life, and reduce the problems associated with, for example, gingivitis and periodontal disease.

Claw clipping

Particularly as dogs get older and less active, wear on the claws is reduced and occasional clipping may be necessary (see Chapter 6 for details). A range of clippers is available (Figure 2.14). Owners should only be encouraged to clip unpigmented claws, as it is impossible to see the vascular and sensitive 'quick' inside black claws. Dew claws are especially prone to overgrowth and should be checked even in young active dogs. Dogs often resent claw clipping, and it is helpful to routinely handle the toes and feet of young dogs to get them accustomed to this.

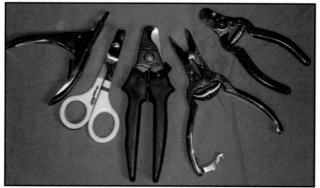

2.14 A range of clippers suitable for clipping a dog's claws.

Bathing and grooming

Owners should not bath their dogs too often as this can affect the oil balance in the skin and coat and predispose to various dermatological disorders. An occasional bath if the dog is smelly or muddy is not usually a problem, and mild veterinary shampoos should be recommended for this. Dogs should be thoroughly dried before being allowed outside especially if young, small or elderly. Details of how to bath a dog are given in Chapter 6.

The amount of grooming attention required by a dog's coat varies tremendously from one breed to another, depending on the coat type (Figure 2.15), and must be an important consideration when deciding on the suitability of a new puppy.

Some breeds, especially the spaniels, often have long hair around the ear openings and around the feet and lower limbs. This should be trimmed short to improve general hygiene but also to discourage lodging of grass seeds. Dogs with excessively long-haired faces (e.g. Shih Tzu, Old English Sheepdog) should have the coat trimmed away from their eyes.

Basic grooming equipment and its suitability are described in Figure 2.16. Full details of grooming processes and equipment are given in Chapter 6.

Sleep and bedding

Just like young children, dogs need regular periods of rest and sleep to maintain their health and good temper. It is important, especially in households with young families, that the dog has an area in which to rest uninterrupted (see 'Preparing for the new arrival' section, above).

A wide variety of beds is available, from the traditional wicker basket to soft fabric 'nests', and choice depends on ease of cleaning, whether or not the dog is destructive, and cost. All beds should be lined or covered with a washable fabric; specialized veterinary

Coat type	Breed examples	Attention required
1. Short	Labrador, Boxer, Dalmatian	Short-bristled brush, slicker or hound-glove once or twice weekly
2. Wire-haired	Terriers	Short-bristled brush or steel comb to remove knots. Many are regularly clipped or stripped professionally
3. Long	Afghan, Old English Sheepdog	Thorough frequent (daily) grooming essential to prevent serious matting. Some are clipped short to obviate this
4. Non-moulting	Poodle, Bichon Frise	Clipped professionally every 6–12 weeks

2.15 Grooming requirements of different coat types.

Equipment	Uses and comments	Short coats [a]	Long coats
Bristle brush	Unlikely to damage coat Useful for cleaning shorthaired dogs and putting finish on longer coats Flexible bristles cannot penetrate thick coats	✓	✓
Pin brush	Useful for longer coats Used gently, will penetrate better than bristles because less flexible and will not damage hair		✓
Slicker brush	Hooks assist in pulling out dead hair Useful for undercoat but care is necessary	✓	
Hound glove	Useful for removing dead undercoat in short-coated breeds	✓	
Rubber-toothed brush	Gentle and well tolerated Useful for general grooming	✓	
Combs	Handled combs generally easier to use, particularly for long periods		✓
Rake comb	Useful for dematting Care necessary Can cause pain and injury to skin		✓
Dematting comb	Used to cut through dense mats Instruction in use essential		✓
Stripping comb	Used principally for trimming terriers	✓	✓

2.16 Basic grooming equipment. [a] Wash leather or piece of silk for final gloss.

bedding is particularly suitable. Larger breeds should be encouraged to sleep in a soft padded bed from the outset (e.g. one with a foam mattress) to prevent development of pressure sores.

Exercise

Suitable daily exercise is essential to a dog's physical and mental wellbeing. The amount, frequency and type of exercise varies widely according to a number of factors.

Breed

Some breeds generally require more exercise than others. For example, Springer Spaniels, Boxers and Dalmatians will often demand longer or more frequent walks than smaller or more sedate breeds such as Cavalier King Charles Spaniels and terriers. The giant breeds and sight hounds are often quite lazy, though the latter may enjoy short periods of hard running.

Age and health

Immature dogs (i.e. less than 12 months old if medium-sized, less than 18 months old if giant breed) should not have prolonged periods of hard exercise, as this may be detrimental to bone and joint development, especially in those breeds predisposed to congenital disorders such as joint dysplasias and osteochondroses. As dogs progress into old age their exercise demands often decline, and shorter periods of exercise given more frequently may be appropriate.

Any dog that is ill or injured may require restricted exercise. Veterinary advice should be sought.

Training

Those dogs that are properly trained to 'come' when called, that are amenable to other dogs and people and that do not chase bicycles, etc. will be more suited to free off-lead exercise, especially in areas frequented by other dogs.

Administration of medication

It can be very difficult to administer medication by mouth to some dogs, especially the smaller breeds. It is a good idea for owners to practise by giving their dogs treats such as yeast tablets, as this will ensure that the dog and the owner are accustomed to the procedure should illness ever require such treatment at home.

Feeding

The dog is classified as an omnivore, which means that it can derive a balanced diet from a wide range of food types of both animal and vegetable origin.

Home-prepared diets

As home-prepared diets are often highly palatable, they are sometimes perceived by owners to be 'better' for their dogs as even the fussiest feeder will accept them. Achieving the correct balance of nutrients (see Chapter 6 for more details) is, however, time-consuming, complicated and expensive. Allowing a pet dog to demand particular foods, or basing a dog's diet on that of the owner, often results in a seriously unbalanced diet.

Commercial dog foods

There is a vast range of commercial dog foods produced by a multimillion-pound pet food industry, many of them being of very high quality as the result of extensive and scientific nutritional research. Proprietary foods are either complete or complementary.

- Complete foods provide all the necessary nutrients apart from water.
- Complementary foods need to be combined with other foods to ensure a complete level of nutrition (e.g. biscuits given with tinned food).

They are available in four main forms:

- **Frozen** foods may be very palatable and only require thawing to prepare. Manufacturers often recommend the addition of a carbohydrate source (usually biscuit). Adequate frozen storage facilities are necessary at home
- **Tinned** foods can be highly palatable and nutritious. They are relatively expensive, especially considering that they contain a large proportion of water (75% on average). They should be refrigerated once opened
- **Semi-moist** foods are similar in palatability but contain only 25% water. They are usually sold in sealed pouches, which should be refrigerated once opened. Special chemical additives designed to prevent drying may cause digestive upsets in some dogs
- **Dry** foods are rapidly becoming the most popular form of food for dogs, as they are relatively cheap and can be stored for long periods without requiring refrigeration. They contain a relatively high density of nutrients and only 10% water. Their main disadvantage is that they are less palatable and attractive, especially to smaller and fussier dog breeds.

Life-stage diets

Life-stage diets are mainly available in the higher quality dry food ranges. They are essentially a series of different diets, each of which is targeted at a different stage in the dog's development, which should ensure that the exact nutritional needs of the dog are closely matched by the diet offered. The various life stages catered for include:

- The growing puppy (separate diets may be available for larger and giant breeds)
- The young/junior dog
- The adult pet dog
- The adult working or performance dog
- The nursing bitch
- Less active/overweight adults
- The senior dog.

It is important to appreciate that dogs reach physical maturity at different ages according to their breed, and this needs to be taken into consideration when switching from a growth or junior diet to the adult diet. For example, a small breed might be mature at 7–8 months of age, whereas a giant breed might not be considered mature until 18–24 months old.

It is essential that all changes in diet are made gradually over 1–2 weeks to avoid digestive upsets.

Prescription diets

A number of pet food manufacturers now produce a range of special diets that are aimed at helping in the management of a number of conditions. These diets are only available through veterinary surgeons and should only ever be fed under careful veterinary supervision. The conditions targeted include:

- Obesity
- Heart disease
- Renal disease
- Gastrointestinal disorders
- Urinary tract disorders
- Liver disease
- Allergic skin disease.

Feeding frequency and amounts

Once the most suitable diet has been chosen by the owner, often with advice from the veterinary team, the frequency of feeding must be decided (Figure 2.17). This will vary according to breed, food type and household routine.

The quantity of food will vary according to:

- Food type
- Method of feeding (i.e. portioned or *ad lib*)
- Breed
- Age
- Activity level
- Health status.

Life stage	Frequency of feeds
Newly weaned puppies	4–6 meals per day
4–6 months old	3 meals per day
9–12 months old	2 meals per day
Adults	1–2 meals per day

2.17 Recommended frequency of meals.

In the first instance, the manufacturer's recommendation on quantities should be consulted, but these may require adjusting – especially with regard to the dog's bodily condition and amount of body fat.

Water

A plentiful supply of clean, fresh drinking water must *always* be available, whatever the diet offered.

Food and water bowls

These can be made from a variety of materials. Factors to consider when selecting bowls include the following:

- Are they of adequate size?
- Can they be cleaned or disinfected adequately and frequently?
- Are they difficult to destroy or break?
- Are they heavy and stable enough to prevent tipping?

In veterinary practices, stainless steel is often the chosen material as these criteria (especially disinfection) are all met, but plastic and ceramic bowls may also be recommended to owners.

Breeding

There is rarely any justification for using a pet male dog for stud purposes, and no owner should contemplate breeding from a bitch unless they are sure that:

- Their bitch is healthy. Apart from good general health, there are a number of health schemes which reduce the risk of inherited diseases in certain breeds (Figure 2.18). There are other schemes unique to certain breeds and administered by their breed societies (e.g. Von Willebrand's disease in Dobermanns). (Note that it is just as important that stud dogs are checked in these schemes before use)
- They are prepared for the hard work, worry and expense that are often entailed in breeding dogs
- They are confident of finding sufficient *suitable* homes for the estimated number of puppies, remembering that some large breeds will give birth to 12–14 offspring. Homing puppies is particularly difficult with crossbred litters

Scheme	Administered by	Breeds	Procedure
Hip Dysplasia Scheme	British Veterinary Association (BVA) and Kennel Club (KC)	Medium and large	Hip X-rays taken in dogs over 12 months of age, scored by panel of expert scrutineers
Elbow Dysplasia Scheme	BVA/KC	Large	Elbow X-rays taken in dogs over 12 months of age, scored by panel of expert scrutineers
Eye Scheme	BVA/KC/International Sheepdog Society	All	Eyes of potential breeding stock examined for number of diseases by specialist ophthalmologists

2.18 Some canine health schemes.

- They have a home and family circumstances suitable to accommodate a bitch and litter of puppies. Small flats, families with very young children or households where everyone is in full-time employment are usually unsuitable environments for dog breeding.

Once all of these considerations have been taken into account, breeding from a suitable bitch can be a very rewarding, pleasurable and educational experience. It is *not* true, however, that:

- Breeding from a bitch once will improve her health for the future
- Breeding from a bitch will reduce her nervousness or excitability
- Breeding from a male dog will reduce his sex drive.

If an owner decides to breed, they should be encouraged to seek reliable information and advice, and veterinary staff should be their first source for this. There are some excellent books that can be recommended to clients. Other more experienced breeders are also often willing to offer advice.

The mating

Owners of bitches should always be advised to go to a knowledgeable breeder with an experienced stud dog, especially if the bitch has not been bred from before.

The timing of mating is important: a bitch's season occurs on average every 6–9 months and lasts for approximately 3 weeks (Figure 2.19). The bitch is only receptive and fertile during oestrus once the vulval bleeding has stopped (usually 10–12 days after the start of the season) and ideally she should be mated every other day until she will no longer accept the dog, though in practice stud dog owners are often reluctant to allow more than two matings. Laboratory tests are available to determine the exact time of oestrus and these may be helpful where a bitch has failed to conceive in previous matings.

The pregnancy

The gestation period of the bitch is *on average* 63 days, but can vary quite normally from 57 to 70 days (larger breeds tend to have longer gestations). Pregnancy diagnosis is ideally performed by a veterinary surgeon:

- By palpation of the abdomen between 21 and 28 days, then again in the last 2–3 weeks of gestation. This may be quite difficult in overweight or nervous bitches
- By ultrasonography from 21–28 days of gestation onwards
- By radiography from 45–50 days of gestation onwards.

Apart from providing a nutritious diet (but avoiding overfeeding) the pregnant bitch does not require any special care. In the last third of pregnancy, it is sometimes helpful to offer smaller more frequent meals and to avoid very boisterous exercise. The bitch should also be introduced to the whelping pen or box at this stage. The whelping area should be:

- In a quiet part of the house but not completely isolated from regular human contact (the early socialization of puppies is an essential factor in developing an acceptable character)
- Kept at a constant and comfortable room temperature and free from draughts
- Large enough to accommodate the bitch and her litter, with some space for puppies to move away from their mother
- Easy to clean and lined with disposable clean bedding material (layers of clean newspaper are ideal).

The whelping

Whelping often occurs at night when the household is quiet. There are three stages of labour:

- First stage:
  - For 12 to 24 hours (up to 36 hours in a first litter) the bitch will become restless and inappetent and begins nesting behaviour
  - A clear mucoid discharge is released from the vulva, which is often licked away by the bitch
  - A fall in body temperature of approximately 1°C occurs at this time and may be measured by experienced breeders to signal that birth is imminent.
- Second stage:
  - Proper straining begins and will last for up to one hour for each puppy (usually longest for the first delivered)

Phase	Average duration	Main signs
Pro-oestrus	7–10 days	Vulva swells (especially in bitch's first season)
		Blood-stained vulval discharge starts
		Male dogs attracted to bitch, but she usually rejects their attention
Oestrus	8–12 days	Vulval discharge becomes less bloody, may become mucoid or cease altogether
		Male dogs attracted to and accepted by bitch
Metoestrus	50–70 days	No external signs present unless pseudopregnancy ('phantom' or 'false' pregnancy) develops, in which case may be mammary swelling, lactation, nesting behaviour and other behavioural changes
Anoestrus	3–4 months	No external signs

2.19   The oestrous cycle of the bitch.

- There may be rest periods of up to one hour between expulsion of puppies, in which straining is not observed
- Normally the bitch will rupture the fetal membranes around each puppy as it is born and will vigorously stimulate it by continued licking
- The umbilical cord will also be severed at this time.
■ Third stage:
- The placenta (or afterbirth) is expelled after each or every other puppy, often with a greenish-brown liquid, and is often eaten by the bitch.

Once whelping is complete, the bitch will often visibly relax and start to feed the puppies. She may take food and/or water, and a toilet break for herself.

Problems during whelping

For members of the veterinary team, one of the most important aspects of breeding is advising clients with a whelping bitch when a problem may be developing. Veterinary advice should be sought when:

■ A puppy is not expelled after one hour of straining
■ The fluid-filled fetal membrane (the 'water bag') has been visible at the vulval opening for 30 minutes without the puppy within being expelled
■ A green discharge is released without the appearance of any puppies
■ The bitch becomes visibly tired and straining becomes weaker
■ The bitch does not appear to have finished whelping but 2–3 hours have elapsed since the last puppy was expelled
■ The second stage of labour has lasted more than 12 hours.

If any of the above occur, the client should be encouraged to telephone their veterinary practice urgently for advice.

The nursing bitch

Contraction of the uterus occurs rapidly after whelping is complete and the uterus usually returns to its normal size within a month. A green or red vulval discharge may continue for 1–2 weeks following whelping, but advice should be sought if this persists or becomes foul-smelling.

Mammary enlargement becomes obvious in the last 2–3 weeks of gestation (earlier in the case of a first litter) and secretion of milk from the teats (milk 'letdown') may be apparent in the first stage of labour in response to hormonal changes. For 2–3 days following birth, the bitch produces a special 'first milk' or colostrum which is a rich source of antibodies and nutrients for the newborn puppies. The bitch will suckle her puppies at regular intervals (every 2 hours for the first few days, gradually becoming less frequent) and semi-solid food can be introduced at 3–4 weeks of age to allow a gradual change from bitch's milk to puppy food over a 2–3-week period, so that weaning is complete by 6–8 weeks of age.

Bitches with their first litter may not appear to take naturally to their maternal duties and may need quiet patient encouragement by their owner to care for their new litter at first.

The young puppies

For the first 3 weeks of life, the bitch and puppies function as a single unit, the dam ensuring that the puppies' requirements for food, warmth, rest and stimulation for defecation and urination are met as far as possible. It is normal for the bitch to be protective of her puppies at this stage, and it is important that they are not disturbed too often, though regular quiet attention from all the family members and other visitors is vital for normal socialization.

Once the puppies' eyes open at 10–14 days old and their hearing develops, they begin to explore and interact with each other and their immediate environment. It is at this stage that the all-important social development begins which will largely determine the dogs' eventual characters.

For more details on breeding and rearing puppies, see the *BSAVA Manual of Practical Veterinary Nursing*.

References and further reading

Bailey G (1995) *The Perfect Puppy*. Hamlyn, London
Fisher J (1991) *Why Does My Dog......?* Souvenir Press, London
Gorman NT (1998) *Canine Medicine and Therapeutics, 4th edn*. Blackwell Publishing, Oxford
Lane DR, Cooper B and Turner L (2007) *BSAVA Textbook of Veterinary Nursing, 4th edn*. BSAVA Publications, Gloucester
Lane DR and Guthrie S (2004) *Dictionary of Veterinary Nursing*. Butterworth-Heinemann, Oxford

Journals

Dogs World, published weekly by Dog World Ltd., Ashford, Kent
Dogs Monthly, published monthly by Ascot House, High Street, Ascot

Useful addresses

Association of Pet Dog Trainers
www.apdt.co.uk

The Kennel Club
1–5 Clarges Street, London W1Y 8AB
www.the-kennel-club.org.uk (includes Discover Dogs)

RSPCA
Wilberforce Way, Southwater, Horsham, West Sussex RH13 9RS
www.rspca.org.uk

3

General care and management of the cat

Jo Masters and Kim Willoughby

> ### This chapter is designed to give information on:
>
> ■ History of the cat and its association with humans
> ■ How a client should select a suitable cat
> ■ Recognition of different breeds of domestic cat
> ■ Basic genetics, including coat colours and patterns
> ■ General care and everyday management
> ■ Routine veterinary care
> ■ Basic nutrition
> ■ Breeding from cats
> ■ Basic understanding of normal behavioural characteristics

Introduction

The cat has recently become Britain's most popular pet: more than 7 million cats share our homes, compared with about 6.5 million dogs. It is almost certainly due to changes in society as a whole that cats have overtaken dogs in popularity, as they seem to be able to cope better than dogs in families where they may be alone for the working day (or have the company of other animals). Despite their reputation for solitude, cats are usually very affectionate companions. The vast majority of pet cats in this country are non-pedigree domestic shorthairs, but pedigree cats are gaining favour and many different breeds are commonly encountered in the veterinary practice.

This chapter gives a general introduction to the choice and care of this deservedly popular pet, from kitten through to adulthood.

History of the domesticated cat

The earliest evidence of the domestic cat is found in Ancient Egypt, where cats were treated as gods, had lavish burial ceremonies and were mummified.

Investigation of these mummified cats has shown that they were very similar to the domestic cat of today, the nearest comparison being the Abyssinian with its short-ticked coat.

During the middle ages the fortunes of the domestic cat in Europe took a downward turn when it became considered a 'witch's familiar'. Cats were burned at the stake alongside witches and even to this day black cats are associated with witchcraft and superstition. These superstitions vary from black cats being a bad omen to giving good luck.

In some Asian countries cats were held in high esteem, giving rise to pedigree breeds such as the Burmese and Siamese, which are still popular today.

The introduction of cats as 'mousers' aboard ships enabled the cat to travel the world, increasing its gene pool and allowing it to adapt to most environments.

Considerations before purchasing a cat

Before acquiring a cat, the practicalities of keeping a pet that may live for 15–20 years must be considered. As with any animal, buying a kitten should not be entered into lightly. All the factors below must be considered before deciding that a cat is a suitable animal for a particular individual or family to keep as a pet.

Cost of keeping a cat

Keeping a cat involves both financial costs and time. These include:

- Feeding – cost of food and time spent
- Equipment (minimal cost in most cases)
- Veterinary care – even routine visits can be expensive
- General attention – playing, grooming, etc. (if there is little company during the day, consideration should be given to keeping two cats)
- Arrangements for holidays – convenience balanced against quality and cost.

Outdoor or indoor cat?

Most pet cats live within the house, usually with access to the outside, but there are alternatives. The following questions need to be considered:

- Does a cat flap need to be fitted? (This may pose a security risk)
- Is the road outside busy? (Risk of road accident)
- Will the cat have free range in the house? (Some cats may be destructive; also toilet arrangements, i.e. provision of a litter tray, need to be made)
- Alternatives: constructing an outdoor run area for the cat; restriction to part of the house only.

Other family members

Other occupants of the house also need to be considered:

- Does everyone want a cat?
- Does anyone have allergies that may be made worse by having a cat in the house?
- Will a cat fit in with other pets?

Many cats end up in rescue centres because a child or other member of the family has asthma or eczema.

Selection of a cat

What kind of cat?

Cats come in many shapes and sizes. Long hair, short hair, curly hair, no hair, highly bred pedigree or local domestic shorthair – all need similar types of care, but some need more than others. For example, longhaired cats need daily grooming while a shorthaired cat may need little more than stroking to keep the coat in good condition.

Unlike the situation with pet dogs, where pedigree animals are popular, for a pet cat many people will choose a non-pedigree domestic shorthair cat. The popularity of pedigree cats is growing, however, and they are now regularly encountered as pets, not just as breeding or show animals.

Prospective owners who plan to show or breed cats will almost certainly want a pedigree cat. In that case they also have to think about how to avoid the production of half-bred kittens, and of the costs associated with breeding and showing.

The advantages of buying a pedigree cat are that some kind of prediction can often be made about its temperament and about what it will look like as it grows. With a non-pedigree kitten, such things are less predictable.

Cat or kitten?

Most people, when they decide they want a cat, will opt for a kitten. Kittens are fun, often very energetic and occasionally destructive. If an owner feels that they may not be able cope with the needs of a growing kitten – and a 'mad half-hour' every night when the curtains are conquered or pot plants tipped over – then perhaps an adult cat will make a better choice. Rescue catteries, such as those run by Cats Protection, always have much more trouble rehoming unwanted adolescent and adult cats than adorable and cuddly kittens. Giving a home to such a cat could save it from a long wait in a cat shelter or even euthanasia.

Which sex?

Should it be a male (tom) or a female (queen) cat? In a pet household both would usually be neutered, and both make good pets. The cost of neutering can be a consideration for owners and it should be borne in mind that males are usually cheaper to have neutered than females. While neutered cats are more likely to put on weight than entire cats, obesity is relatively uncommon.

Real differences between the sexes show themselves in entire cats (Figures 3.1 and 3.2).

- Toms become 'butch' as the secondary sex characteristics develop, getting large and often stocky, with a broad neck.
- Behaviour usually considered inappropriate for pets may develop, such as spraying urine around the house or staying out all night, fighting with the other local bruisers while seeking out the ladies.
- Entire males maintain larger territories than neuters, which can put them more at risk from road accidents and infectious diseases.

3.1   Tom cat characteristics.

- Entire queens are capable of producing litters of kittens at regular intervals, and it can be hard to tell, especially with a non-pedigree cat, when she is in season, or even when she is pregnant, until it is too late.
- Rescue centres have many pregnant cats and kittens as a result of unwanted pregnancies, where the owners cannot find homes for the kittens and no longer want the cat now that she has become a 'problem'.
- Even breeders of pedigree cats sometimes have difficulty selling kittens, and so breeding kittens intentionally should not be entered into lightly.

3.2   Queen cat characteristics.

Where to get a cat

It is preferable to get a kitten from either a private house, a breeder (Figure 3.3) or a cat rescue society (Figure 3.4). In this way, the new owner can learn a bit about the home background of the cat and can often, in the case of a kitten, see the mother. It can be established whether the kitten is used to children or dogs, and the temperament of individual kittens can be assessed in a home environment. With a pedigree cat it may be possible to see the father as well, but it should be remembered that many breeders do not keep their own stud cat and the queen may have travelled a long way to be mated.

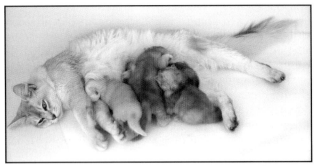

3.3 A litter of pedigree kittens (Tiffanies) will often have homes arranged even before their birth. (© Alan Robinson.)

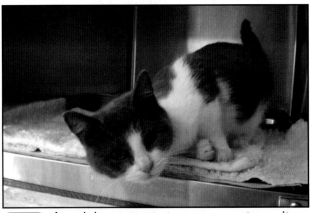

3.4 An adolescent cat at a rescue centre waits for a home.

Choosing an individual cat

A potential owner may have decided that they prefer a male or female kitten, or one of a particular colour, but often they will choose a non-pedigree cat or kitten by instinct, because that ginger one looks 'nicest', or the little black and white one has a sweet expression.

Pet quality

With a pedigree cat, the breeder will know which cats are 'pet quality' and which are suitable for showing or breeding. This does not imply that pet quality kittens are inferior in any way, other than in terms of the defined breed description in the official 'standard of points' against which cats are judged at shows.

Cat clubs

Where the owner is looking for a cat to show or to breed from, cat clubs and magazines can be valuable

resources for locating a particular breed. Most areas have mixed-breed local clubs and there are nationwide breed clubs. These can be contacted via the registering bodies (Governing Council of the Cat Fancy or the Cat Association of Britain; see 'Useful addresses' at the end of this chapter) or by purchasing one of the cat magazines widely available in newsagents.

It is also useful for the prospective owner to visit a local cat show to meet breeders and see the cats at first hand. Lists are available from the registering bodies.

Home visits

Vendors, especially pedigree breeders or rescue catteries, might want to 'vet' prospective owners before they let them have a cat. Many rescue societies like to perform home visits to ensure that their animals are going to good homes, and breeders usually want to meet owners at least once to decide on their suitability before selling them a pedigree kitten.

Selecting a kitten

Unless the potential owner is knowledgeable about cats, it is advisable that someone who is more experienced should go with them to look at or collect a kitten. They should expect to be able to see the whole litter, and the queen, in most circumstances.

It is likely that they will not meet the kittens until they are around 6–8 weeks old, when kittens should be bright and active, curious about strangers and playing with each other and the queen. Kittens that have been reared in the house with human company usually make better pets than those reared in catteries, and are familiar with ordinary household objects such as vacuum cleaners.

A simple health check is suggested in Figure 3.5.

While non-pedigree kittens often leave their mothers at around 8 weeks of age, pedigree kittens are usually at least 12 weeks old. All kittens should be fully weaned and (mostly) litter trained before they move to a new home – the queen usually trains the kittens (see 'Kitten development and behaviour', below).

Paperwork

Before being sold, pedigree kittens should be vaccinated against at least cat 'flu and enteritis (see below) and a written pedigree, registration transfer certificate and record of vaccination should be supplied at the time of purchase. Many pedigree cat breeders also supply kitten insurance as a kitten 'cover note', valid for 6 weeks or so after purchase.

General condition:
- Bright, alert and responsive. Kittens should be curious and should respond to being stroked by purring, rubbing or pushing against your hand
- Weight. Pick the kitten up. It should feel plump and not bony or clammy. The whole litter should be of a similar size. The kitten should not feel limp or floppy; there should be good muscle tone. Kittens should not be pot-bellied
- Movement. The kitten should move easily, with no signs of loss of balance or difficulty walking or jumping.

3.5 Basic health check for a kitten. (continues) ▶

Examination for problems:
- Eyes and nose should be clean and free of any discharge. The third eyelid (haws) should not be visible in the corner of the eyes. The kitten should not sneeze or cough. All these can be signs of infectious respiratory disease, which may be problematic to treat
- Ears should not be waxy or irritated. This can be a sign of ear mites (watch the kitten for shaking the head or scratching)
- Teeth should be white and clean; gums should not be excessively red or inflamed. The front teeth should meet, though this is not always the case, especially with longhaired cats of Persian type
- The coat should be clean and show no signs of hair loss, sore patches, scaliness or irritation. Check for parasites such as fleas
- The area under the tail should be clean with no sign of faecal staining on the surrounding hair. Sometimes worms may be seen around the anus. The cat should not have diarrhoea. Always check the sex of the kitten or cat
- The kitten should have no obvious deformities. Check for hernias at the umbilicus (navel), for kinks in the tail, that the ribcage feels normal and not flattened, and that the back and limbs feel normal
- Take the cat or kitten to a veterinary surgeon for a full checkover within a few days to ensure all is well.

3.5 (continued) Basic health check for a kitten.

Cat breeds

Governing bodies

The majority of the pedigree cat world in the UK is regulated by the Governing Council of the Cat Fancy (GCCF, founded in 1910) in much the same way as the Kennel Club regulates dog breeders. It recognizes new breeds, maintains registers of pedigree cats, runs shows (see 'Activities with cats', below) and sets out the rules by which breeders affiliated to it should behave. The GCCF produces various publications, including the breed descriptions against which cats are judged at cat shows, known as the 'standard of points'. It also organizes the Supreme Show (the 'Crufts' of the cat fancy).

The Cat Association of Britain is a much smaller group affiliated to the Fédération Internationale Féline (FIF), which organizes shows and recognizes breeds in a similar way.

Breed recognition

'Breed recognition' means that the particular governing body will accept kitten registrations for that breed and will allow them to be exhibited at shows. For a new breed to be recognized, a group of breeders must demonstrate that they are committed to the breed, that there is sufficient interest in it and that it is sufficiently different from other breeds. The new breed can then progress through a process that involves registering a minimum number of cats and kittens and demonstrating their merits at shows before 'full recognition' is granted.

Cat breeds are subdivided into breed sections, in much the same way that dogs are divided into groups, e.g. working and toy. The breed sections into which the recognized cat breeds are divided are:

- Longhair
- Semi-longhair
- British
- Foreign
- Burmese
- Oriental
- Siamese.

In addition, some other breeds are present but not recognized.

Popular breeds

Figures of kittens registered (1997, supplied by GCCF) demonstrate that the most popular are the well established breeds: Persian 8443 (Figure 3.6a); Siamese 4873; British Shorthair 4287; Burmese 3327; and Birman 2216 (Figure 3.6b). Some of the more recently recognized breeds are also becoming popular, notably the Maine Coon (1296) and Bengal (1222) (Figure 3.6c).

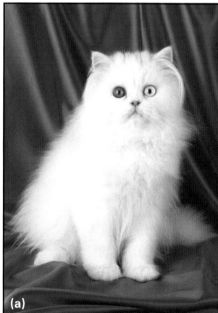

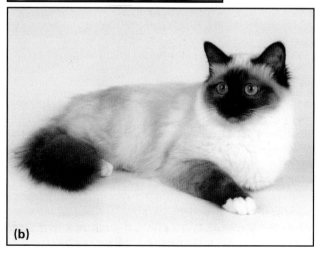

3.6 (a) Odd-eyed white Persian. (b) Seal point Birman. (© Alan Robinson.) (continues) ▶

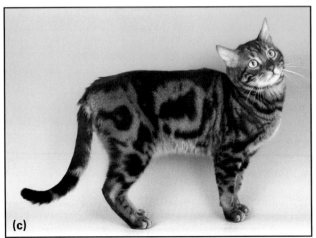

3.6 (continued) **(c)** Brown marbled Bengal. (© Alan Robinson.)

Other breeds

Other breeds are very uncommon, but include a longhaired version of the Manx known as the Cymric, and a longhaired rex known as the Selkirk Rex. There is also a hairless cat called the Sphynx and a cat with folded-over ears, the Scottish Fold. In other countries, notably North America, other breeds are also seen, including a cat known as the 'Munchkin', which has short, dachshund-like limbs.

Coat colours and patterns

The majority of pedigree cats are described by a combination of their colour (e.g. blue, seal point, silver tabby) and their 'type' or breed (e.g. Oriental, Persian, Burmese). Thus a full description of a cat might be, for example, 'silver tabby British Shorthair' (see Figure 3.10b), 'blue point Siamese' (see Figure 3.15c) or 'brown tabby and white Maine Coon' (Figure 3.7), though some breeds can be only one specific colour (e.g. Korat – blue).

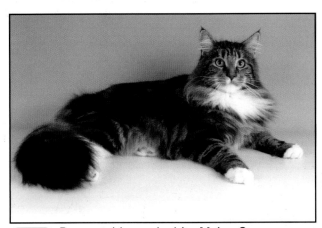

3.7 Brown tabby and white Maine Coon. (© Alan Robinson.)

It is useful to be able to recognize the more common breeds and to be able to have at least an educated guess at their colour, though some of them are definitely not easy for the amateur (even breeders

get it wrong sometimes and have to re-register kittens). A very good way to pick up the different colours and breeds is to visit a local show or, even better, to help with 'vetting-in' at a show early in the morning, when all the cats are examined before going into the show hall. Show managers are usually delighted to be offered extra help at 7.30 am.

Basic genetics

Genetic material (genes) is arranged in structures called **chromosomes**, which are present in the nucleus of every body cell of the cat. These chromosomes are present in pairs: there are two copies of every gene in most cells. There are two exceptions to this general rule:

- The sex chromosomes – males have one X and one Y chromosome and females have two X chromosomes
- The reproductive cells (eggs and sperm) – only one 'set' of genes is present, so that when these fuse to become a fertilized egg (and eventually a new kitten), two copies are present: one set inherited from the father and one from the mother.

Individual genes may be described as **dominant** or **recessive**. Where a gene is dominant, a single copy on either of the two chromosomes ensures its expression, whereas if a gene is recessive, both copies must be of the recessive gene for it to be expressed. (In a genetic context, 'expressed' means that that character will be produced.)

By convention, the symbols used for gene names are written in italics. Symbols for dominant genes are written in capital letters; symbols for recessive ones are in lower case letters. The example in Figure 3.8 demonstrates this principle.

Genetic makeup	Basic colour	Genes that can be passed to offspring
BB	Black	*B* (black) only
Bb	Black	*B* (black) or *b* (brown)
bb	Brown	*b* (brown) only

3.8 Genetics example 1. Note that black (*B*) is dominant to brown (*b*).

Where both copies of a gene are the same (e.g. *BB* or *bb*), the genetic makeup is known as **homozygous** and the cat can pass on only that gene to any kittens. Where the cat has one of each (e.g. *Bb*), it is called **heterozygous** and the cat can pass on either gene; the cat might be described as a black cat 'carrying' brown, for example. Where a dominant gene is present, it is usual to write this as '*B-*', rather than writing *BB* or *Bb*, and this will be done in this section.

The genetics of coat colours are the same for every cat, be it domestic pet or pedigree. The fundamental genes, colours and patterns are listed in Figure 3.9 and are briefly described below. For more detail, consult the References and further reading.

Gene (symbol)	Effect	Gene (symbol)	Effect
Agouti (*A*)	Tabby expression	Non-agouti (*a*)	Self-colour
Mackerel (*T^m*)	Striped (or spotted) tabby	Abyssinian (*T^a*) Blotched (*t^b*)	Abyssinian tabby Blotched (classic) tabby
Black (*B*)	Black	Brown (*b*) Light brown (*b^l*)	Dark brown (chocolate) Medium brown (cinnamon)
Not orange (*o*)	Normal colour	Orange (*O*) (red, ginger) (sex-linked)	All pigment altered to orange
Dense (*D*)	Dense colour	Dilute (*d*)	Dilutes colour (e.g. black to blue; brown to lilac)
Full colour	Colour over whole cat	Burmese (*c^b*) Siamese (*c^s*) Albino (*c*)	Burmese colour restriction Siamese colour restriction, blue eyes White coat, pink eyes
Normal pigment (*i*)	Full pigment development	Inhibitor (*I*)	Pigment suppression of some parts of hair shaft; also known as silver gene
Normal colour (*w*)	Allows expression of all other colour genes	Dominant White (*W*)	White coat; eyes blue, orange or odd-eyes Associated with deafness
Normal colour (*s*)	No white spots	White spotting (*S*)	White patches or spots – expression variable

3.9   Genes affecting coat colour. Dominant genes are shown in upper case, recessive in lower case.

Coat patterns: tabby and self-coloured

The 'tabby' pattern of a cat is controlled by two genes. All cats have tabby (*T*) genes but whether or not they are expressed is dependent on the agouti (*A*) gene, which determines the banding of pigment on the hair shaft. Agouti (*A*) allows banding and is dominant to non-agouti (*a*). All tabby cats are therefore *A-* (remember, that means *AA* or *Aa*) and all non-tabby (i.e. 'self-coloured') cats are *aa*.

There are three tabby patterns:

- Abyssinian: no stripes as such but a broad ticking of the coat, like rabbit's fur (Figure 3.10a)
- Blotched: the so-called classic tabby with wide stripes (Figure 3.10b)
- Mackerel: the tiger stripe, where the stripes are narrower and tend to break into spots (Figure 3.10c).

The tabby genes form a 'gene series' in which mackerel is dominant to abyssinian, which is itself dominant to blotched. An example of the influence of these genes is shown in Figure 3.11.

Basic coat colours

The basic coat colour genes are:

- Black (*B*)
- Brown (*b*) (also sometimes called chocolate)
- Orange (*O*)
- Dominant white (*W*).

A further light brown gene (*bl*) is also seen, which is uncommon even in pedigree cats. The black and brown genes behave as expected (see Figure 3.8), provided that neither the orange nor the white gene is present.

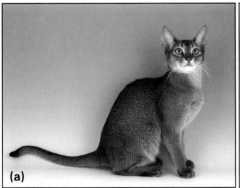
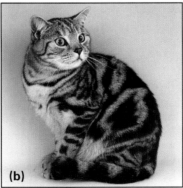
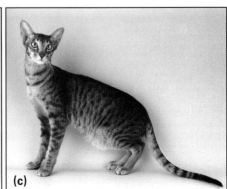

(a)   **(b)**   **(c)**

3.10   Tabby patterns. **(a)** Usual Abyssinian (ticked) tabby pattern. **(b)** Blotched (classic) tabby pattern in a silver tabby British Shorthair. **(c)** Mackerel (spotted) tabby pattern in an Oriental Blue spotted tabby. The stripes tend to break into spots; this feature is sought after in pedigree cats. (© Alan Robinson.)

Genetic makeup	Coat pattern and colour
A– T^m– B–	Mackerel tabby, black stripes
aa T^m– B–	Black self
A– $T^a T^b$ bb	Ticked tabby, brown tips to hairs
aa $T^a T^b$ bb	Brown self

3.11 Genetics example 2.

Orange

The orange gene (Figure 3.12) is a special case because it is on the X chromosome.

Genetic makeup	Coat pattern and colour
A– $T^m T$– B– $X^o Y$	Ginger mackerel tabby male
aa T^m– B– $X^o X$	Tortoiseshell (ginger and black) female
A– $T^b T^b$ bb $X^o X^o$	Ginger classic tabby female
aa $T^a T^b$ bb $X^o X$	Chocolate tortoiseshell female

3.12 Genetics example 3.

- A male cat has only one X chromosome. If this carries the orange gene he will be orange (ginger), regardless of the other basic colour genes present, because orange prevents the expression of the basic colours.
- A female cat has two X chromosomes. If the combination is $X^o X^o$ she will be ginger, but a combination of $X^o X^-$ (i.e. one X chromosome has orange, one does not) leads to 'tortoiseshell', which is a mixture of ginger and black (Figure 3.13).

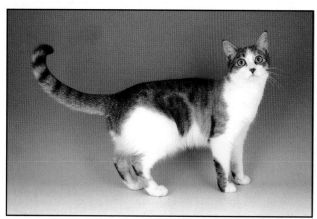

3.13 Tortoiseshell tabby and white Domestic Shorthair. Note the tabby markings on the black areas in addition to the ginger. (© Alan Robinson.)

That is why almost all tortoiseshell cats are female. Very occasionally, male 'torties' are seen, but most are sterile, as they have a chromosomal abnormality.

A further effect of the orange gene is that, very often, tabby markings are produced on a ginger cat (or ginger patches on a tortoiseshell one), whether or not the agouti (*A*) gene is present. Tortoiseshell cats can also be tabby, known as 'tortie-tabby', where the black is also tabby (Figure 3.14).

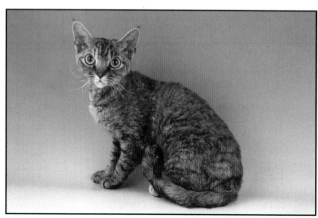

3.14 Tortie-tabby Devon Rex. (© Alan Robinson.)

White

Dominant white (*W*) is a very special gene that prevents expression of all other colours (including orange) and produces an all-white cat, with eyes of blue or amber, or even one of each (see Figure 3.6a). This gene is also associated in many cats with deafness, due to a deformity in the cochlea in the inner ear.

Modifying genes

The basic colours of black, brown and orange (in their self-coloured, tabby or tortoiseshell forms) can be modified further by a number of genes, the most important of which are the dense (*D*) and dilute (*d*) gene pair, and the colour series gene (*C*), which controls the Siamese and Burmese colour restrictions.

Dilute and dense genes

The dilute gene is a recessive one that dilutes the main colour. The various permutations of the basic colour with the dilute gene produce the three dilute colours, blue (*B-dd*), lilac (*bbdd*) and cream ($X^o X^o dd$), as well as the blue–cream tortoiseshell pattern ($X^o X^- B-dd$).

Colour series gene

The colour series gene (Figure 3.15) produces:

- Full colour (*C*): colour develops over the entire cat
- Burmese restriction (c^b): colour is lightened over the body, and though darker on the 'points' (face, ears, feet and tail) it is not as dark as the genetic colour
- Siamese restriction (c^s): the body is very pale with darker points, and the eyes are blue
- Albino (*c*): the most recessive gene in the series, pink-eyed albino, not to be confused with dominant white (although both cats are white, the albino has pink eyes and is not associated with deafness).

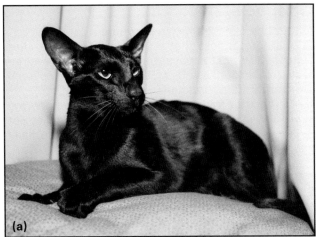

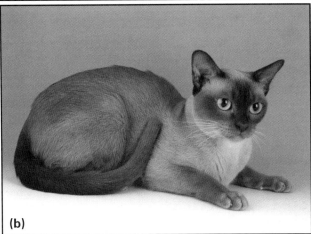

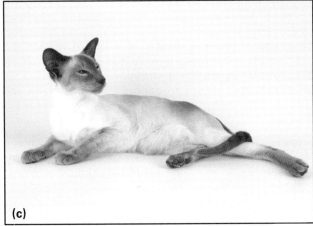

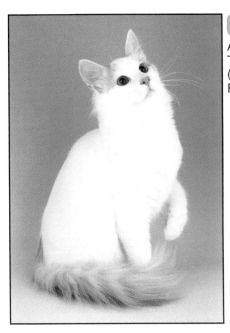

3.16
Auburn Turkish Van. (© Alan Robinson.)

3.15 The colour series gene. **(a)** Oriental Black. **(b)** Chocolate Burmese. The influence of the Burmese gene modifies the brown gene from all-over brown to brown only at the points. **(c)** Blue-point Siamese. The influence of the Siamese gene modifies the colour genes so that they are only developed at the points. (© Alan Robinson.)

Other genes

White spotting gene

The white spotting gene is a common one that controls white patches. It has variable expression, from only a small white bib, or perhaps just one white toe, through a cat with quite a lot of white (see Figure 3.13), to the cat that has only very small amounts of normal colour, often restricted to the ears and tail – for example, a cat such as the Turkish Van (Figure 3.16).

Inhibitor or silver gene

The only other colour gene that might be encountered is the inhibitor (*I*) or silver gene, which suppresses colour on parts of the hair shaft. This gene is dominant but has some variable expression. Cats with the silver gene can be described as silver (see Figure 3.10b), shaded, smoke, shell or tipped, or given other names depending upon the breed being described, and the basic cat colour. For example, a silver-tipped British Shorthair is a genetically black cat with the silver gene. The cat looks white, with a small amount of black tipping to the hair. Though this gene is quite rare in the domestic shorthair population, smoke non-pedigree cats are seen now and again.

Preparation for a new arrival

While in some cases a stray quite literally walks in off the street, in most cases people make a conscious decision to have a cat and some preparations need to be made for the new arrival. The basic equipment required includes:

- Cat carrier
- Bed and bedding
- Food and water bowls
- Litter box
- Scratching post
- Toys.

Cat carrier

A suitable box in which to transport the kitten or cat is essential (Figure 3.17). A cardboard box picked up from the local supermarket checkout is not acceptable as a carrying box. Some more substantial corrugated cardboard carriers are available from pet shops or veterinary surgeries that are satisfactory for relatively short-term use, but they are not secure if left unattended and cannot be cleaned adequately. Similarly designed plastic versions are available, which are a little better. More

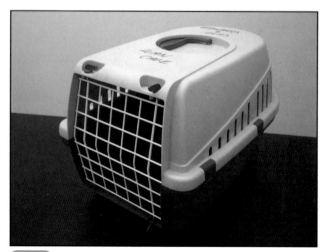

3.17 Cat carrier.

substantial carriers are more durable and range from traditional wicker baskets (also difficult to clean) to more sophisticated designs made from covered wire, plastic or fibreglass.

Points to bear in mind concerning the design of the carrier include the following:

- It is easier to get a cat into and out of a top-opening container than a side-opening one
- Good visibility is usually desirable for both owner and cat, but some cats prefer being able to hide in a solid-sided carrier
- The carrier should be easy to clean (some have removable trays to make cleaning of in-transit 'accidents' easier).

Beds and bedding

A cardboard box can make a very suitable bed: it has the advantages of low cost, ready availability, ease of redesign (holes can be cut out at appropriate places) and hygienic disposal. A more permanent basket of wicker, plastic or fibreglass may be more aesthetically pleasing, and the plastic versions are easy to clean. Polystyrene bead 'bean bags' are warm and comfortable, but can be too much like a litter box for some cats.

Whatever the basic bed, warm bedding such as a towel, blanket or purpose-designed pad will be much appreciated – cats spend a lot of time sleeping and a comfortable bed may help to reduce the time they spend sleeping on chairs or their owner's bed.

Feeding equipment

Ceramic, plastic or metal feed bowls are perfectly suitable for home use. Disposable bowls are available but are really needed only in catteries. As cats often have food left out for *ad lib* feeding and often prefer wide, shallow bowls, it is wise to have a feeding mat or tray under the bowl to minimize mess.

Plastic caps are useful to seal cat food cans after use until the next meal. For general hygiene reasons, cat bowls should be washed separately from (or at least after) the general washing up. A fork or spoon for use with cat food should be kept separate from the family cutlery.

Litter box

A litter box is necessary even where a cat has access to outdoors, unless that access is permanent. Litter boxes are almost always made from plastic and are easy to clean and disinfect. Some designs are covered, or incorporate air-fresheners.

Lining litter trays with purpose-designed liners or even newspaper can help to make cleaning easier. Soiled litter should be removed at least twice daily, using a scoop.

Cat litter is available in many forms:

- Mineral-based types in both 'clumping' (i.e. clumps when wet) and 'non-clumping' varieties
- Those based on sawdust or newspaper pellets
- Sand or peat
- 'Reusable' litters.

'Reusable' litters are based on plastic pellets or other inert material that can be cleaned after use; these usually require a special type of tray through which urine can drain into a lower chamber.

Pregnant women should avoid cleaning litter trays or should use gloves, due to a risk of *Toxoplasma* infection, which may be harmful to the unborn child. Pregnant women should also wear gloves when gardening, as it is possible that the flowerbed has been used as a cat latrine at some point.

Scratching post

It is a good idea to give a cat or kitten somewhere to scratch, in an effort to dissuade it from scratching the furniture. Scratching posts can be bought from pet stores, or pieces of bark or carpet may be mounted on a wall or other vertical surface. Usually cats are very happy to use these items when they know where they are. Sometimes the addition of catnip may be encouraging.

Toys

A wide variety of toys is available and most of them involve some kind of chasing or hunting activity – balls, mice, furry toys, toys dangling on the end of a 'fishing line' and so on. Some toys are very popular with individual cats, while others are never played with. A cardboard box with cut-out holes to hide in and jump out of can provide a lot of fun for a cat (or, even better, for two cats).

Some cats enjoy a lot of attention and will play with their owners for hours, even retrieving objects such as balls of silver paper; others ignore all toys and refuse to play with humans. Pedigree cats, especially the Foreign, Siamese and Burmese types, are often very playful and need time set aside for play.

General cat care

Compared with dogs, cats need less 'maintenance' in terms of walks, grooming, etc. However, they do still need time, effort and money spent on them. The costs of feeding are generally lower than for a dog, but costs of boarding (for holidays), veterinary visits and so on are not so different.

Grooming

Coat

Most cats groom themselves quite adequately and do not need their owner to groom them, other than regular stroking to make sure that there are no grass seeds stuck to their fur and keeping them free from parasites. However, longhaired or semi-longhaired cats need regular (daily) grooming to keep their coats in good condition. Without this, unmanageable and uncomfortable mats of hair will result. Longhaired kittens should be groomed with a wide-toothed comb from as young an age as possible.

It is important to groom all over and not just where the cat will allow it. The problem areas are usually along the back of the thighs, under the tail and under the axillae and chin. If mats develop, they may need to be cut or clipped out, which may have to be done under sedation or general anaesthesia and should not be attempted by the inexperienced.

Even in a shorthaired kitten, weekly use of a flea comb is wise – to give an early warning of parasites – and may be beneficial at times of moulting to help to prevent the development of a hairball (an accumulation of hair in the stomach). Hairball causes retching and occasionally more serious illness, and can require veterinary treatment ranging from the use of mild laxatives to surgery in severe cases. A soft-bristle brush or rubber brush is used by many people to groom shorthaired pedigree cats, giving them a final shine with a silk handkerchief to keep them looking their best.

Eyes and ears

Apart from the coat, the grooming routine should include inspection of the eyes and ears for evidence of any discharge or other problems. In certain cats, especially where the skin is pale, the eyes may naturally look pinkish but if there is any concern a veterinary opinion should be sought. Where a cat has deep-set eyes (e.g. a Siamese), it is not uncommon for a drop of mucus ('sleep dust') to form at the corner of the eye.

Any breed with a short nose (e.g. Persian, Exotic) may suffer from tear overflow and subsequent staining of the face. This should be bathed and dried carefully, or inflammation may result. A little petroleum jelly may help to prevent tear staining.

Claws

A cat's claws may need attention. The claw grows from the inside and older layers are removed by scratching to reveal the sharp new claw underneath. A scratching post should be provided so that a cat can exercise the claws, but it may be necessary to clip them occasionally to prevent scratching on furniture or to stop the claws getting caught on soft blankets. Some older cats have joint problems, which prevent them from keeping their own claws in order, leading to overgrowth.

It is not hard to clip a cat's claws, but most cats will object at first and so help may be needed. Gently squeezing the toe will extrude the claw and the sharp point can be safely cut off using claw clippers (Figure 3.18).

- It is often easier to sit with the cat on your knee.
- The claw can be extruded by gentle pressure on the toe.
- The point can be simply cut with sharp nail clippers.
- Do not cut above the point, as the tender quick will be damaged.
- In older cats, or cats without the opportunity to scratch and exercise their claws, the claws may be quite layered in appearance.

3.18 Clipping a cat's claws.

Playing

Most cats like to play and interact with their owners in some way and some time should be set aside to play with the cat every day. The sorts of toy that are available have been described above. Probably the best toy is another cat, but an attentive owner willing to throw a toy mouse or ball, or dangle something just out of reach, is usually appreciated. Many cats like to retrieve, play hide-and-seek, or to be chased in fun.

Outdoor access

Most cats will need outdoor access (Figure 3.19). Going outside gives them exercise, the ability to hunt and the opportunity to eat grass, which most cats will do. It also allows them to interact with other cats on common ground and to establish a territory of their own, which they can mark as they feel fit.

Outdoor access can be controlled by the owner opening a door or window, or can be via a cat flap.

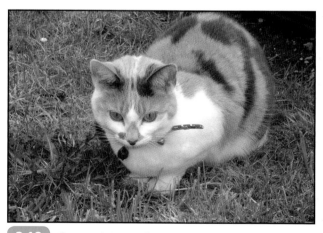

3.19 Cats enjoy outdoor access.

Cat flaps

Cat flaps can have some disadvantages, the most significant of which is that other cats may be able to get in, depending upon how sophisticated the flap is, and this may be a threat to the resident cat. Most of the time, however, cat flaps are very satisfactory. They can be locked at night; they can allow one-way traffic only; and some are electronically operated by a magnet on the cat's collar to prevent unwanted visitors.

Whether a cat has a flap or whether the owner controls outside access, a litter box should still be available for emergencies.

Risks

There are three main hazards with outdoor access:

- Risk of being hit by a car
- Risk of injury by another cat
- Risk of unwanted pregnancy.

Many cats are injured or killed on the road before their first birthday and this can be hard to prevent. In some cases, injured cats are never reunited with their owners if they are not easily identifiable and so a cat with outdoor access should either wear a collar or have other identification, such as an implanted microchip.

The risk of injury from other cats arises because cats fight each other to maintain their territories. Cat bites suffered during fights frequently become painful abscesses needing antibacterial therapy.

As for the risk of unwanted pregnancy, pet cats are usually neutered to prevent this and pedigree cats intended for breeding are not usually allowed unrestricted outdoor access.

Provision for holidays

It is important to stress to an owner that holiday arrangements must be made for a cat. Options include pet-sitters and boarding catteries.

Pet-sitting

Often, holiday arrangements will involve simply making sure that a friend or neighbour has a key and is willing to come into the house to feed the cat and clean the litter tray, preferably twice daily, and also, if possible, to play with the cat and provide some social interaction. This system has the advantage of cheapness and that the cat is not removed from its home environment. An added extra is the security for the holidaying owner of having someone in the house every day. Where a neighbour is not available, there are commercial companies that provide pet-sitting or house-sitting services.

Boarding catteries

An alternative for holidays is to put the cat into a boarding cattery. Catteries can be found by looking in the telephone directory or by asking friends, local veterinary surgeons or cat rescue groups for recommendations. All boarding catteries have to be inspected by the local council, but some are better than others. The Feline Advisory Bureau has a system of inspection that is very stringent and they publish a list of approved catteries (see 'Useful addresses'). It should always be possible for an owner to inspect a cattery before booking a place for their cat.

There is wide variety in cattery design, from entirely indoor cages to chalets with outdoor runs, and a broad range in between. Basically, catteries should have individual housing for each cat or household, with sufficient space for sleep and exercise, availability of food, water and a litter box, and heat in the winter. Premises should be clean, and cattery managers should insist that cats boarded with them should have current vaccination certificates against feline enteritis and cat 'flu (see below). Chapter 5 describes cattery construction and management in more detail.

Veterinary attention

Routine veterinary attention includes:

- Vaccination
- Control of internal and external parasites
- Neutering
- Pet identification (tattooing, microchip implantation)
- Consideration of purchase of pet insurance to cover veterinary fees for illness or accident.

Vaccination

There are various vaccines available for cats in the UK (Figure 3.20). These diseases are either common, serious, or both, and some form of vaccination is considered necessary for all cats. Vaccination is discussed in greater detail in the *BSAVA Manual of Practical Veterinary Nursing*, and only a brief summary is presented here.

Available in the UK:
- Feline infectious enteritis (FIE; feline panleucopenia; feline parvovirus)
- Feline herpesvirus (FHV-1; feline viral rhinotracheitis, FVR)
- Feline calcivirus (FCV)
- *Chlamydophila felis*
- Feline leukaemia virus (FeLV).

Available elsewhere in Europe, or in the USA:
- Feline coronavirus (FeCoV; feline infectious peritonitis, FIP)
- *Bordetella bronchiseptica*
- Rabies.

3.20 Cat vaccine components.

Feline infectious enteritis

Feline infectious enteritis is a viral disease, causing depletion of white blood cells (panleucopenia) and thus suppression of the immune system. It also causes severe damage to the lining of the intestine. This disease is often fatal and affected cats may die within 24 hours or less of becoming ill, though not all affected cats will die. If a pregnant queen is infected (or if she is vaccinated with a live vaccine while pregnant) the virus may damage the kittens within the womb, causing brain damage – specifically, cerebellar hypoplasia. Kittens with cerebellar hypoplasia cannot walk properly and may have fits or visual problems.

Cat 'flu

So-called cat 'flu is caused by two respiratory viruses: feline herpesvirus and feline calicivirus. Both viruses cause a raised temperature and nasal discharge, but cats often have slightly different clinical signs depending on which virus is involved.

Feline herpesvirus causes quite a severe illness, usually featuring conjunctivitis and rhinitis, with discharge from the nose and eyes. More severe cases may have pharyngitis and tracheitis, causing drooling of saliva.

Feline calicivirus usually has milder effects. It does not commonly cause the severe conjunctivitis associated with feline herpesvirus, but is usually associated with mouth ulcers. Occasionally feline calicivirus can cause a lameness syndrome, with a high temperature and shifting lameness, most common in young kittens.

Both viruses produce carrier cats after primary infection, which means that recovered cats may transmit the disease to other cats, despite appearing healthy. In addition, some cats never recover fully from cat 'flu and have chronic ocular or nasal discharges for life. It is rarely fatal in healthy adult cats, but young kittens and cats with immunodeficiency (e.g. infected with feline leukaemia virus or feline immunodeficiency virus, or on anti-cancer treatment) may die.

Chlamydiosis

Chlamydophila organisms primarily cause conjunctivitis in cats. Chlamydiosis (feline pneumonitis) can be difficult to resolve and may cause problems in breeding catteries, with young kittens being affected most often and most severely.

Feline leukaemia virus (FeLV)

Feline leukaemia is a fatal disease of cats that attacks the white blood cells, causing tumours and other diseases associated with derangement of the immune system. Usually young cats are affected, and an infected queen will transmit the virus to all of her kittens through the placenta, while they are still in the uterus. A blood test is available for FeLV; it may be used to diagnose the disease, to eliminate the infection from catteries and to screen cats before vaccination or at rescue catteries before rehoming.

Combined routine vaccinations

Combined feline enteritis and cat 'flu vaccines are the most commonly advised, but more owners are now choosing to have cats vaccinated against feline leukaemia virus and *Chlamydophila*. Some manufacturers produce these in a form that allows them to be combined with the more routine vaccinations. Vaccination is usually carried out at 9 and 12 weeks of age, though this regimen may be altered in some circumstances. Booster vaccinations are recommended annually by all manufacturers. For further information on these diseases and vaccination regimens see the *BSAVA Manual of Practical Veterinary Nursing*.

Worming

Cats can play host to a variety of internal parasites, including roundworms, tapeworms and lungworms. Parasites are discussed more fully in the *BSAVA Manual of Practical Veterinary Nursing*, but a brief résumé is given here.

Roundworms

Roundworms can cause problems in young kittens and routine worming, using a product suitable and safe for kittens, is usually advised. Unlike puppies, kittens are not born with roundworms but they can be infected by the queen early in life.

Tapeworms

Tapeworms can be transmitted by fleas or by consumption of infected prey. Cats can become reinfested regularly and may need repeated treatment by either tablet or injectable drugs.

Lungworms

Lungworms are quite common but rarely cause major disease, though they may be responsible for some cases of mild coughing. Only drugs available from a veterinary surgeon will be suitable to control lungworm infestation.

Fleas

Fleas are very common in cats, and it is an unusual cat that does not pick up fleas at some stage. Fleas commonly cause skin disease, which can be severe and may need veterinary treatment. There is a peak in flea numbers in the summer, but fleas can be a problem all year round with centrally heated houses. It is usually necessary to treat a cat for fleas at least through the summer months.

There are various control measures. The simple application of insecticide preparations to the coat is common and these are available as sprays or spot-on style products. An oral preparation that breaks the flea's life cycle is also popular; it can be given in food or by injection.

Where a flea problem is present, it may be necessary to use a spray in the house to kill larvae in the carpet and prevent reinfestation. The control of parasites is also discussed in the *BSAVA Manual of Practical Veterinary Nursing*.

Neutering

It is usual to neuter cats not intended for breeding. This has the advantage of preventing the birth of unwanted kittens and also of altering the less socially acceptable habits of the entire cat.

- Queens that are not neutered will come into season around every 3 weeks and can have unpredictable behaviour, including aggression and spraying of urine around the house
- Entire males can be aggressive and will often spray in the house after sexual maturity.

Spraying is a form of territory marking and can be difficult to stop once the behaviour has become established, as the cat will return to the marked area to reinforce the signal.

Neutering is usually carried out from around 5 months of age, though some advocate earlier neutering. For both sexes, general anaesthesia is required. Routine surgical procedures are covered in the *BSAVA Manual of Practical Veterinary Nursing*.

- Male cats are castrated, having both testes removed via the scrotum (Figure 3.21)
- Female cats have a complete ovariohysterectomy (i.e. the ovaries, oviducts, uterus and cervix are removed) in a procedure usually termed 'spaying'.

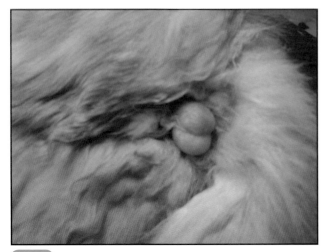

3.21 Preparing a cat for castration.

Spaying can be carried out by a flank or midline incision (Figure 3.22). A midline incision is often suggested for Siamese cats, as the coat tends to regrow darker in a shaved patch.

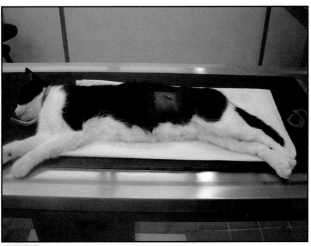

3.22 Wound site after a flank spay.

There are many local names for neutering and veterinary staff should not be surprised if an owner asks about the best age to 'dress' a cat, or when male cats should be 'doctored'. 'De-sexing' is a term routinely used in Antipodean countries and can be confusing.

A practice's clients will often have been given differing information by friends and family on the subject of neutering and may require advice to put them at ease before a cat neutering is carried out. Commonly asked questions regarding cat neutering include the following.

Would it be better for my cat if I allow her to have a litter first?

There is no scientific evidence to prove that cats that do not have litters suffer psychologically from not having the opportunity to have kittens. An owner who allows their cat to have a litter puts her at risk from disease transmission from the tom, as well as possible complications from carrying and giving birth to the litter. The owner will have the responsibility of finding good homes for all the kittens and, as cat rescue societies will report, there are too many cats looking for homes already without adding to the problem.

Will my cat change in personality after he/she has been neutered?

The basic personality of the cat will stay the same. Once it does not feel the need to reproduce, it may stay at home more and become more affectionate to the family. All in all it will become a better pet.

Will my cat become fat after being neutered?

It is true that neutering of animals does slow their metabolism, therefore effectively they will require less food than before. However, cats generally do not suffer from major obesity problems, and if an individual does have an issue in later life there are many dietary regimes that can be used to reduce weight.

My cat hasn't been 'calling' or in season and she is 6 months old. Do I have to wait before I can have her neutered ?

It is usually recommended to have a cat neutered between the ages of 5 and 6 months to prevent unwanted pregnancies. This is regardless of whether a season has been noticed or not. It is common for owners not to be aware when their cat is in season, especially if she is free to roam.

My tom cat doesn't spray in the house and is a very friendly much loved pet. Why should we have him neutered ?

As the tom cat matures he will start to mark and defend his territory much more. He will also start to roam far and wide to look for females. This will lead to a likelihood of cat fights (leading to injuries and disease transmission) and road accidents (major injuries and possibly death). Spraying around the house is likely to develop with the cat, and the responsibility of preventing unwanted litters should be taken into account. To ensure a long life for a much loved family pet, neutering is the best option.

Microchipping

As already mentioned, cats that are free to roam are independent spirits and can easily become injured or lost. Collars can be used but are not tolerated by some individuals and are frequently lost by others. The best way to ensure permanent identification of the cat is the implantation of a microchip. If the cat is found without an owner it can be scanned and quickly identified, as the owner's details are kept on a national database. Veterinary practices, the RSPCA and most cat charities will have access to a scanner.

The microchip is implanted under the cat's skin, usually between the shoulder blades (Figure 3.23). It is released via a large needle (which the cat may object to). It is common practice to microchip the cat when it is under general anaesthetic for neutering.

Once chipped, the cat will retain this identification for life.

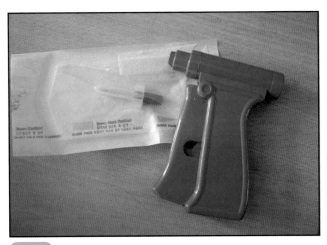

3.23   Microchip and implanter.

Insurance

Cats are often very important family pets and their owners will wish them to have the best care available if they become ill or are injured. To this end most cat owners will benefit from having pet insurance. As cats cannot be controlled like dogs, they do suffer from more accidental injuries (such as road accidents) as well as general disease conditions, and treatment bills can mount up.

Veterinary practices can advise clients on appropriate insurance companies or clients may wish to seek their own. Clients should be advised that insurance is not available on pre-existing conditions; therefore the earlier they can get their cat insured, whilst it is healthy, the better.

Illness and injury

To describe in detail every illness and injury that can be suffered by a cat is beyond the scope of this chapter, but common examples are described below.

Cat bite abscesses (CBAs)

Even neutered cats will fight with others, especially in areas where the cat population is high. Cats have a high level of oral bacteria, which become inserted into their opponent's skin via teeth during a fight. The resulting puncture is very small and heals quickly, trapping the bacteria inside. Pus accumulation soon develops as part of the inflammatory process and a painful swelling appears – the abscess. If left it is likely that the abscess will rupture on its own, but only after the cat has endured a period of intense discomfort, and it may not drain sufficiently to enable healing to take place.

Most cat bite abscesses require veterinary treatment, to be lanced and either free drained or have a drain placed in the remaining crater. Usually this needs to be done under a general anaesthetic and the cat will require antibiotics postoperatively.

Road traffic accidents (RTAs)

Roaming cats are often brought into the practice after an RTA. Injuries can vary from straightforward fractures, to prolapsed eyeballs and facial trauma and of course death.

Many cats that suffer an RTA will have pelvic injuries. Cats with pelvic injuries that are stable may only require cage rest in order to heal. Other injuries may require complicated orthopaedic surgery. Soft tissue injuries can look dreadful initially (e.g. degloving injuries) but cats are extremely good healers and can do very well eventually.

Rupture of the diaphragm can occur after being squashed during an RTA and these patients are likely to require thoracic surgery once they have been stabilized.

Facial injuries may require the cat to be tube fed whilst healing is taking place. This can be a complicated procedure but once a routine is established it is often well tolerated by the cat.

A cat presented to the surgery after an RTA should firstly be assessed for shock (see Chapter 8). It should be kept in a kennel that is warm and quiet and should have veterinary attention as soon as possible.

Parasitic infestation

As mentioned above, fleas are extremely common in cats and are the causative agents for most cat skin disease. Less commonly, cats can also suffer from mites and lice. A diagnosis needs to be made by the veterinary surgeon before a treatment regime can be started.

Ear mites are extremely common but the cat may not exhibit clinical signs. If scratching of the ears is seen, the veterinary surgeon will need to examine the cat to make a diagnosis.

Infectious diseases

Hopefully most patients in the practice will have been vaccinated again the most common feline infectious diseases, i.e. cat 'flu, feline enteritis and feline leukaemia. However, there are others that can be a problem, including the following (all of which carry a poor prognosis for the cat):

- Feline infectious peritionitis (FIP) – a viral disease affecting the peritoneum
- Feline infectious anaemia (FIA) – caused by *Mycoplasma haemofelis*, a blood parasite
- Feline immunodeficiency virus (FIV) – cat 'Aids', affecting the abilities of the immune system.

Geriatric cats

Cats that are over 10–12 years of age can be classed as geriatric. Geriatric cats require a warm secure environment in which to spend their days. They do not tolerate change as easily as they would have when younger and may seem more lethargic. They may benefit from being fed a geriatric-compliant diet, which they will find easier to digest and utilize.

Older cats may stay in and sleep more than their younger counterparts and, as an owner may expect, can suffer from more diseases than when they were younger. Arthritic changes can occur, especially with cats that have suffered injuries, and they may resent being handled. The owner needs to consider the welfare of the pet at all times and ensure that the cat has a good quality of life. Although some cats will live healthily until they are in their late teens or older, most cats will reach the end of a good life at around 14–15 years of age. If the quality of the cat's life has diminished in any way owners should seek the advice of the veterinary surgeon, who may advise euthanasia.

Common diseases seen in older cats include dental disease, hyperthyroidism, renal failure and diabetes mellitus.

Dental disease

Tooth extractions and dental scaling are likely to be required as the cat gets older. Calculus forms on the teeth and is seen as a build-up of a hard white/yellow substance. Cats will suffer from halitosis, inability to eat and salivation. Dentistry under general anaesthetic will need to be carried out at the practice.

Hyperthyroidism

This is a common condition of the geriatric cat. Problems that may be noticed by the owner include loss of weight (despite an increase in appetite), diarrhoea, staring coat and bad temper. This condition can be diagnosed by blood test and treated either medically with drugs, or surgically to remove the affected thyroid gland or glands.

Renal failure

Older cats are prone to kidney disease in later life. This is diagnosed by blood test and treatment includes management with low-protein diets, many of which are commercially available.

Diabetes mellitus

The management of a diabetic cat can be difficult for many owners. It is hard to control the food intake of an animal that is allowed to roam freely and may not be happy as a house cat. Cats do not tolerate being injected with insulin by their owner as easily as dogs and some owners may not wish to follow this line of treatment. It should be remembered that sometimes the diabetes is transient, but if owners are not prepared for the commitment required they may resort to euthanasia.

The Pet Passport scheme

The Pet Travel Scheme (PETS) has been developed to allow certain pet species (including cats and dogs) to be able to travel from the UK to other countries and return without the need for quarantine. This enables pet owners to take their pets abroad on holiday or to live in another country knowing that they will be able to return easily to the UK.

The procedure for obtaining a pet passport (Figure 3.24) for a cat is not complicated but does take time. Owners are advised to start the procedure at least 8 months before requiring the passport. Before starting, the owner needs to check with the Department for the Environment, Food and Rural Affairs (Defra) as to whether the country to which they are travelling is included in PETS. The veterinary practice may have some advice on this but it is best for the owner to double-check first.

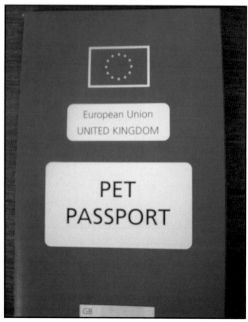

3.24
UK pet passport.

Whilst some dog owners may enjoy taking their dog away on holiday with them, for most cat owners this is not practical. Cats do not enjoy travel (and most are not used to it) and will initially be very stressed by new surroundings. If the cat escapes or roams away from the owner's base, there is very little chance of getting it back. The Pet Passport scheme is useful for owners who will be living abroad temporarily but will be prohibitive for most owners who only wish to have a holiday break.

Contact details for the Pet Passport scheme are listed at the end of this chapter.

Feeding cats

It is important to recognize that cats have very specific nutritional needs, different from those of dogs, humans and other omnivores. This is because cats are true carnivores and must have a high proportion of meat or other animal tissues in their diet. It is therefore necessary to consider carefully what to feed a cat and to recognize that table scraps are unlikely to be adequate.

Macronutrients

The macronutrients are protein, fat and carbohydrate.

Protein

Protein requirement, in both quantity and quality, is one of the most important nutritional differences between cats and dogs. Proteins are made up of chains of amino acids, some of which are essential (i.e. have to be consumed in their final form) and some of which are non-essential (i.e. can be synthesized by the cat).

Being strict carnivores, cats have an absolute requirement for meat in their diet. The cat is unable to synthesize certain amino acids (taurine and arginine) found only in animal protein sources and cannot meet these needs from protein of non-animal sources. If these amino acids are not available in sufficient quantity, deficiency diseases will occur:

- Taurine deficiency causes serious eye and heart problems
- Arginine deficiency causes grave metabolic disease.

The cat's reliance on protein does not stop with the supply of essential amino acids. Though protein is usually regarded as a 'body-building' food, most important in growth, pregnancy and lactation, cats also rely on protein to meet part of their energy needs. The protein part of a feline diet should therefore comprise at least 30–40% of the dry matter of a complete food for a healthy cat, which is twice as much as a dog needs. Cats cannot get enough protein from dog food and their special amino acid needs mean that they cannot tolerate a vegetarian diet either.

Fat

Fat is another important factor in the feline diet, accounting for about 10% of intake. Fat is important not only as a concentrated energy source but also as a source of essential fatty acids, and is another reflection of the cat's status as a carnivore. Omnivores can synthesize arachidonic acid from its precursor, linoleic acid, but the cat cannot and it needs animal fat in the diet.

Fat is also a valuable source of the fat-soluble vitamins A, D and E, and the cat requires animal-sourced vitamin A, being unable to produce it from carotene (the vegetable source) as omnivores can. Furthermore, fat makes a diet palatable to cats and is often used in this way by pet food manufacturers.

Carbohydrate

The remainder of the cat's diet will often come from carbohydrate, a useful source of energy and bulk, and which may also include micronutrients, depending on the source (e.g. B vitamins from wholegrain wheat). As carnivores, cats can survive relying largely on protein and fat for energy sources, but carbohydrates can be useful at times of nutritional stress and are usually present in commercially prepared foods. Starch sources (e.g. cereals) must be pre-cooked before being fed to cats.

Micronutrients

The micronutrients are vitamins and minerals.

Vitamins

Cats require an animal source of vitamin A, found in fat, but it is important that they do not receive too much vitamin A, as this can lead to skeletal disease. Excessive vitamin A consumption usually occurs in cats with a high consumption of liver and so feeding liver should be restricted to (at the most) a once-a-week treat, if it is fed at all.

Vitamin E can also cause problems for cats as it can be destroyed in contact with some fish oils, leading to the painful deficiency disease pansteatitis (yellow fat disease), where the body fat of the cat becomes inflamed. Feeding cats on a diet with a high proportion of oily fish is therefore to be discouraged, and this includes excessive use of some commercially available products sold as 'complementary' foods.

A further problem with fish is that it can contain an enzyme that destroys the vitamin thiamine (vitamin B1), causing thiamine deficiency and leading to neuromuscular disease. High levels of some preservatives in brawn-type foods can also break down thiamine and cause thiamine deficiency.

Another vitamin compromised in cats is pyridoxine (vitamin B6), for which cats have a high requirement. The other vitamins will usually present no cause for concern in a varied diet.

Minerals

The most important minerals are calcium and phosphorus, which must be present in the diet in the correct proportions to allow for healthy bone growth and maintenance. A cat hunting for itself in the wild and consuming the small bones of rodents or birds naturally provides itself with a balanced source. It is important to remember that lean meat will not provide this balance and supplementation will often be needed if a homemade diet is fed.

Over-supplementation is as dangerous as under-supplementation and the amounts of any extra calcium and phosphorus given must be calculated properly. Other minerals will usually be present in sufficient quantities in a varied diet.

Water

Water is a basic requirement, essential for all body processes. Cats can concentrate their urine a great deal if required, but water must always be available. The use of dried foods increases the cat's need for water; this is discussed below.

Milk

Most cats like milk and it is a valuable source of calcium, protein, fat and vitamins.

Some cats, as they reach adulthood, are unable to digest milk properly. They lack an enzyme in the intestine that breaks down lactose (the milk sugar) and this can lead to diarrhoea. Special cat milks are available that may help to prevent this problem.

For kittens at weaning, a queen's milk replacement is usually preferable to cow's milk. Some cat breeders suggest the use of goat's milk, though this may not be readily available.

Basic nutritional requirements

Nutrition for various stages of the cat's life, including for some disease states, is described in more detail in Chapter 6.

- In general terms, an active adult cat has a calorie (energy) requirement of approximately 85 kilocalories (kcal) per kilogram bodyweight, falling to around 70 kcal/kg for a cat that is less active.
- Growing kittens and pregnant queens have higher calorie requirements than this: approximately 100 kcal/kg.
- Lactating queens have the highest requirements of all: up to 250 kcal/kg at peak milk production (around 2–4 weeks after kittening).

Although these daily feeding requirements are expressed as energy, it should be remembered that protein is an important source of energy for cats and that these requirements must be met with a diet balanced for macro- and micronutrients. The higher energy requirements for kittens and pregnant or lactating queens are most easily met by increasing the quantity of fat in the diet, as it is a more concentrated form of energy. Inspection of most prepared foods intended for this group of cats will usually show an increased fat content to help meet the energy requirements without adding extra bulk, as might be the case if carbohydrate sources are used.

Feeding habits

Cats do not tend to have 'meals' in the same way as dogs or humans do, and are more likely to return to their bowl for a snack at a number of stages during the day. Fed in this way (*ad lib*), cats rarely become overweight. In the occasional case of an overweight or even obese cat, some form of calorie restriction has to be practised.

Types of diet available

The choice is basically between commercially available foods and homemade diets. Although the choice of fresh feeding is uncommon, it is preferred by some breeders.

Fresh (homemade) diet

With a homemade diet it is very important to ensure that no deficiencies or excesses are produced. It can be difficult to achieve a balanced diet, though the cat will often supplement the supplied diet by hunting if outdoor access is allowed.

It is beyond the scope of this chapter to formulate homemade diets but in general terms:

- Three parts of an animal-derived protein food (meat, fish, eggs, cheese) to one part of carbohydrate (cooked rice, bread, potatoes) will be adequate if combined with a vitamin/mineral mix
- It is usually necessary to give full-cream milk to cats on homemade diets in order to help to meet their calcium needs, though a calcium supplement can also be used
- It is important to remember the general advice about avoiding excesses of liver and fish, to prevent nutritionally related diseases.

Commercially manufactured diet

There is a wide variety of commercial cat foods. They may be presented as canned, semi-moist or dry, and may be either complete (designed to be fed as the entire diet) or complementary (designed to be used as part of a balanced diet). It is common for cats to be fed a mixture of different foods, with perhaps the canned food being given as meals, and dry or semi-moist food left out during the day.

Canned foods

Canned foods remain the most popular in the UK. Similar in nutritional terms to the canned foods are the premium 'tray' foods – individual portions, cooked in a foil tray.

- Most complete canned foods are around 75–80% water, with a balanced mix of protein (around 8%), fat (around 5%) and carbohydrate, and a certified quantity of vitamins and minerals.
- An average adult cat (around 4 kg bodyweight) requires approximately one can (400 g) per day.
- It is usually necessary to supply a fresh serving at least twice daily when using canned food as it tends to dry out, lose palatability and become at risk of spoiling.
- A food designed for adult cats will usually be sufficient for the needs of pregnant and lactating queens, though of course larger quantities will be required.
- Also available in cans are kitten diets, which are higher in fat, protein and vitamins, and which are also eminently suitable for use with pregnant or lactating queens, having a higher calorie content in a smaller volume.
- After weaning, kittens should still be fed at least three times a day until around 5–6 months old and should have access to milk or milk substitute.

Dried foods

Dried foods are the next most commonly used foods. They are usually designed as complete diets.

- The major difference in nutritional terms is the percentage of water, which is less than half the water content of a canned food. A cat on a dried food diet must drink extra water (or milk) to make up the difference.
- While canned foods usually rely on animal protein sources alone, some dried foods contain vegetable protein in addition.
- Around 100 g of complete dried food, along with about 200 ml of water, is sufficient for an adult cat weighing 4 kg.
- Dry food has the advantage that it does not appreciably spoil through the day, though the highly palatable fat on the surface does diminish with time.
- Dry food is better for the cat's teeth and gums, and will help to reduce tartar build-up.
- Dry food should be introduced gradually into a cat's diet and may be soaked with water, milk or gravy at first. Changing abruptly to dry food before the cat has had a chance to adapt to increased drinking habits may result in the formation of crystals in the urine, which can be life-threatening.
- Kitten dry food formulations are also available, as are some 'senior' diets with lower energy concentrations to help to prevent obesity in the less active older cat, and with lower protein, which may assist in lessening the effects of renal failure, a common problem in older cats.

Semi-moist foods

Semi-moist foods have never really gained much popularity in the UK. With a dough-like texture, they are similar to true dry foods in their advantage of convenience and in the requirement for additional water consumption.

These foods can contain a preservative, propylene glycol, which may cause anaemia by reducing the lifespan of feline red blood cells. Although this is not common, problems may be seen where there is underlying disease.

Complementary foods

All the foods above have been described from the point of view that they are complete, as are most of the cat foods generally available. There are also some complementary foods available, which are designed to be fed as part of a balanced diet, or as part of a homemade diet. As long as they are used as they are intended, there is unlikely to be any problem in feeding complementary foods, but some owners do not realize that these food are not intended as complete diets and this can cause problems.

Perhaps the best known of these are the high-fish canned foods, which can cause pansteatitis due to lack of vitamin E (see above). It is important that owners examine the labels of cat food and use the contents as directed.

Another type of complementary food, rarely fed except by cat breeders, is 'brawn', a high-meat product usually produced in a plastic sausage-like skin. Most of these foods are not complete and may contain high levels of sulphur dioxide as a preservative, which can destroy thiamine and cause thiamine deficiency.

Breeding

It is not usually advisable to breed intentionally from non-pedigree cats; there are so many cats crowding cat shelters that producing more kittens will generally be discouraged by veterinary surgeons or rescue societies.

Reproduction is covered in more detail in the *BSAVA Manual of Practical Veterinary Nursing* but is summarized briefly here.

Signs of oestrus

The queen is seasonally polyoestrous (i.e. comes into heat, or on call, many times during a breeding season). When 'on call' she will usually rub against items of furniture, especially marking with the side of her face. If she can find a low chair or table, she will often rub her back along that.

The cardinal sign of calling is lordosis, where the back is flexed downward to push the vulva upward, and she may attempt to entice other cats to mount her, regardless of their sex or ability. This performance is usually accompanied by a loud and persistent yowling call, and she may lie writhing on the ground on her side or back, crying in a most alarming manner. It is not unusual for owners to fail to recognize the signs of calling and to ring the veterinary surgeon for advice, believing the cat to be in pain.

Breeding season

The breeding season for cats in the UK is from around March to September, though there is individual variation within this and some queens will call all year round, especially pedigree cats of Foreign or Oriental type.

Puberty

The queen will usually reach puberty at between 6 and 15 months, though this depends on breed, date of birth and weight. Cats of the Foreign, Oriental or Siamese type are more precocious; British and Persian cats tend to reach puberty later. Kittens born early in the year may come into call that summer or autumn, while they are little more than kittens themselves.

Males are generally fertile by 5–6 months of age, but there is similar breed variation in the development of appropriate sexual behaviour.

Mating

Where an owner intends to breed from a cat, it is generally advised that the animal should be at least 12 months old and at most 4 years old at mating. The novice breeder can get a lot of help and advice (at times contradictory) from other cat breeders. It is often a good idea to contact the original breeder for advice on selection of stud etc., but local or national cat clubs are also valuable sources of information about the location of suitable males.

It is usual for a queen to be taken to the stud cat within the first few days of her starting to call, and for her to remain with him for a week or more. The stud owner will usually observe mating.

It is important that queens are mated frequently, as the stimulation of mating is required to induce ovulation. If a cat is not mated, she will call for around 10 days. After successful mating(s) and ovulation, she will usually come off call within 2–3 days. The gestation period is around 63 days.

Obviously an entire queen, whether pedigree or not, who gets out while on call will make her own arrangements for selection of a male and frequency of mating. There will often be a number of entire males queuing up outside the owner's house awaiting an escape by a calling queen.

Pregnancy and parturition are covered in the *BSAVA Manual of Practical Veterinary Nursing*.

Kitten development and behaviour

As kittens usually spend the first few months of their lives with the queen, a great deal of the behavioural influence comes from her and from her owners.

Neonates

At birth, a kitten is blind, mostly deaf (eyes and ears open around 10–14 days) and unable to regulate its own body temperature. It can crawl along the queen's abdomen, seeking a nipple, treading to assist in milk 'letdown' and often purring, surprisingly loudly. An individual kitten often has a preference for a particular nipple, and those nearest the back are most favoured. Happy, feeding kittens are quiet; cold or hungry kittens vocalize to let the dam know their distress.

For the first month after parturition the kittens are largely immobile, remaining in the nest feeding. The queen stimulates them to urinate and defecate by licking the perineal area, and either consumes the waste or removes it from the nest for disposal elsewhere. Should the queen feel threatened, she will carry the kittens to another nest, by the scruff of the neck – a reflex relaxation of the kitten makes this safe for both queen and kitten and this is a useful method of restraint in later life.

Contact with the mother during the first month is very important for normal behavioural development of kittens. If the mother dies a foster mother is best, but if this is not possible, quality human contact and handling for at least 20 minutes a day will help to reduce potential problems. More detail on the care of neonatal kittens is given in the *BSAVA Manual of Practical Veterinary Nursing*.

Weaning

As kittens become more mobile at around the end of the first month, they start to leave the nest and the queen starts to become slightly more resistant to their demands for feeding. She presents them with solid food and teaches them how to bury their faeces and urine.

From this age the normal social contact between kittens matures rapidly as recognition and play behaviour patterns develop. The kitten can already discriminate between the calls of the queen and other kittens, and those of a potential threat such as growls or sudden unexpected sounds. The senses of vision and smell are also well developed, and weaning on to solid food can start. In free-ranging cats, the mother will start to bring in prey at this stage and though it will be many weeks before the kitten is a competent predator itself, it will learn through observation and play.

Play behaviour

Play behaviour is a prominent feature of kittens, presumably linked to refining their social and predatory skills, but some patterns seem to have no special function and might perhaps be assumed to be fun. The types of play seen in kittens and cats are often segregated by behaviouralists into social play, object play, locomotor play and self-directed play.

Social play

The patterns used in social play alter as the kittens grow older and more experienced. This form of play starts in the nest and peaks at between 9 and 14 weeks. Kittens will dance sideways, 'bat' at each other with forepaws, lie on their backs, raise themselves on to their haunches, and chase and pounce on each other in a highly ritualized way, all the while with a variety of facial expressions, yowls and growls.

Kittens seem to be able to separate this play from true aggression, and while one or other may be dominant at some times, this position may be rapidly reversed, even in the same encounter. Young kittens will often interact in this way as a 'gang' of three or more but as they get older often only two kittens are involved in more direct stand-offs. At around 18–20 weeks, actual aggression becomes more common, as does sexual behaviour from the males.

Object play

Object play incorporates some of the features of social play, even though the interaction is with an inanimate object or prey. Kittens will investigate unknown objects intensively (thus the saying, 'Curiosity killed the cat') by observation, sniffing and gentle touching, perhaps from a 'safe' distance and retreating quickly afterwards, and will eventually – especially if the object is small – culminate with batting, chasing and pouncing on it. Kittens will frequently pick up suitably sized objects using one or both paws, for biting or mouthing, and will toss them into the air for further pursuit.

Object play may be better developed in a single kitten, or in hand-reared kittens, where the opportunities for social play with other kittens are unavailable.

This facet of play becomes more important than social play at around 16 weeks and may be driven by the weaning process. Its persistence seems to depend upon the individual temperament of the cat: some cats will happily play with objects all their lives; others will ignore them after they have grown out of kittenhood. This play is usually considered desirable by owners and can be encouraged by a variety of cat toys.

Cats are slightly unusual in also using a scoop behaviour to capture an object from a confined space (e.g. a box or from under a chair) by reaching the paw in as far as possible in order to retrieve it. Several toys are designed to exploit this behaviour pattern.

Locomotor play

Locomotor play includes what many owners think of as a kitten's 'mad half-hour' of running about, wild eyed, over many unsuitable objects. A large scratching post may help to divert a kitten from the rival attractions of the curtains or the top of the bookshelves, but even adult cats will indulge in this and send cups or lamps flying, apparently for no good reason. This behaviour is thought to be self-rewarding, i.e. it is just fun.

Self-directed play

Self-directed play is typified by the kitten that chases its tail or bites its feet. Again, this seems to be purely motivated by fun, rather that having any great purpose. Most cats seem to grow out of these behaviours.

Isolated kittens

A kitten weaned early and reared in isolation (for example, as part of a programme to reduce the level of an infectious disease in a cattery) can suffer as a result of the failure of normal socialization with other adult cats and people. Such kittens need careful handling to ensure that they grow up well balanced.

Activities with cats

Unlike dogs, cats are not usually taken for walks in the country or on the beach, nor do they attend training classes or similar. Cat-orientated activities revolve around playing with owners or suitable toys and, for a few cats, going to cat shows.

Games

It is quite easy to train a tractable cat in some simple activities that can be fun for both owner and cat.

Many cats will retrieve objects and will respond to commands similar to those given to dogs ('Sit!', 'Paw!' etc.) in return for an edible reward. Cats will play hide-and-seek, or other chasing games, with people. Most will 'help' their owners around the house – by lending a paw with tasks such as brushing the floor or getting between their owner and the computer screen. Some cats like to watch television and there are even videos available for cats to watch.

Cat shows and clubs

Going to cat shows is not solely the domain of the pedigree cat, as there are classes for non-pedigree ('household pet') cats too. Unlike dogs, neutered cats can also be shown and have their own classes.

Cat shows are mostly run by local cat clubs and lists of shows may be obtained from the GCCF or Cat Association of Britain offices (see 'Useful addresses'). As well as running shows, most cat clubs organize social events, which can be a good way for owners to meet others with similar interests.

The rules for showing are quite strict and the novice is well advised to attend at least one show before considering showing their own cat. All cats are checked on entry to the show hall by a veterinary surgeon, who screens for infectious diseases and veterinary defects. The cats are then 'penned' in cages in which only very specific objects (plain white feed bowl, water bowl, litter tray, blanket) are allowed. The cat is identified only by a number, to ensure impartiality of judging.

Usually, a cat or kitten may be entered in an 'open' class, where it competes against others of the same breed, and then may enter further classes for mixed breeds (e.g. 'Any variety Foreign kitten').

- When a pedigree cat is adult (and entire), it competes for a Challenge Certificate (CC) in the open class. If it wins three of these, the cat becomes a champion.
- Champions may compete for a Grand Challenge Certificate (GCC) in a mixed-breed open class for champions of their breed group; in a similar way, a cat with three GCCs is a grand champion.
- Many clubs also run a best-in-show competition.

The major show in the British cat world is the GCCF Supreme Show, where cats compete for top honours. Here, in addition to the normal classes, there is a special class for grand champions to compete for UK Grand Challenge Certificates. As this show only takes place once a year, just two UK GCCs are needed to become a UK grand champion.

The system outlined for entire cats is exactly mirrored by one for neuters, in which the competition is for premier, grand premier, etc.

Although the GCCF is the major registering body in the UK, there are others and these may have different procedures. They may recognize further breeds, or variants of established breeds (in terms of colour or pattern), and have different show rules and awards. For example, the Cat Association of Britain allows Sphynx to be shown, permits decoration of pens and has different judging procedures.

References and further reading

A number of cat magazines are available from newsagents, with articles for those interested in cats. These can be very useful and informative for both clients and professionals, and a good source of information on pedigree cat breeders in specific geographical areas.

Bradbury JWS (1992) *The Behaviour of the Domestic Cat.* CAB International, Wallingford, Oxon

Mullineaux E and Jones M (2007) *BSAVA Manual of Practical Veterinary Nursing.* BSAVA Publications, Gloucester

Pedersen NC (1991) *Feline Husbandry.* American Veterinary Publications Inc., Goleta, California

Robinson R (1991) *Genetics for Cat Breeders, 3rd edn.* Butterworth-Heinemann, Oxford

Taylor D (1989) *The Ultimate Cat Book.* Dorling Kindersley, London

Turner T and Turner J (1994) *Veterinary Notes for Cat Owners.* Stanley Paul, London

Walter S (1980) *The Book of the Cat.* Pan Books, London

Wills JM and Simpson KW (1994) *The Waltham Book of Clinical Nutrition of the Dog and Cat.* Butterworth-Heinemann, Oxford

Useful addresses

Pedigree cat organizations

Pedigree cat clubs may be local or national. These associations maintain lists of affiliated clubs. Many breed clubs operate a rescue scheme for pedigree cats.

Governing Council of the Cat Fancy
5 King's Castle Business Park, The Drove, Bridgwater, Somerset TA6 4AG
Telephone: 01278 427575
www.gccfcats.org

Cat Association of Britain
Mill House, Letcombe Regis, Oxon OX12 9JD
Telephone: 01235 766543

Fédération Internationale Féline
www.fifeweb.org

Other organizations

Feline Advisory Bureau
Headquarters: Taeselbury, High Street, Salisbury, Wiltshire SP3 6LD
Telephone: 0870 742 2278
www.fabcats.org

The FAB is a charity that supports a number of veterinary surgeons working in the field of feline medicine at a number of the veterinary schools in the UK. It publishes a quarterly journal with articles of general and veterinary interest, and organizes meetings for breeders and veterinary surgeons. It also runs a boarding cattery inspection service and publishes a guide to catteries.

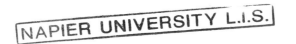NAPIER UNIVERSITY L.I.S.

Association of Pet Behaviour Counsellors
PO Box 46, Worcester WR8 9YS
Telephone: 01386 751151
www.apbc.org.uk

The APBC is a network of behavioural counsellors who, on referral from a veterinary surgeon, can give advice on the management of pet animals exhibiting inappropriate behaviour.

Cat shelters

Two major groups run cat shelters in the UK; numerous small organizations are also involved. Look in the telephone directory for local shelters. Veterinary surgeons often have lists of local groups.

Cats Protection
Headquarters: 17 Kings Road, Horsham,
West Sussex RH13 5PN
Telephone: 01403 221900
www.cats.org.uk

A charity basically for cat rescue, CP can also sometimes provide support to owners in financial difficulty over neutering of their cats. It publishes leaflets about cat care and infectious diseases.

Royal Society for the Prevention of Cruelty to Animals (RSPCA)
Headquarters: Wilberforce Way, Southwater, Horsham, West Sussex RH13 9RS
Telephone: 0870 3335999
www.rspca.org.uk

PETS

For more information about the Pet Travel Scheme and current requirements, contact:
PETS helpline: 0870 241 1710; fax: 01245 458749; email: pets.helpline@defra.gsi.gov.uk; visit: www. defra.gov.uk/animalh/quarantine/pets/index.htm

4

General care and management of other pets and wildlife

Anna Meredith, Sharon Redrobe and Elizabeth Mullineaux

This chapter is designed to give information on:

- The species of animals kept as exotic pets, and their advantages and disadvantages as pets
- Basic biology, anatomy and husbandry requirements of exotic pets
- How to handle and determine the sex of exotic pets and wildlife safely and humanely
- How to recognize the signs of pain and disease in exotic pets and wildlife
- How to administer basic medication to exotic pets and wildlife

Introduction

Pets other than cats and dogs are extremely popular and their numbers are on the increase. The rabbit is now the third most popular mammalian pet in the UK. In addition to small mammals, many people keep birds, reptiles, amphibians, fish and invertebrates as pets. In many veterinary practices, these so-called exotic pets make up a significant proportion of the patient caseload and some practices now offer specialist expertise in exotic pets.

The expectations of the owners for the level of knowledge and care that these animals should receive is also increasing. The aim of this chapter is to provide guidance as to the suitability of the various species as pets and to give a broad introduction to their general husbandry and care.

Abandoned, injured and sick wild animals are also commonly presented for veterinary attention. The requirements and behaviour of wildlife are extremely varied and often differ very significantly from those of domestic animals. This chapter describes the techniques for caring for wildlife patients, including emergency first aid for the wildlife casualty.

Exotic pets: considerations before purchasing

The main types of pet that are generally available are listed in Figure 4.1.

Unfortunately, a lot of pets are purchased on impulse and without any prior thought or planning. This can lead to welfare and disease problems and

Group	Examples
Mammals	Rabbit, guinea pig, chinchilla, hamster, gerbil, rat, mouse, ferret
Birds	Parrot, budgerigar, canary, finch, pigeon
Reptiles	Snake, lizard, tortoise, turtle, terrapin
Amphibians	Frog, toad, salamander, axolotl
Fish	Goldfish, tropical fish
Invertebrates	Stick insect, spider, snail

4.1 Types of exotic pet available.

unwanted animals, as owners are not aware of their special requirements. Research and advice from knowledgeable sources should always be sought before acquiring a new pet. Veterinary nurses are often approached for advice on this subject. Points that should be considered include the following:

- The reason for wanting a pet – companionship, special interest, children's pet, education. A reptile would not be suitable for someone wanting a close companion with a lot of interaction
- Facilities and space available – a garden is desirable for rabbits, guinea pigs or ferrets, whereas very little space is required for invertebrates
- Financial aspects – costs of housing, feeding and veterinary care. Vivarium set-ups for reptiles can be very expensive, whereas a pet hamster is very cheap to keep
- Amount of spare time available – parrots need a lot of individual attention from an owner who is at home most of the time, whereas fish require very little attention
- Other pets already kept – some species may be incompatible or must be kept apart, such as small mammals and cats

- Human health risks – many people are allergic to the hair and dander of small mammals, and there are several zoonotic diseases that can be passed on to owners from pets, such as psittacosis from parrots and pigeons and salmonellosis from reptiles.

When choosing a pet, it is useful to consider the advantages and disadvantages of the species available (Figures 4.2 and 4.3).

Mammals

The mammals are haired endothermic ('warm-blooded') animals that bear live young and suckle them. The small mammals kept as exotic pets share the basic mammalian features of the dog and cat but with some important differences, especially in dentition, gastrointestinal tract and female reproductive tract anatomy.

Rabbits

Rabbits belong to the Order Lagomorpha (rabbits and hares), the members of which have distinct anatomical differences from the Rodentia. All pet rabbits are the same species and are descended from the wild European rabbit *Oryctolagus cuniculus*.

Mammal	Advantages	Disadvantages
Mouse	Small, cheap, clings to handler	Smells, tends to be more active at night
Rat	Intelligent, responsive, sociable, clings to handler	
Gerbil	Odourless, active during day	Difficult to handle, easily dropped
Hamster	Odourless	Nocturnal, can bite, easily dropped
Chipmunk	Active during day	Easily stressed, difficult to handle, best kept outdoors
Guinea pig	Rarely bites, active during day	Can be nervous
Chinchilla	Extremely attractive	Destructive, often dislikes being handled
Rabbit	Generally docile, good house pet	Occasionally aggressive or nervous and difficult to handle Larger breeds difficult for young children to handle
Ferret	Highly intelligent, responsive, entertaining	Smells, needs a lot of attention, good escape artist

4.2 Pet mammals: advantages and disadvantages.

Species	Advantages	Disadvantages
Birds	Very responsive, trainable, talk (psittacines) 'Guard dogs' (geese) Provide eggs (poultry)	Require a lot of attention (psittacines) Can be noisy and destructive (psittacines) Can be aggressive (geese)
Reptiles	Quiet, low maintenance once initial vivarium equipment set up, non-allergenic	Equipment expensive, some species dangerous, do not respond to owner, diet can be unpleasant to owner
Amphibians	Quiet, low maintenance, non-allergenic	Handling not advised, often very inactive
Fish	Quiet, soothing to watch, low maintenance	No direct interaction

4.3 Other pets: advantages and disadvantages.

Points to consider when choosing rabbits

- There are over 80 breeds or varieties of rabbit, ranging in size from 1 kg to 10 kg or more. Many pets are crossbred (Figure 4.4).
- Rabbits have traditionally been kept outside, but do make very good house pets and can be litter-trained.
- Rabbits are highly sociable but two males (bucks) will fight.
- Rabbits are diurnal (more active at dawn and dusk).
- Rabbits are generally docile if handled regularly. Large rabbits can be difficult for young children to handle, and incorrect handling can damage the animal's spine.
- Rabbits should be vaccinated every 6 months against myxomatosis and annually against viral haemorrhagic disease. This expense should be borne in mind before purchase.

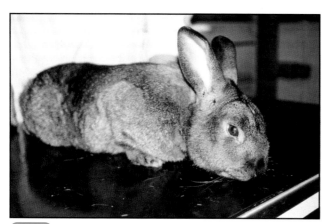

4.4   A crossbred rabbit.

Biological data: rabbits

Average lifespan	6–10 years
Sexual maturity	3–6 months
Oestrus	Induced ovulation (Jan–Oct)
Gestation	28–32 days
Average litter size	2–7
Weaning age	6 weeks
Adult weight	1–10 kg
Body temperature	38.5°C

Anatomy and physiology

Dentition

- The dental formula is 2/1, 0/0, 3/2, 3/3.
- Rabbits have a second small pair of incisors ('peg teeth') directly behind the first pair in the upper jaw.
- Rabbit teeth are not pigmented and the enamel should appear smooth and creamy white.
- The upper incisors possess a single vertical groove.
- There is a large diastema between the incisors and the cheek teeth, with cheek folds drawn across it.
- Both incisors and cheek teeth are open rooted and grow constantly throughout life.
- Incisors grow at approximately 3 mm/week, and cheek teeth at approximately 3 mm/month.
- The mandible is narrower than the maxilla.
- The upper lip is cleft.

Skeleton

The rabbit skeleton is lightweight, making up only 7–8% of bodyweight (compared with 12–13% in dogs and cats). Rabbit bones are brittle and easily broken, making orthopaedic surgery more challenging.

Limbs and feet

The hindlegs are long and the metatarsal area is in contact with the ground at rest. The feet have no bare footpads and are completely covered in hair. There are four toes and a dewclaw on the forefeet and four toes on the hindfeet.

Tail and ears

The tail or 'scut' is short and curves upwards over the rump. The ears are large and upright, except in lop breeds. The ears are an important site for heat regulation. Female rabbits develop a large fold of skin under the chin, known as the dewlap.

Digestive tract

- The rabbit's digestive tract has a simple large stomach, a long small intestine, a very large sacculated caecum and a long colon.
- Rabbits produce two types of faeces: soft mucus-covered caecal pellets (caecotrophs), which are produced at night or in the early morning and eaten directly from the anus (caecotrophy, coprophagy); and hard dry faecal pellets, which are not eaten.
- Bacterial fermentation of food takes place in the caecum (hind gut fermentation).

Urination

- Rabbits excrete excess dietary calcium in the urine and it is normal for the urine to contain crystals.
- Normal urine can vary in appearance from thick and turbid to clear, and range in colour from pale creamy yellow through to a deep red, depending on the diet of the rabbit.
- Reddish urine is often mistaken as containing blood; a urine dipstick will test for the actual presence of blood.

Sexing

The anogenital distance is similar in male and female rabbits. The sex of a rabbit can be determined by looking at the shape of the genital opening: it is round in the male (buck) and the penis can be protruded with gentle pressure from above. After sexual maturity the testicles in the male can easily be seen lying on either side of the penis in scrotal sacs. In the female (doe) the vulva is a V-shaped slit.

Behaviour

- Rabbits have poor displays of greeting behaviour, pain and fear due to their prey status.
- Scent is much more important than sight and each animal has an individual scent profile. They can distinguish between familiar and unfamiliar humans, and between human genders.
- Rabbits are highly social. In the wild they live in warrens of 70 or more individuals, broken down into small groups of 2–8. They will spend a lot of time engaged in mutual grooming and lying together.
- Does are more territorial than bucks and as they reach sexual maturity they may become aggressive towards the owner and other animals. Does may also bite, dig and chew flooring and household items, spray urine and mount other rabbits. If outdoors on soil the doe may excavate deep tunnels.
- Socialization of young rabbits is often overlooked.
- A well-socialized pet rabbit will beg for treats, 'hum' and circle the owner, stand on its back legs and lick the owner's hands and arms.
- Rabbits are inquisitive and enjoy exploring. Picking up objects with the teeth and throwing them is common, as is exploratory chewing.
- A rabbit in pain will be immobile with a hunched posture, and may grind its teeth and show increased aggression. Thumping with the hindleg is an alarm call. Fear elicits either complete immobility or a flight response, often with frantic attempts to escape and screaming.
- Rabbits have not been bred for positive behaviour traits and behavioural problems are common. Individual rabbits have distinct 'personalities', from timid to aggressive. In general, smaller breeds tend to be more highly strung.
- Aggression is generally learnt (the owner leaves the rabbit alone if it behaves aggressively). Other causes are territorial behaviour, boredom, pain, improper socialization and negative association (a previous aversive or traumatic situation). Behavioural aggression can be successfully treated in many cases using similar techniques to those used in dogs.

Housing

Rabbits are social animals: they should never be kept singly. They can be kept in small groups, but not bucks together as they will fight. Rabbits should not be kept with guinea pigs, as rabbits tend to 'bully' guinea pigs. Many rabbits are now kept as house pets and they can be trained to use a litter tray.

Rabbits are generally hardy animals but need protection from extremes of weather. Most pet rabbits are housed in commercial or homemade wooden hutches, but these are often far too small.

- A hutch should be high enough for the rabbit to stand upright on its hindlegs and long enough to allow the rabbit to perform at least three hops from end to end.
- A separate solid-fronted nesting area and a mesh-fronted day living area should be provided, bedded with wood shavings and hay or straw.
- Outdoor hutches should be raised off the ground.
- If it is outside, a waterproof roof and a louvered panel to cover the mesh-fronted area in bad weather should be provided.
- Rabbits need the opportunity to exercise and to graze. Hutch-kept rabbits frequently suffer from osteoporosis due to inactivity. The hutch should be placed within an enclosure, or a separate ark or run should be provided.
- Rabbits will burrow, so precautions should be taken to prevent escape.
- When outside, a shelter or drain-pipe should be provided as a bolt-hole. Rabbits are susceptible to overheating and stress.
- House rabbits need a secure cage or pen where they can be kept when unsupervised. Care should be taken to prevent house rabbits from chewing electrical cables or toxic house plants such as *Dieffenbachia* (dumb cane).

Nutrition

Feeding the correct diet to rabbits is fundamental to maintaining health, particularly of the dental and gastrointestinal systems. Based on current knowledge, the following recommendations are made:

- The best diet for rabbits is one that mimics as closely as possible their natural grass-based diet in the wild. Grass is approximately 20–25% crude fibre, 15% crude protein and 2–3% fat. The bulk of the diet of the pet rabbit should consist of grass (fresh or freeze-dried) and/or good quality meadow/timothy hay, and this should be available at all times. Hay can be fed from racks or nets to minimize contamination and increase the time spent feeding
- Green leafy foods are also important and a variety should be fed daily to rabbits of all ages. They should be introduced gradually to weanling rabbits. Wild plants can be given if available (e.g. bramble, groundsel, chickweed, dandelion). All green foods should be washed before feeding
- Commercial concentrate rabbit diets are not essential if *ad lib* hay, grass and greens are available. Commercial rabbit diets can be too low in fibre and too high in protein, fat and carbohydrate. However, many owners like to feed these diets for convenience. They should not be fed exclusively or *ad lib*, and it must be emphasized that hay or grass should always be available and make up the bulk of the diet. Pelleted diets prevent selective feeding of high carbohydrate items. *A good general rule is to feed a maximum of 25 g of high-fibre pellets/kg bodyweight per day.* Overfeeding of concentrated diets is a significant factor in gastrointestinal and dental disease, and can also lead to obesity, boredom and behavioural problems
- Fruit should be regarded as a treat item and fed in limited quantities only, as it is high in simple sugars and may lead to gastrointestinal disturbance. High-fat or high-carbohydrate/starchy

items should be avoided completely. These include commercial 'treats', beans, peas, corn, bread, breakfast cereal, nuts, seeds and chocolate
■ Sudden changes in diet must be avoided. Any change in diet should be made gradually over several days or weeks, starting with small amounts of the new item and gradually increasing them, whilst making a corresponding decrease in the unwanted item if necessary. Hay should always be available, especially for weanling rabbits. A sudden change in diet and lack of fibre combined with the stress of movement is a significant cause of morbidity and mortality in young rabbits over the period of weaning and moving to a pet shop or new owner. When purchasing a rabbit it is important for a new owner to be informed of the rabbit's diet so that any changes can be introduced gradually
■ Frosted or mouldy food, and lawnmower clippings, should not be fed as these can lead to severe digestive disturbances
■ Dietary supplements consisting of vitamins and minerals are not generally necessary if the correct diet is fed
■ Fresh drinking water must be available at all times. Drinking bottles are easier to keep clean than water bowls and avoid wetting the dewlap, which can lead to a moist dermatitis.

Handling and general care

Rabbits should never be picked up by the ears. The correct way to handle a rabbit is to grasp the scruff of the neck firmly with one hand and use the other hand to support the body, either by placing it along the underside of the body, or by placing it over the rump and holding the rabbit against the handler's body. The rabbit's head can be tucked into the crook of the arm (Figure 4.5). Incorrect handling may allow the rabbit to kick out or twist, which can result in damage to its spine.

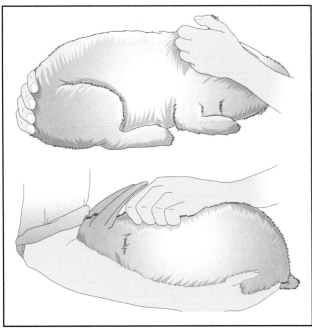

4.5 Handling a rabbit. It is important to support the body.

When putting a rabbit down, the hind end should be placed down first and the scruff released last.

Rabbits enjoy being groomed and this is essential in longhaired breeds. The perineum of outdoor rabbits should be checked twice daily for soiling in warm weather, as fly-strike is common.

Breeding

Does do not have regular oestrous cycles, but can show long periods of oestrus when ovarian follicles are constantly developing and regressing. The vulva is purple and congested when in oestrus.

Rabbits are reflex ovulators, i.e. ovulation is triggered by copulation or sometimes if mounted by another doe. A non-fertile mating results in a pseudo-pregnancy of about 17 days. Breeding is simple: if a receptive doe is taken to the buck, mating will rapidly occur.

The young are altricial and it is normal for the doe to enter the nest box only once or twice a day to nurse them.

Veterinary care

Pain, distress and discomfort are all difficult to assess in rabbits, particularly in the hospital environment, where excessive background noise may prevent the rabbit from relaxing. Rabbits are nervous, sensitive animals and are less likely to show visible signs of pain than dogs and cats, because in the wild they would be predated on.

Practical ways of minimizing stress in rabbits in the hospital environment are as follows:

■ Have a separate waiting area away from cats and dogs, or keep rabbits in the car until called
■ Use a separate consulting room or have consultations at different times of day, ensuring that the room has been thoroughly cleaned after predator species
■ Have a separate hospitalization area out of sight and preferably sound of predator species
■ If using dog/cat kennels, clean thoroughly first to remove odours
■ Co-hospitalize with a companion wherever possible
■ Provide a hide box in the kennel
■ Use separate outer clothing
■ Always talk calmly and avoid sudden movements
■ Provide a familiar diet (even if unsuitable) and water presentation
■ Avoid sudden changes in diet
■ Provide a litter tray if the rabbit is used to this
■ Use sedation if appropriate
■ Handle correctly and always place on a non-slip surface
■ Covering the eyes has a calming effect
■ Minimize handling and keep interventions as short as possible.

General supportive care

Rabbits should be weighed daily. Feed intake and faecal and urine output should be noted daily.

It is essential to hospitalize the sick rabbit in a quiet area away from barking dogs and the smell of dogs, cats and ferrets, to reduce external stressors and to allow the rabbit to express normal behaviour. General therapy consists of fluid replacement, analgesia, gastrointestinal motility drugs, oxygen administration (if indicated), probiotics, vitamins and provision of a high-fibre diet.

Fluids (Figure 4.6) may be given via the following routes: intravenous, intraosseous, intraperitoneal, subcutaneous or orally by syringe feeding or via a nasogastric tube. Daily maintenance fluid requirements are 75–100 ml/kg/day.

The marginal ear vein, jugular vein, cephalic vein and lateral saphenous vein can all be used for i.v. catheter placement. Long-term use of the marginal ear vein may cause sloughing and sedation may be required for the jugular vein. An Elizabethan collar can be used to prevent the rabbit from chewing or removing the catheter but will prevent caecotrophy and may be stressful. Use of a topical local anaesthetic cream ('EMLA') is recommended prior to placement.

Intraosseous catheters may be placed into the top of the trochanter of the femur parallel to the long axis of the femur, using an 18–23 gauge, 1–1.5 inch needle.

Oral administration can be achieved via the drinking water, by mixing with small amounts of food (e.g. 'Milupa' baby food), by syringe or dropper if the substance is palatable, or by gavage using a polyethylene catheter or commercial gavage needle. Rabbits tolerate syringe feeding well and recently commercial high-fibre diets have become available for this purpose.

Rabbits also tolerate nasogastric tubes well. Placement is as for the cat:

1. Use a local anaesthetic gel and a 5–8 FG catheter.
2. Measure from the nares to the caudal end of the sternum.
3. Elevate the head and insert tube into the ventral nasal meatus, aiming ventrally and medially.
4. Check the placement radiographically, since rabbits do not cough if the tube is placed in the trachea.
5. Glue the tube to the fur on the head and place an Elizabethan collar if necessary.

Guinea pigs
Points to consider when choosing guinea pigs

■ Three main types of guinea pig are kept as pets, but a huge number of breeds and varieties exists:
  – The English has a short smooth coat (Figure 4.7)
  – The Abyssinian a longer rough 'rosetted' coat
  – The Peruvian is longhaired, requires daily grooming and is mainly kept for showing purposes.
■ Guinea pigs are generally very docile and almost never bite, but tend to be nervous and easily startled.
■ They are highly sociable animals and should not be kept singly. Groups of females can be kept together, or two or more males, as long as they are not within sight, sound or smell of females. Males can be castrated or vasectomized and females spayed.

Route	Volume	Advantages	Disadvantages	Suggested fluids
Oral (nasogastric tube, syringe feeding)	10–15 ml/kg q8h	Simple, non-sterile solutions Prevents ileus and bloat	Slow, variable absorption Tracheal intubation possible	'Lectade', baby foods (e.g. fruit 'Milupa'), soaked ground pellets, 'Supreme Recovery Diet', 'Oxbow Critical Care Diet', probiotics
Subcutaneous injection (scruff, flank)	Up to 60 ml/kg in two sites	Large volume Simple technique	Slow absorption Sterile solution Predisposes to hypothermia	Isotonic
Intraperitoneal injection	50 ml slow injection	Rapid absorption Simple technique	Aseptic Painful technique Risk of peritonitis and adhesions	Isotonic
Intravenous injection (marginal ear vein)	Maintenance: 2–4 ml/kg/h Shock dose: 100 ml/kg over 60 minutes	Rapid rehydration Large volumes Easy catheter placement, well tolerated	May chew through drip line Painful unless local anaesthetic cream used	Crystalloids and colloids
Intraosseous catheter (femur, tibia)	Maintenance: 2–4 ml/kg/h Shock dose: 100 ml/kg over 60 minutes	Rapid rehydration Large volumes Easy access if vascular collapse	Aseptic procedure Requires anaesthesia (local, general)	Crystalloids and colloids

4.6 Fluid therapy for rabbits (using smallest possible needle/catheter gauge).

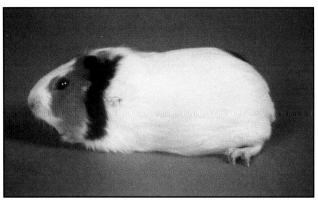

4.7 An English guinea pig. (Courtesy of Paul Flecknell.)

Biological data: guinea pigs

Average lifespan	4–7 years
Sexual maturity	8–10 weeks (male)
	4–5 weeks (female)
Oestrus	Every 15–16 days
Gestation	60–72 (average 65) days
Average litter size	2–6
Weaning age	3–3.5 weeks
Adult weight	750–1000 g
Body temperature	38–39°C

Anatomy and physiology

Guinea pigs are rodents of the suborder Hystricomorpha, which also includes chinchillas.

Teeth and jaws

- Guinea pigs are gnawing mammals, and they possess chisel-shaped curving incisors for gnawing and flat cheek teeth for chewing.
- The temporomandibular joint is adapted so that the mandible can move forward and back to allow either gnawing or chewing, and from side to side.
- The dental formula is 1/1, 0/0, 1/1, 3/3 and the enamel is creamy white.
- The mandible is wider than the upper maxilla.
- Cheek folds are drawn across the diastema (gap between the incisors and cheek teeth) to separate the front and the back parts of the mouth.
- The incisors and cheek teeth have open roots and grow continuously throughout life.
- The upper lip is cleft.

Digestive tract

- The digestive tract of guinea pigs consists of a simple stomach, long small intestine, a large sacculated caecum where bacterial fermentation of plant material occurs (hind gut fermentation) and a long colon.
- Guinea pigs practise coprophagy (the eating of faeces), which enhances the uptake of vitamins B and K.

Reproductive system

- Female guinea pigs have separate vaginal and urethral openings (Figure 4.8).
- The vaginal opening is usually only patent when the animal is in oestrus.
- After mating, a vaginal plug is formed which persists for 1–2 days. Its presence is used by breeders to show if mating has taken place.
- Both males and females have two inguinal nipples.
- Male guinea pigs have an open inguinal ring and can retract the testicles into the abdomen.

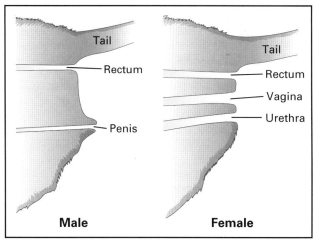

4.8 Perineal openings in male and female rodents.

Toes

Guinea pigs have four toes on the forefeet and three toes on the hindfeet.

Skin

Guinea pigs have a glandular area in the midline above the tail, which produces a greasy secretion. This is more prominent in males.

Sexing

The sex of a guinea pig can be determined by looking at the conformation of the genital opening. In the male (boar) a circle of tissue is present through which, when pressure is exerted above it, the penis can be extruded. The female (sow) has a Y-shaped opening. The anogenital distance is similar in males and females.

Housing

Guinea pigs are highly social grassland dwellers and should be kept in single-sex groups, pairs or harems. They are not hardy animals and cannot tolerate wet weather well.

A wide range of wooden hutch designs is available:

- The best types have two compartments – one mesh-fronted and one solid-fronted, for a nesting area
- Wood shavings and hay make ideal bedding
- To avoid damp, hutches should be raised off the ground if outside

- Guinea pigs need exercise and the opportunity to graze:
  - In summer a movable run or ark should be provided; this should be covered to prevent predation and should have a shelter (the hutch, a box or an old piece of drain pipe) to give a bolt-hole if the animal is startled
  - In winter the hutch should be moved indoors or into a garage and an indoor run with wood shavings can be provided.

Nutrition

Guinea pigs have an absolute dietary requirement for vitamin C. They need 10 mg/kg bodyweight per day, rising to three times this in pregnancy. Commercial guinea pig diets are often supplemented with vitamin C, but the shelf-life is short and cool dark storage conditions must be provided.

- A commercial mix or pellet should be fed, well supplemented with good quality hay and a variety of greenfoods (e.g. groundsel, fresh grass, dandelion, cow parsley, broccoli).
- Roughage or fibre in the form of hay or grass is essential for dental and gastrointestinal health.
- *Ad lib* water should be provided from a drinking bottle.
- Fruit should be regarded as a treat item and fed in limited amounts.

Handling

Guinea pigs very rarely bite but are often nervous and easily startled. A rapid, smooth approach to handling should be adopted.

- The guinea pig should be grasped around the shoulders and lifted clear of the cage or box (Figure 4.9)
- The hindquarters should be supported with the other hand (Figure 4.9).

Breeding

It is essential to breed female guinea pigs young, ideally at about 12 weeks old. After the age of 1 year, the pubic symphysis fuses and if guinea pigs are bred for the first time after this they will experience difficulty in giving birth (dystocia): an emergency Caesarian operation may be required.

Female guinea pigs come into oestrus every 15–17 days, and will arch their back (lordosis) when receptive. An obvious vaginal plug is present after mating.

Approaching parturition can be detected by feeling separation of the pubic symphysis. The gap widens to approximately 2 cm, 24–36 hours before birth. At birth, the young are fully furred and have eyes and ears open (precocious).

Veterinary care

Guinea pigs are nervous patients and all measures should be taken to minimize stress when hospitalized, as for rabbits. The principles of nursing care are the same as for rabbits.

As guinea pigs have an absolute dietary requirement for vitamin C, it should always be supplemented in sick individuals; this can be done via the drinking water. Provision of a high-fibre diet is also vital.

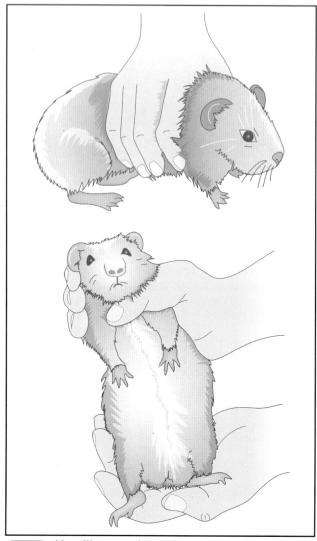

4.9 Handling a guinea pig. It is important to support the hindquarters.

General nursing care includes:

- Daily weighing
- Close monitoring of urine and faecal output
- Provision of heat
- Oxygen supplementation if respiratory distress
- Housing away from predators and excess noise
- Provision of a quiet nest box with nesting material
- Minimal handling and cleaning out
- *Ad lib* water by a familiar route
- Provision of tempting food (e.g. moist mashes, baby food)
- Co-hospitalization with a cage mate possible.

Chinchillas

Points to consider when choosing chinchillas

- Chinchillas are very attractive with beautiful soft fur, fluffy tail and large whiskers (Figure 4.10).
- Chinchillas often resent being handled.
- They are mainly nocturnal and spend most of the day asleep.
- They have a tendency to gnaw and be very destructive.

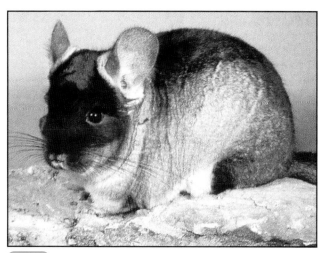

4.10 Chinchilla. (Courtesy of Anna Meredith.)

Biological data: chinchillas

Average lifespan	10–15 years
Sexual maturity	8 months
Oestrus	Every 30–35 days (Nov–May)
Gestation	111 days
Average litter size	2–3
Weaning age	6–8 weeks
Adult weight	350–500 g
Body temperature	38–39°C

Anatomy and physiology

This is very similar to the guinea pig (see above). Differences from the guinea pig are:

- Chinchilla incisors have pigmented enamel
- Females have 3 pairs of nipples
- Chinchillas have five toes on the forefeet and four toes on the hindfeet.

Sexing

Sexing chinchillas is by anogenital distance. Confusion can arise as female chinchillas have a large urethral process, which can be confused with a penis.

Housing

Female chinchillas are aggressive to each other and so they should be kept singly, or with a male as a breeding pair. Housing for chinchillas must be indoors.

- Wire cages are best, as chinchillas will gnaw through other materials.
- Cages should be as large as possible (at least 2 m x 2 m x 1 m).
- A nest box must be provided and plenty of branches to gnaw.
- Chinchillas must have a daily dustbath in order to keep the fur in good condition.

Nutrition

Chinchillas are essentially grassland dwellers and should be fed grass-based chinchilla pellets and good quality hay, supplemented with leafy green vegetables. High-sugar treats, such as raisins, should be avoided as these can cause tooth decay.

Handling

Chinchillas often dislike being handled and wriggle violently when restrained.

- They should be grasped gently but firmly around the shoulders, with the bodyweight supported with the other hand.
- Rough handling can lead to a condition known as fur-slip, where large chunks of fur fall out.

Breeding

Chinchillas will form monogamous pairs, or can be kept in a harem system with a male having access to several separate females. Oestrus occurs every 30–50 days, and is shown by an open vulva and mucoid vaginal discharge. A large vaginal plug is present after mating. Gestation is very long at 111 days. The young are precocious.

Veterinary care

As for guinea pigs.

Rats

Points to consider when choosing rats

Rats (Figure 4.11) are increasingly popular pets, among adults as well as children.

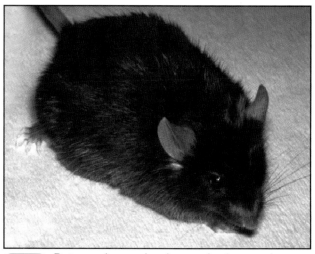

4.11 Rats are becoming increasingly popular as pets. (Courtesy of Paul Flecknell.)

- Rats cling on to the handler and so are unlikely to be dropped.
- They are sociable, highly intelligent and responsive and will learn to recognize their owner.
- Most rats are docile and rarely bite.
- Rats are naturally more active at night, but if handled frequently they often adapt to their owner's timetable.
- Rats can become very tame and will interact with the owner, for example sitting on the shoulder.

Biological data: rats

Average lifespan	3 years
Sexual maturity	6 weeks
Oestrus	Every 4–5 days
Gestation	20–22 days
Average litter size	6–12
Weaning age	21 days
Adult weight	250–600 g
Body temperature	38°C

Anatomy and physiology

Dentition

- The dental formula is 1/1, 0/0, 0/0, 3/3, and the enamel covering the front surface of the incisors is orange–yellow to reddish.
- The incisors grow continuously but the cheek teeth do not.

Digestive tract

- Rats have a simple stomach, long small intestine, large non-sacculated caecum and long colon. They are not hind gut fermenters.
- Rats are coprophagic.

Skin

Rats have sparsely haired tails.

Toes

Rats have four front toes and five hind toes.

Sexing

Sexing is by anogenital distance (greater in the male) and the presence of nipples (6 pairs) in the female. An obvious scrotum and testicles are visible in the mature male.

Housing

Commercial metal cages and glass or plastic tanks are suitable for rats.

- Wooden cages should be avoided, as rats will gnaw.
- Cage mesh must be small enough to prevent escape of young if breeding animals are kept (one wire per 1.5 cm).
- The cage should be as large as possible and enough space should be provided for cage furniture, such as branches, tubes, ladders, exercise wheels (solid rather than open, to prevent tail injuries).
- A nest box should be provided. A deep layer of wood shavings makes suitable bedding, plus shredded paper, hay or straw as nesting material. Cotton wool-type bedding should be avoided as it can become impacted in the stomach if ingested.
- Rats enjoy the opportunity to exercise out of the cage, but this should always be under supervision.

Nutrition

Rats are omnivorous opportunists. A commercial rodent mix makes a suitable diet, consisting of carbohydrate-type seeds/grains (wheat, maize, oats, barley) and higher fat-type seeds and nuts (sunflower, peanuts) plus biscuit, locust bean and dried rolled peas. This can be supplemented with fruit and vegetables, household scraps and dog biscuits.

Water should be provided *ad lib* from a water bottle with nipple, attached to the side or roof of the cage.

Handling

- Rats can be grasped gently around the shoulders and lifted out of the cage or box, with the thumb placed under the mandible to prevent biting (Figure 4.12).
- If the animal is large or pregnant, the bodyweight should be supported with the other hand.
- If, for example, an intraperitoneal injection is to be given, the tail can be held with the other hand to steady the animal.
- A fractious animal can be scruffed as described below for the smaller rodents, but many rats resent this if they are not used to it and will vocalize.
- Rats can also be lifted on to the sleeve by grasping the very base of the tail and lifting gently. They should not, however, be suspended by the tail.

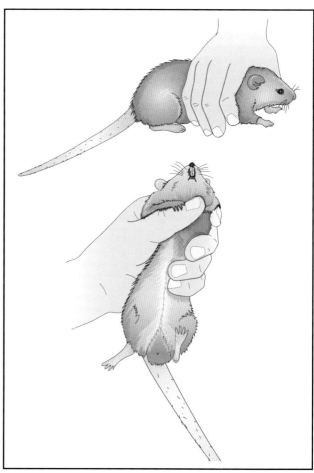

4.12 Handling a rat. The thumb is placed under the mandible to prevent biting.

Breeding

- Oestrus occurs approximately every 4 days.
- A visible vaginal plug is formed after mating. This acts to prevent mating by another male, and prevents leakage of semen. The vaginal plug falls out after 12–24 hours.
- Newborn rats are blind and naked (altricial). The mother should not be disturbed for the first 2–3 days after parturition or she may eat the young.
- Female rats have a post-partum oestrus and so can become pregnant almost immediately after parturition.
- Breeding in rats is easily achieved simply by placing male and female together, or keeping them as a pair or harem.
- The vaginal opening is patent when the female is in oestrus. Mating invariably occurs at night.
- Males can be castrated to prevent breeding or enable males to be kept together.

Mice
Points to consider when choosing mice

- Small and easy to keep.
- Good climbers and cling on to the handler, therefore unlikely to be dropped by small children.
- Male mice have a distinctive strong smell, which can be unpleasant.
- Although they are social animals, male mice often fight if kept together, so a breeding pair or harem, or two or more females, should be kept.
- More active at night.
- Can bite if not handled frequently.

Biological data: mice

Average lifespan	2–2.5 years
Sexual maturity	3–4 weeks
Oestrus	Every 4–5 days
Gestation	19–21 days
Average litter size	5–10
Weaning age	18 days
Adult weight	20–40 g
Body temperature	37.5°C

Anatomy and physiology

As for rats. Sexing is by anogenital distance (greater in the male) and by the presence of nipples in the female.

Housing

As for rats. Bars should be 1 cm to prevent escape of young.

Nutrition

As for rats.

Breeding

As for rats. The vaginal plug persists for up to 2 days in mice.

Handling

Mice are often not used to being handled and so care should be taken not to get bitten.

- The mouse should be grasped firmly by the base of the tail and lifted out of the cage or box (Figure 4.13a).
- It can then be placed on a rough surface, such as a towel or the sleeve.
- If gentle traction is maintained on the tail the animal will grip the rough surface and try to pull away, making it remain stationary and enabling a visual examination to be undertaken.
- For additional restraint, such as for injection, the scruff is grasped between the thumb and forefinger of either the same hand or the other hand (Figure 4.13b). Sufficient scruff must be grasped to prevent the mouse turning its head to bite.

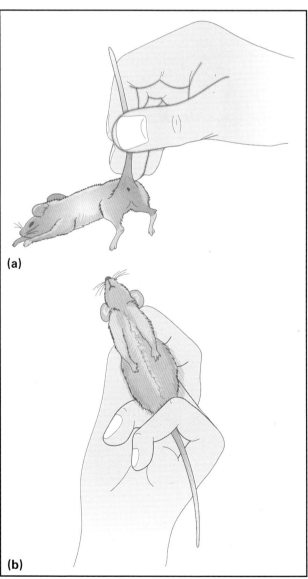

4.13 Handling a mouse. **(a)** Grasping the base of the tail. **(b)** Grasping the scruff.

Hamsters

Points to consider when choosing hamsters

Three species of hamster are kept as pets:

- Golden or Syrian hamster:
  - Many varieties exist, including longhaired and satin-coated
  - Solitary and should be kept singly
  - Mainly nocturnal
  - Can often bite, especially if roused from a deep sleep during the day
  - Easily dropped and injured
  - Hibernates at temperatures below about 5°C, and will become torpid (aestivation) at very high temperatures.
- Russian (dwarf) hamster:
  - About half the size of Syrian hamsters, with a very round body shape
  - Naturally grey coat with black tips to the hairs, a dark stripe down the back and a pale underside, but different varieties now exist (e.g. albino). The tail is very short
  - Can be very aggressive if not handled frequently and easily dropped
  - Social and, unlike Syrian hamsters, should be kept in female groups or breeding pairs or harems
  - Does not hibernate.
- Chinese (dwarf) hamster:
  - Similar to Russian hamster but with longer tail and more elongated body shape
  - Social and does not hibernate.

Biological data: hamsters

Average lifespan	**1.5–2 years**
Sexual maturity	**6–10 weeks**
Oestrus	**Every 4 days**
Gestation	**Syrian: 15–18 days**
	Russian/Chinese: 19–22 days
Average litter size	**3–7**
Weaning age	**21–28 days**
Adult weight	**Syrian: 110–150 g**
	Russian/Chinese: 20–40 g
Body temperature	**38°C**

Anatomy and physiology

As for rats. Significant differences are:

- Hamsters have large cheek pouches
- Hamsters have scent glands on their flanks, which are often pigmented and become hairless with age
- Tail is short and haired
- Females have 6–7 pairs of nipples.

Sexing

The mature male has very large obvious testicles. Otherwise anogenital distance can be used to sex hamsters.

Housing

Cages suitable for mice are appropriate. Modular systems comprising tubes and living spaces, mimicking burrows, are also popular. Cotton wool-type products should be avoided as nesting material, as they may become impacted in the pouch.

- Russian and Chinese hamsters are highly social animals and should be kept as single-sex groups (females best, as males may fight), breeding pairs or harems.
- Syrian hamsters should be kept singly.
- Syrian hamsters will hibernate at temperatures below 5°C and aestivate at very high temperatures, so are best kept at 19–23°C.

Nutrition

As for rats and mice. Hamsters tend to hoard food in the nest box, so perishable items must be removed regularly.

Handling

Before handling it is necessary to ensure that the hamster is awake, or gently wake it up, otherwise it may be startled and bite. Some hamsters resent being handled and can be quite aggressive, especially Russian and Chinese hamsters.

- A docile hamster can be cupped between two hands (Figure 4.14) and gently lifted and rolled on to its back if necessary.
- For true restraint, the loose scruff should be firmly grasped between the thumb and forefinger (it is a myth that scruffing a hamster tightly will cause its eyes to pop out).
- There is a lot of loose skin around the scruff in hamsters due to the presence of cheek pouches. If insufficient skin is grasped the hamster will be able to turn its head and bite.
- The bodyweight can be supported with the other hand in large or pregnant individuals.

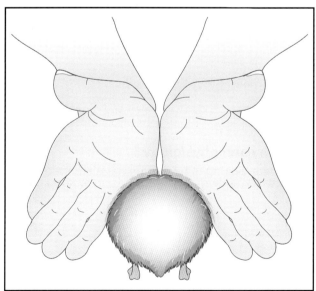

4.14 A docile hamster can be cupped between two hands.

Breeding

Syrian hamsters should be supervised for breeding, as the female can be very aggressive towards the male. A neutral cage is used, or else the female is placed in the male's cage.

Female hamsters produce a copious vaginal discharge post-ovulation (day 2 of the oestrous cycle) which should not be mistaken for a bacterial infection.

Breeding in Russian and Chinese hamsters is easily achieved simply by placing male and female together, or keeping them as a pair or harem. The vaginal opening is patent when the female is in oestrus. Mating invariably occurs at night.

Gerbils

Points to consider when choosing gerbils

- Attractive and entertaining.
- Active in the day, when they are constantly arranging and rearranging their bedding, digging and gnawing.
- Produce very little urine and are almost odourless.
- Social animals and form monogamous pairs.
- Two males can be kept together if litter mates, otherwise a breeding pair or two females should be kept.
- Rarely bite but can be difficult to handle, and can leap vertically into the air if startled.
- Do not cling to the handler and can easily be dropped.
- Incorrect handling can lead to sloughing of the tail skin (see 'Handling').

Biological data: gerbils

Average lifespan	2–3 years
Sexual maturity	10–12 weeks
Oestrus	Every 4–6 days
Gestation	24–26 days
Average litter size	3–6
Weaning age	21–28 days
Adult weight	70–120 g
Body temperature	38°C

Anatomy and physiology

Generally as for rats, except that:

- Gerbils have a large hairless scent gland on the ventral abdomen (more obvious in males)
- The tail is haired
- There are 4 pairs of nipples
- Gerbils have five toes on the forefeet and four toes on the hindfeet.

Sexing

Sexing is by anogenital distance.

Housing

Gerbils can be kept in a 'gerbilarium' – a glass or plastic tank with a close-fitting wire mesh lid or plastic cover, half-filled with a mixture of peat and sawdust or shavings. Sand, although 'natural', is not a good substrate as it causes abrasions to the nose.

- Nest material should be provided and wood to gnaw. Insides of toilet rolls and other pieces of cardboard are also gnawed with relish.
- The tank should be kept out of direct sunlight, as it can overheat.
- The gerbils will spend a great deal of time creating a system of burrows that they will constantly rearrange. This system only needs to be cleaned out two or three times a year, as very little urine is produced.
- The only disadvantage with a gerbilarium is that the occupants can be difficult to catch.

Nutrition

Gerbils are largely herbivorous, although they may take the occasional insect in the wild. They should be fed a commercial rodent mix supplemented with small amounts of fresh fruit and vegetables.

Handling

Gerbils do not tend to bite. They must *never* be held by the tail, as the skin is very delicate and can easily be pulled off.

- To restrain a gerbil, first capture it using cupped hands, or place the whole hand over the back of the gerbil and hold it gently around the shoulders, with the thumb under the mandible.
- Alternatively, grasp the scruff as for the mouse (Figure 4.15).

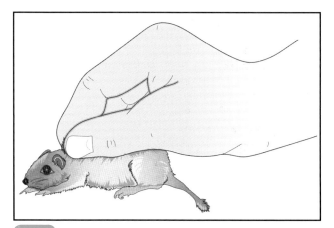

4.15 A gerbil can be grasped by the scruff.

Breeding

- Oestrus occurs approximately every 4 days.
- The vaginal opening is patent when the female is in oestrus. Mating invariably occurs at night.
- Breeding in gerbils is easily achieved simply by placing male and female together, or keeping them as a pair or harem.
- Newborn gerbils are blind and naked (altricial). The mother should not be disturbed for the first 2–3 days after parturition or she may eat the young.

- Gerbils have a post-partum oestrus, and so can become pregnant almost immediately after parturition.
- Gerbils form monogamous pairs and the male will assist with the rearing of the young.
- Males can be castrated to prevent breeding or to enable males to be kept together.

Veterinary care of small rodents

Rats, mice, hamsters and gerbils are similar in their nursing requirements.

Routes of administration

Routes for drug administration are listed in Figure 4.16.

- Intravenous drug administration is difficult but possible using the sites listed in Figure 4.16; however, in practice it is generally avoided.
- The oral route is often the most practical as repeated injections can cause local reactions and pain, and make even the most tractable animal difficult to handle. Paediatric suspensions, mixed with jelly or jam, sweetening solutions with ribena, etc. are all useful aids to cooperation.
- In-water medication is not advisable as intake is often insufficient and is difficult to monitor.
- Subcutaneous administration can be in the scruff or flank.
- Intramuscular injection should be avoided if possible as it is painful, and absorption is usually just as good via the subcutaneous route.
- Other routes are:
  - Intraperitoneal – caudal abdomen; take care to avoid intestines and bladder
  - Intraosseous – useful for fluid administration in severely debilitated animals. The largest bore spinal needle possible is passed through the trochanteric fossa using an aseptic technique. Alternatively, it can be passed through the tibial crest into the tibia. The catheter should immediately be flushed with heparin once in place in the marrow cavity, as clotting occurs rapidly. The needle can be taped or sutured in place.

Fluid therapy

Maintenance fluids for rodents are approximately 50 ml/kg bodyweight/day. As a general rule:

- Mouse-sized: 2–3 ml s.c.
- Gerbil/hamster: 3–4 ml s.c.
- Rat-sized: 10 ml s.c.

Warmed lactated Ringer's solution or saline is appropriate in most cases. Amino acid/electrolyte/vitamin solutions are also useful.

Nutritional support

Nutritional support is essential for long-term critical care and must be instituted quickly (within 12–24 hours) whenever a rodent becomes anorexic. Hypoglycaemia occurs rapidly in these animals, which have a high metabolic rate.

Assisted feeding can be by syringe, which is usually well tolerated, or by gavage. If by gavage, care should be taken to ensure that the tube is not bitten. Metal ball-ended commercial gavage tubes are available.

- Baby food, puréed fruit and vegetables may all be used.
- Probiotics seem to be beneficial and can be added to the feed.
- Multivitamin supplementation (especially B and K) should be given where caecotrophy is absent.

General nursing care

This includes:

- Daily weighing
- Close monitoring of urine and faecal output
- Provision of heat
- Oxygen supplementation if respiratory distress
- Housing away from predators and excess noise
- Provision of a quiet nest box with nesting material
- Minimal handling and cleaning out
- *Ad lib* water by a familiar route
- Provision of tempting food (e.g. moist mashes, baby food)
- Co-hospitalization with a cage mate if possible.

Ferrets

Points to consider when choosing ferrets

- Originally domesticated and bred for hunting rabbits.
- Highly intelligent and entertaining pets that require a lot of attention from and interaction with their owner and regular exercise.
- Have the disadvantage of a very distinctive smell that many people find unpleasant. This is particularly strong in the male and although neutering will decrease the odour slightly, it is a myth that a ferret can be 'de-scented', as the odour is from the sebaceous gland secretions rather than the anal sacs.

Species	Subcutaneous	Intramuscular (quadriceps)	Intraperitoneal	Intravenous
Mouse	Scruff, 2–3 ml	0.05 ml	2–3 ml	Lateral tail vein, 0.2 ml
Hamster, gerbil	Scruff, 3–4 ml	0.1 ml	3–4 ml	Not practicable
Rat	Scruff, flank, 5–10 ml	0.3 ml	10–15 ml	Lateral tail vein, 0.5 ml

4.16 Drug and fluid administration in small mammals.

- Ferrets need a lot of attention and regular exercise. They can be trained to be taken for walks on a harness and lead.

Biological data: ferrets

Average lifespan	5–7 years
Sexual maturity	6–9 months
Oestrus	Induced ovulation (Feb–Sept)
Gestation	42 days
Average litter size	2–6
Weaning age	8 weeks
Adult weight	0.5–2 kg
Body temperature	38.8°C

Anatomy and physiology

Ferrets are carnivores and belong to the Order Mustelidae. They have a typical carnivorous dentition similar to cats and dogs.

- The dental formula is 3/3, 1/1, 3/3, 1/2.
- Ferrets have long backs, small rounded furred ears, short legs and a medium-length furred tail. All four feet have five toes.
- The digestive system is similar to other carnivores, with a simple stomach and no caecum.
- Ferrets possess a pair of anal sacs that secrete an unpleasant-smelling liquid.

Sexing

Male ferrets (hobs) have the preputial opening on the underbelly, as in the dog. The testicles are obvious in the breeding season (February–September). In the females (jills) the vulva is present just below the tail.

Housing

Ferrets are solitary in the wild, but single-sex pairs and groups or breeding pairs can be kept.

- Ferrets can be kept outside in a hutch, pen or shed, or inside as a house pet.
- If kept outside, they must be sheltered from direct sun in the summer as they are very prone to heat stress. In the winter a garage or shed is more suitable.
- If kept inside, they must still have a secure pen or cage where they should be secured when the owner is out of the house (ferrets are very inquisitive and destructive).
- Bedding of woodshavings and straw is suitable, or blankets inside. Cat beds or 'igloos' are suitable. Hammocks are greatly enjoyed.
- Ferrets are very clean, despite their strong odour, and will use a litter tray.

Nutrition

Ferrets are true carnivores and their diet should consist of a good quality cat food; both wet and dry foods are readily accepted. Commercial dry ferret foods are also available. Dry diets lead to less skin odour. The diet can be supplemented with fresh dead mice, rabbits or chicks if available.

Handling

- Tame ferrets can be held around the shoulders, with the other hand supporting the bodyweight (Figure 4.17).
- Fractious or aggressive animals can be grasped by the tail and drawn backwards. At the same time they are grasped firmly around the shoulders, with the thumb under the chin and the forelegs crossed to prevent biting.

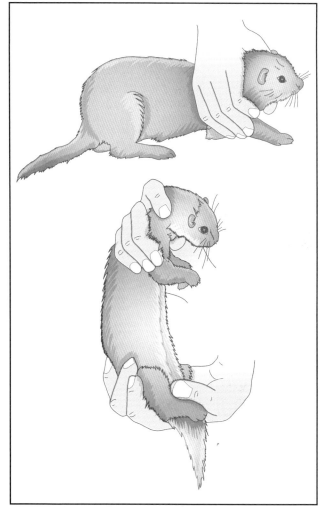

4.17 A tame ferret can be grasped around the shoulders with the other hand supporting the body. Additional measures are required for aggressive animals (see text).

Breeding

- The breeding season in ferrets is from spring to autumn. Jills in oestrus will have a swollen vulva. Mating can appear quite violent and last for up to 3 hours.
- Ferrets are reflex ovulators. If unmated they will stay in oestrus for many months and this can lead to health problems, such as anaemia and hair loss. It is best to spay non-breeding jills, or mate them to a vasectomized hob (known as a hobble). Treatment can be given for persistent oestrus with an injection of a progestagen or chorionic gonadotrophin.

Veterinary care

Supportive care

Fluid therapy requirements are calculated as in dogs and cats, with maintenance of 75–100 ml/kg bodyweight/day. Subcutaneous fluids are resented by ferrets and the animal should be scruffed prior to injection by this route. The skin over the neck is extremely tough and a 23 or 21 gauge needle should be used. In debilitated animals intravenous or intraosseous routes should be used.

Nutritional support may be provided in anorexic animals by syringe-feeding Hill's a/d diet liquidized with electrolyte solutions such as 'Lectade', giving 2–5 ml 3–4 times daily.

Drug administration

Drugs may be given orally and should be directly administered rather than mixed in food. Medication may be mixed with food items, such as peanut butter, to encourage the ferret to take them. Intramuscular injections should be given into the quadriceps or hamstring muscles in the hindlimb.

Birds

Anatomy and physiology

Birds are vertebrate endothermic animals with a high metabolic rate and body temperature (40–42°C). They are adapted for flight in several ways:

- The presence of feathers
- A lightweight skeleton (Figure 4.18) – the bones have thin cortices and some contain an air sac (pneumatic bones). The skull weight is reduced by containing air-filled sinuses and having no teeth

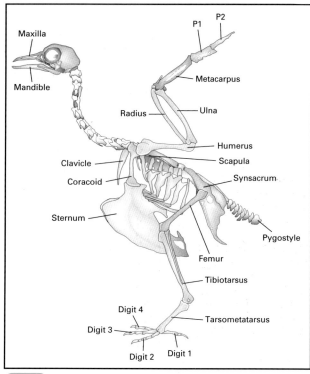

4.18 A simplified bird skeleton.

- Fusion of some of the vertebrae to provide body rigidity. The neck remains flexible to allow the bird to reach all parts of its body with the beak
- A large sternum (keel) for attachment of powerful flight muscles.

Feathers

Feathers (Figure 4.19) are made of keratin and can be divided into:

- Flight feathers on the wings and tail, which are rigid and long
- Contour feathers on the body, neck and head, which are short
- Down feathers and filoplumes that lie under the contour feathers and provide insulation.

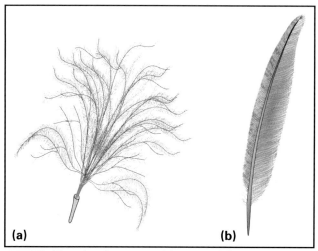

(a)   **(b)**

4.19 Two basic types of feather. **(a)** Down. **(b)** Contour or flight.

Feathers are moulted and replaced usually once a year in most species, but up to three times a year in some (e.g. budgerigars). Growing feathers contain a blood vessel in the shaft and are protected by a keratin sheath.

Pelvis

The pelvis of birds has an open pubis rather than a symphysis, to allow passage of a large egg.

Beak

The beak consists of bone covered in cornified keratin. In psittacines there is a hinge joint (craniofacial hinge) between the upper beak and the skull, allowing greater movement of the upper beak in relation to the lower than in other species.

Ear

Birds have no external ear.

Feet

Birds have four digits on their feet:

- In psittacines, the outer two point backwards and the middle two point forwards
- In most other species the outer three digits point forwards and the inner digit points backwards

- In ducks and geese the three forward-pointing digits are webbed
- Cockerels have a sharp, backward-pointing horny spur above the foot, which is used in fighting.

Digestive tract

There are two significant features of the bird digestive system (Figure 4.20) that are different from mammals:

- The crop, which is used to store food. It is present in some species, such as psittacines and pigeons, and absent in others
- The gizzard, which has a thick muscular wall and is used for grinding food.

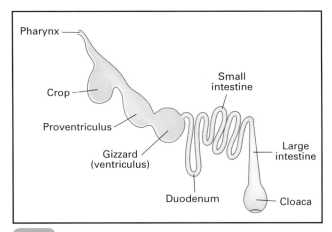

4.20 The digestive tract of a bird.

Bird droppings consist of three portions: brown–green faeces, white urates and liquid urine (Figure 4.21). The colour of the faeces depends on the diet of the bird.

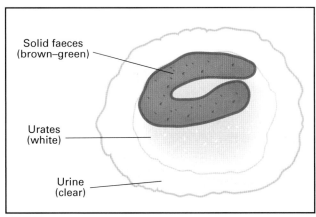

4.21 The parts of a normal bird dropping.

Respiratory system

The avian respiratory system (Figure 4.22) is much more efficient than that of mammals and consists of paired lungs plus a system of air sacs that act as 'bellows'. This allows oxygenated air to flow through the lungs in both inspiration and expiration.

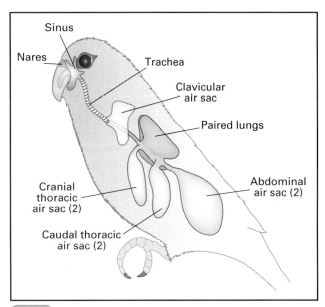

4.22 The respiratory system of a bird.

Psittacine birds

The term psittacine is generally used to refer to members of the Order Psittaciformes. Popular species include the budgerigar, cockatiel, lovebird, parrot and cockatoo.

Points to consider when choosing psittacines

- Psittacines are kept:
  - Indoors in or out of cages as pets
  - Outdoors in aviaries as breeding or exhibition specimens.
- All psittacines are highly intelligent and social, and can be very destructive.
- Some species, including budgerigars, African Grey parrots, cockatoos (Figure 4.23) and Amazon parrots, can be taught to talk.
- The larger species in particular make very demanding pets, require a great deal of attention and companionship, and should not be left alone for long periods. They are therefore not suitable pets for people who go out to work all day.

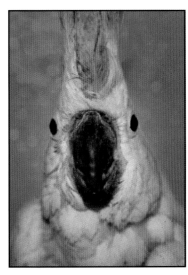

4.23 A Sulphur-crested Cockatoo. (Courtesy of Sharon Redrobe.)

- The larger species of parrot can live for 40–50 years or longer.
- Hand-reared British birds make the best pets. Birds that are not hand-reared can be very difficult to tame and can inflict a painful bite.
- Pet parrots kept singly often form a strong pair bond with one member of the household and become aggressive towards other family members.

Sexing

Many species are monomorphic, i.e. the male and female look the same. For these species determination of sex is carried out either surgically, by visualizing the internal gonads via an endoscope, or by DNA analysis of a blood sample or plucked feather. Most psittacines have to be sexed in this way.

- In the budgerigar, the cere can be used to distinguish the sexes. The cere is a fleshy structure at the base of the upper beak, containing the nares. The male has a blue cere and the female a pinkish-brown cere.
- In the cockatiel, the male has brighter red cheek patches and the female has pale bars on the underside of the tail feathers.

These differences are only reliable in the wild-type variety of these species.

Housing

Most psittacines should be kept in breeding pairs, but a single hand-reared bird makes the best pet.

Aviaries

A garden aviary should be in a quiet secluded location, facing the sun, with shelter from prevailing wind.

- Minimum dimensions for a flight should be 1.8 m long by 1.8 m high by 0.9 m wide.
- Height should be as great as possible to minimize stress on the birds, and width must allow two birds to pass each other easily in flight.
- Welded mesh of appropriate size on a treated wooden or metal framework is ideal.
- Earth floors should be avoided and concrete flooring should be used for ease of cleaning. Shingle or bark chippings are also suitable.
- Shallow baths or a misting system should be provided for bathing.
- If multiple flights are placed side by side, double mesh is essential to prevent pairs fighting.
- An inside shelter must always be accessible. This can be a box-like structure at the top half of the back section of the flight, or a full indoor shed.
- To encourage roosting at night, perches in the shelter should be higher than those in the flight.
- Birds only feed during daylight. To avoid reduced food intake on short winter days, artificial light should be provided to give a 12-hour light period.

Cages

Even if an indoor bird is allowed free run of the house, it will need a cage to provide a territorial area where it feels safe and in which it can be secured when the owners are not present.

- A cage should be large enough to allow the bird to beat its outstretched wings and to have its tail clear of the floor when perching (this is required by law under the Wildlife and Countryside Act 1981).
- At least two perches, of differing sizes, should be provided. Branches of any deciduous tree (e.g. fruit trees or willow) are ideal and the bird will enjoy stripping the bark.
- Sandpaper-covered perches should be avoided, as they can cause foot sores and do little to keep nails worn down.
- The cage should be situated at or above human head height, away from strong sunlight and excessive draughts.
- Birds should also be kept away from cigarette smoke and overheated Teflon pans, as these fumes can kill.
- Cages should be cleaned daily.

Psittacines are highly intelligent, inquisitive and social birds and require a lot of attention if kept singly.

- Toys can be provided but should not be so densely packed as to interfere with the bird's movement around the cage. Note that male budgerigars can become sexually bonded to one toy, or to their own reflection in a mirror.
- Chains are to be avoided as the animal can get caught and suffer serious injury.
- A bath in the form of a shallow dish or a daily misting encourages preening and good feather condition and is greatly enjoyed.

Nutrition

Malnutrition is the commonest cause of disease in caged psittacines. The most important requirement is to feed as varied a diet as possible. Psittacines can be very fussy and conservative eaters: it is important to mix different food items in one bowl so that preferential selection of one item (e.g. sunflower seeds or peanuts) is minimized. These high-fat seeds are nutritionally unbalanced, and eating only these items can lead to serious nutritional disease (hypovitaminosis A, metabolic bone disease).

- Feed several times a day.
- Removing food and replacing it later stimulates interest and relieves boredom.
- To avoid faecal contamination, food bowls must be placed higher than perches.
- At least three types of vegetables, three types of fruit and five types of seed should be offered daily.
- Treats can be offered occasionally (e.g. fruit cake, biscuits, brown bread, breakfast cereal).

Suitable food items are listed in Figure 4.24. Alternatively, complete pelleted diets are now available for many species. These are a useful option for owners who have many birds to feed, or who do not have the time to prepare a homemade diet. However, they are expensive and lacking in variety for the bird.

Type	Examples
Seed mixture	Wheat, oats, canary seed, millet, buckwheat, groats
	Millet sprays are often preferred during the moult and by debilitated birds
	Budgerigars should be fed a good proprietary seed mixture containing an iodine supplement
Oil seeds	Sunflower seed, linseed, rape seed, hemp seed
	These should be rationed and should not exceed 20–30% of the diet, or obesity and nutritional deficiency will occur
Fruit	Any fruit except avocado
	Birds will have their favourite type
Vegetables and greenfood	Carrots, celery, beetroot, alfalfa, broccoli, watercress, lettuce, groundsel, chickweed, dandelion, dock
Pulses	Haricot beans, soya beans, green peas, mung beans, chick peas, black-eyed beans
	Fed soaked, cooked or sprouted
Peanuts	Must be fit for human consumption and form only a small part of the diet
Bones and household scraps	Often enjoyed as an occasional treat by larger species
Rawhide chews	Enjoyed by larger species
Cuttlefish bones	A good source of calcium
	Ignored by some species and enjoyed by others
Vitamin/mineral supplements	A good avian supplement will prevent any deficiencies, but overzealous use can cause damaging excesses

4.24 Suitable food items for psittacine birds.

Handling

All birds are more easily handled in dim light. For security, always make sure that all windows and doors in the room are closed before the cage or box is opened. If the bird is in a cage:

- Toys and perches should be removed from the cage if possible, so that the bird is more accessible
- It is often easier to approach the bird from the bottom, by tilting the cage off its base, rather than putting the hand in through the small side door.

The use of thick gloves should be avoided, as the handler's sense of touch is diminished and too much force can be exerted. Instead, thin cloths or towels are very useful for masking the hand and for wrapping around the wings to prevent flapping.

Caught birds must never be squeezed, as restriction of movement of the sternum and abdomen can result in asphyxiation. A bird should never be held around the chest, as this can hinder its respiration.

- Small birds can be grasped in one hand, with the head between the first and second finger (Figure 4.25).
- Larger psittacines should be grasped firmly from behind, using a towel or cloth, around the mandible and neck. Tilting of the cage usually makes the bird grab on to the side with its beak, making this procedure easier. With the other hand, the towel is wrapped around the body.

Breeding

Provision of an appropriate nest box will stimulate breeding behaviour in most species. In a flock situation, sufficient nest boxes must be provided for every pair – and preferably more than this so that the birds have a choice of box.

- Increasing day length in the spring is the normal stimulus to breeding behaviour, but some species will breed all year round.
- The most common reason for failure to breed is that the pair is of the same sex.

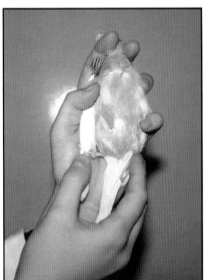

4.25

Holding a budgerigar in one hand. (Courtesy of Sharon Redrobe.)

- Pairs of birds kept in cages without a nest box rarely breed.
- Psittacines form strong pair bonds, especially the larger species.
- Eggs are generally laid daily, or every other day, until the clutch is complete.
- Removal of the eggs will stimulate the laying of another clutch.

Passerine birds

Passerines are the perching birds, which include canaries and finches.

Points to consider when choosing passerines

- Male canaries are kept for their attractive singing.
- Other finches are best kept in pairs or in flocks in aviaries.
- These birds are rarely very tame.

Sexing

Some species show sexual dimorphism (e.g. finches). In others, behavioural differences can be used; for example, male canaries sing.

Housing

Most commercially available cages for birds are far too small. All birds are fitter if kept in aviaries.

- Mixed species can be kept together in an enclosed outdoor area or a covered flying area with a shed for shelter.
- Aviaries should have a double safety door.
- Suitable plants in pots encourage insect life.
- Perches of different heights and diameters should be provided – natural branches are best.
- Shallow (1 cm) water bowls for bathing should be provided early in the day.
- Some aviculturalists fit timed sprinkler systems in their aviaries.
- Water for drinking should be provided in column containers to prevent contamination.
- Food containers should be above floor level and never under perches.
- Healthy birds can withstand a wide range of ambient temperatures as long as fluctuations are not rapid.

Many passerines are kept indoors in cages (e.g. male canaries, which sing well) and these should always be as large as possible.

- Minimum dimensions must allow full extension of the wings, and the tail should be clear of the floor when perching. Cages should be as large as possible to allow horizontal flight between perches.
- Sandpaper-covered perches should be avoided, as these predispose to foot problems and do nothing to keep nails worn down.
- Cages should be placed well above ground level, preferably at human head height.
- Birds only feed during daylight and so artificial light should be provided to prevent reduced food intake on short winter days. A 12-hour light period is suitable.

All housing, whether cage or aviary, must be easy to clean:

- Perches should be kept scrupulously clean, using soap and water, mild disinfectant solution or dilute chlorine bleach, and thoroughly rinsed
- Cage-bottom coverings and food and water containers should be cleaned daily
- The whole cage or aviary should be thoroughly cleaned once a month.

Nutrition

Birds are conservative feeders and will only eat foods they recognize or on which they have become imprinted. Therefore changes in diet must be introduced gradually.

Seed-eaters

- Finches and canaries are seed-eaters. Seed of appropriate size should be provided, i.e. millet, canary seed, rape seed and hemp. Husks should be removed daily.
- Grit must be available at all times to ensure proper functioning of the gizzard. Grit must be of appropriate size and consist of two types: soluble (oyster shell, egg shell) and insoluble (quartz, igneous stone).

Variety is essential in providing a good balanced diet for passerine species, and lack of variety is the most common cause of malnutrition.

- At least six different food items should be offered daily.
- In addition to as many different seed varieties as possible, green food (lettuce, watercress, alfalfa, chickweed, dandelion, parsley), sprouted seeds, vegetables and fruit should be offered.
- 'Softfood', 'eggfood' and 'condition' or 'tonic' food are commercially available and can be fed at a ratio of 1:3 with the seed mixture.
- Complete diets are now widely available, and inexperienced owners often find these diets easier to use.

Insectivores and frugivores

- Insectivores (e.g. mynahs) usually need live food, such as mealworms, crickets and fruit flies. Commercial insectivore preparations are available.
- Frugivores (fruit-eaters) and nectar feeders (e.g. toucans, sunbirds and hummingbirds) need a variety of ripe fruit and/or syrupy fluids such as evaporated milk and honey with added vitamins, minerals and a little animal protein. Commercial liquid diets are also available.

Domestic fowl

Chickens, ducks and geese are sometimes kept as pets.

Points to consider when choosing domestic fowl

■ These species must be kept outside, with a secure house or pen to protect them from predators at night.
■ Geese can be used as guard animals and are very long-lived (20 years or more).
■ Ducks and geese will require access to water to swim on.
■ All three species have the advantage of providing eggs for consumption.

Handling

Domestic fowl can be lifted around the body, holding the wings against the body and then supporting the neck below the head.

Veterinary care of birds

Birds are very good at hiding signs of disease. This phenomenon is sometimes called the 'preservation reflex': a sick bird in the wild would be predated or harassed by other members of the flock. It is only when the bird can no longer compensate that an owner actually recognizes that something is wrong, and at this stage any disease process may be very advanced. It is for this reason that signs of illness, however slight, must be taken seriously in a bird and veterinary advice sought promptly.

■ Sick birds should be maintained at a high ambient temperature (approximately 28°C), without draughts.
■ Incubators are very useful – additional oxygen should be provided for birds with severe respiratory disease or those in shock.
■ Perches should be lowered.
■ Perching birds feel most secure if the cage is at shoulder height.
■ Dim lighting and a quiet environment reduce stress.
■ Birds should never be in visual contact with potential predators (e.g. cats).
■ Very tame species (e.g. parrots) will respond to human attention, but wild birds should be handled and disturbed as little as possible.

Force-feeding and fluid therapy

Birds have a high metabolic rate and must be force-fed if they are not eating voluntarily. It should be remembered that birds will only eat when it is light: at least 12 hours of light per day need to be provided to ensure that a bird is eating sufficiently to fulfil its metabolic requirements.

■ Force-feeding is achieved by crop tubing (as described below for administration of medicines).
■ Commercial enteral nutrition products are available.
■ Commercial dog or cat liquid diets can be used for carnivorous species.
■ Vegetable baby foods or human high-calorie invalid formulas are suitable for seed- and fruit-eaters.

■ Low-fat products are preferable if hepatic function is compromised.
■ Probiotics are very useful in sick or stressed birds.
■ Baby birds will require feeding every 1–2 hours, or whenever the crop is empty.
■ Baby birds must not be overfed, as crop stretching or stasis will occur.

Suggested volumes and frequencies for common species are shown in Figure 4.26.

Species	Amount per feed (ml)	Times/day
Finch	0.1–0.3	Six
Budgerigar	0.5–1.0	Four
Cockatiel	1.0–2.5	Four
Amazon parrot	5.0–8.0	Two

4.26 Volume and frequency for force-feeding birds.

Fluid therapy

■ The daily fluid requirements of birds are a minimum of 50 ml/kg/day (5% bodyweight).
■ Birds tolerate blood loss much better than mammals, and similarly can tolerate bolus treatment of relatively large volumes of fluid.
■ Percentage dehydration can be difficult to gauge in birds, but it can safely be assumed that any sick bird will be 10% dehydrated.
■ Fluids must always be warmed to 30–35°C.

Administration of medicines

Tablets or liquids can be incorporated into the food, but additions are often detected and uneaten, and accurate dosing is difficult. Figure 4.27 suggests routes of administration.

Route	Site	Notes
Oral	By tube into crop	
Subcutaneous	Axilla, lateral flank, interscapular area	Avoid large volumes
Intramuscular	Pectoral muscles	
Intravenous	Jugular, brachial, medial metatarsal vein	Care with haemostasis after withdrawal of needle
Intraosseous	Distal ulna, proximal tibia	Avoid pneumatic bones
Nebulization	Bird placed in tank with nebulizer attached	For treatment of respiratory disease

4.27 Routes of administration of medicines in birds.

Gavage or crop tubing

1. An assistant restrains the bird.
2. Place a gag between the upper and lower beak.
3. Insert a flexible tube or rigid metal tube with a rounded tip from the left side of the beak and down the oesophagus on the right side of the neck, into the crop.

Reptiles

Reptiles can be divided into three main groups: snakes (Figure 4.28), lizards (Figure 4.29) and chelonians (tortoises, turtles and terrapins) (Figure 4.30). In general tortoises are terrestrial, terrapins are semi-aquatic and turtles are aquatic. There are exceptions to this; for example, the Americans tend to refer to all chelonians as turtles.

Points to consider when choosing reptiles

- Reptiles have very specialized husbandry requirements, which can be expensive.
- While many people find reptiles attractive and fascinating, they are not interactive or 'cuddly' pets, and only tolerate being handled.
- Although some owners would claim to have a strong relationship with their reptile, this is largely anthropomorphism, but in some species in particular (such as tortoises) distinct personalities can be observed.
- Strict attention to hygiene must be observed if reptiles are kept as pets, as they can carry *Salmonella* in their faeces.
- Some species can grow very large. For example, the green iguana when mature can be up to 1.8 m in length, and the larger snakes can grow to about 4.6 m (e.g. Burmese python). These facts must be borne in mind when buying a small juvenile, especially in terms of the size of the housing they will require.
- Some people find the dietary requirements of reptiles unpleasant to deal with (e.g. dead rodents for snakes, insects for lizards).
- Large lizards can inflict deep scratches with their claws and can lash out with their tail. Large snakes can constrict around a handler's limbs or neck.
- All reptiles can bite.

Anatomy and physiology

Reptiles differ significantly from mammals and birds in that they are ectothermic ('cold-blooded'). This means that they are unable to generate body heat and so they rely on an external heat source and behavioural means to regulate their body temperature.

Reptiles have a dry skin that is folded into scales (Figure 4.31). All reptiles shed their skin periodically in a process known as ecdysis. The pattern of shedding depends on the species.

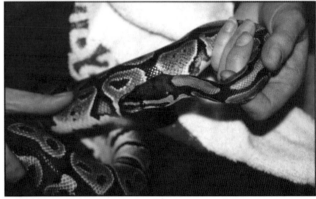

4.28   A Royal python. (Courtesy of Sharon Redrobe.)

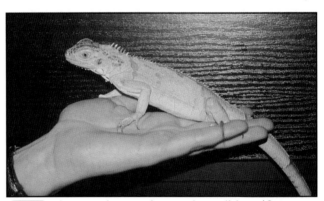

4.29   A green iguana in good condition. (Courtesy of Sharon Redrobe and reproduced from *BSAVA Manual of Exotic Pets, 4th edition*.)

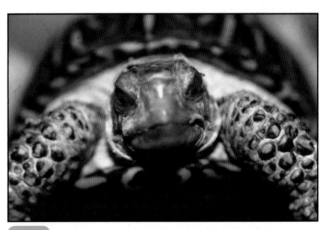

4.30   A box turtle. (Courtesy of Sharon Redrobe.)

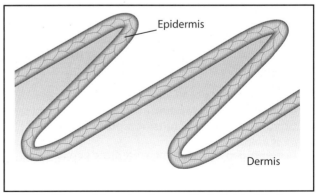

Epidermis

Dermis

4.31   The epidermis of a reptile is folded to form the characteristic scales.

The cloaca is the common opening of the digestive, reproductive and urinary tracts. Reptiles produce droppings with three components: faeces, white urates and, in some species, urine.

Housing

Reptiles are not social animals and most pet species are best kept singly, as the presence of other reptiles can be stressful if insufficient space is provided.

Environmental stress (including inadequate husbandry) predisposes an animal to infection, by immunosuppression. Thus, a knowledge of the reptile's basic environmental requirements is vital in the prevention of many diseases. Most diseases of reptiles in the UK are caused by an incorrect diet or incorrect housing conditions.

Figure 4.32 shows a typical vivarium set-up for a reptile. The exact configuration will depend on the species. Vivarium dimensions vary with species:

- Arboreal species require height
- Terrestrial species require floor area
- Aquatic species require water and basking platforms.

Items that can be ingested (e.g. small stones, gravel, corncob bedding) should be avoided. Newspaper is perhaps the best substrate as it is digestible, cheap and disposable. Other options include washable carpet squares or artificial turf.

A few items of safe cage furniture might include large stones, stable 'caves' or hides, secured branches that can take the weight of the reptile, and non-toxic non-injurious plants.

Water

A body of water is required for aquatic and semi-aquatic species, with adequate filtration and heating.

Drinking water should always be available to all reptiles in a form that is acceptable to them. For example, chameleons will only lick droplets, but tortoises need to immerse their mouth and nose and so should be placed in shallow water three times a week.

Temperature

To be able to thermoregulate, reptiles require the provision of a range of temperatures. This range is known as the preferred optimum temperature zone (POTZ). The preferred body temperature (PBT) is the optimum temperature for the functioning of the reptile's systems (e.g. movement, feeding, digestion, reproduction, immunocompetence).

The two types of heat source are:

- Primary – for background/ambient heat (this should not be a light source). A heat pad or ceramic heater (attached to a thermostat) is used
- Secondary – specific 'hot spot' areas with a higher temperature for basking or to provide a temperature gradient. An overhead incandescent bulb, a ceramic heater or an infra-red bulb is used.

Monitoring is vital to check the range of temperatures. Maximum/minimum thermometers and thermostats are essential.

Lighting

Timers are required for the maintenance of a stable photoperiod. Suitable photoperiods (light/dark) are:

- Tropical species: summer 13 h/11 h; winter 11 h/13 h
- Temperate species: summer 15 h/9 h; spring/autumn 12 h/12 h; winter 9 h/15 h.

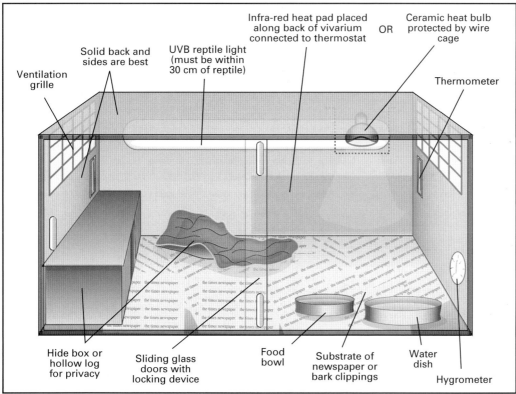

4.32

A vivarium suitable for a reptile. (Adapted from *BSAVA Manual of Reptiles, 2nd edn.*)

Ventilation grille

Solid back and sides are best

UVB reptile light (must be within 30 cm of reptile)

Infra-red heat pad placed along back of vivarium connected to thermostat   OR   Ceramic heat bulb protected by wire cage

Thermometer

Hide box or hollow log for privacy

Sliding glass doors with locking device

Food bowl

Substrate of newspaper or bark clippings

Water dish

Hygrometer

The wavelength of the light is also a factor:

- UVA (320–400 nm) stimulates agonistic and reproductive behaviour in lizards
- UVB (290–320 nm) is important for the conversion of provitamin D3 to previtamin D3 in the reptile skin, and is therefore important for calcium metabolism.

The broad-spectrum light must be placed within 30 cm of the reptile in order to expose the animal to sufficient UVB. UVB output is generally lost after 6 months and so the bulb must be regularly replaced, even if the visible light appears normal.

Humidity

- A relative humidity of 50–70% is tolerated by most species. Some, such as iguanas, require higher humidity.
- A humid chamber may be provided for ecdysis.
- Humidity should not be increased at the expense of ventilation.

Nutrition

Preferred food items for various species of reptile are shown in Figure 4.33.

Snakes

Anatomy and physiology

Snakes have an elongated slender body shape (Figure 4.34).

- Snakes have no visible limbs. Some species have vestigial skeletal pelvic girdles and hindlimbs (e.g. boas, pythons).
- Snakes have from 150 to 400 vertebrae, each articulating with a pair of ribs as far as the cloaca. In the tail the ribs are small and fused to the vertebrae.
- Snakes have no sternum.
- The lower jaw has no mandibular symphysis and the upper and lower jaw are only loosely connected, enabling a snake to have a very large gape and to swallow prey that is larger than its head.

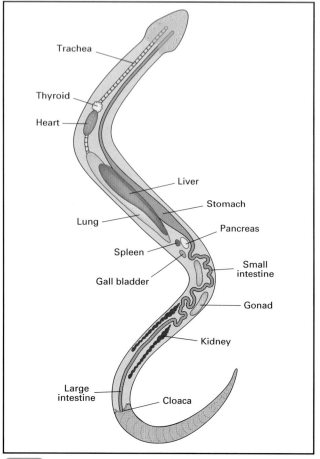

4.34   The internal organs of a snake.

- Snakes have backward-pointing teeth. Only venomous snakes have fangs.
- Snakes have no eyelids but have a clear scale of skin over the surface of the eye, known as the spectacle.
- Snakes shed their skin all in one piece, including the spectacles, starting at the head. About 4–7 days before shedding they will appear dull and cloudy, as a layer of milky fluid is secreted between the old and new layers of skin. This will then clear again just before shedding.

Reptiles	Families	Preferred foods
Snakes	Boas, pythons, ratsnakes, gopher snakes, bull snakes, vipers	Warm-blooded prey (e.g. rodents, birds)
	Garter and water snakes	Fish, frogs, earthworms, slugs
	Racers and vine snakes	Lizards (fed killed)
Lizards	Horned lizards	Ants (small crickets)
	Green iguanas	Dandelions, watercress, alfalfa, etc.
	Monitors	Raw eggs, pinkies, rodents, birds, fish
	Geckos, anoles, skinks, chameleons	Appropriately sized crickets, fruit flies, waxworms
Chelonians	Turtles and terrapins	Earthworms, small whole fish, pinkies, green vegetables
	Tortoises	Flowers, succulents, grass, cucumber, frozen mixed vegetables, fresh fruit

4.33   Preferred foods for reptiles.

Sexing

Several methods can be used to sex snakes:

- Sexual dimorphism (rare)
- Length of tail (longer in the male)
- Probing
- Popping (hatchlings) – the finger is rolled gently up the tail towards the cloaca to evert the hemipenes.

The most reliable of these methods is probing. An aseptic lubricated probe is passed gently into the cloaca, pointing towards the end of the tail. In the male the probe passes into the hemipenis (Figure 4.35) to a length of six to eight subcaudal scales. In the female it will only pass to a length of two to four scales. It is important to check both hemipenis orifices: a plug of smegma may sometimes block them, preventing the probe from entering.

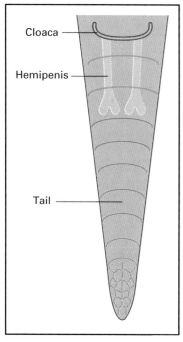

4.35 The tail of a male snake, showing the position of the hemipenes.

Nutrition

All snakes are carnivores and in captivity are fed on rodents of appropriate sizes (usually purchased frozen) or rabbits.

- It is illegal and inhumane to feed live vertebrate prey, even to an anorexic animal. Food may be bloodied, warmed and wiggled to encourage feeding.
- Some snakes (e.g. constrictors) prefer to eat in a small dark box.
- Small adult snakes should be fed once or twice a week.
- Juvenile snakes should be fed three times a week.
- Large snakes should be fed once every 2–4 weeks.
- Snakes should not be handled when they have recently eaten, as they may regurgitate.

Handling

Snakes should always be transported in an insulated, warm, dark and secure box or bag.

- Snakes should be grasped by the head first, with thumb and second finger behind the occiput and the forefinger on top of the head (Figure 4.36).
- The body must then be supported. Never lift the head and let the bodyweight dangle as snakes have a single occiput which can be easily dislocated.
- Avoid squeezing the body too hard, as bruising can lead to debility or even death. The ribs of snakes are easily broken.
- The teeth of a snake are angled caudally, so resist pulling rostrally if bitten. Pulling the hand out of the snake's mouth can result in a deeper bite or loss of the snake's teeth into the wound. This can lead to a foreign body reaction in the handler or osteomyelitis of the jaw in the snake.
- Snakes should never be placed around the neck. This is bad practice and can be dangerous – even fairly small specimens can constrict strongly.
- Always handle large snakes with the help of an assistant.

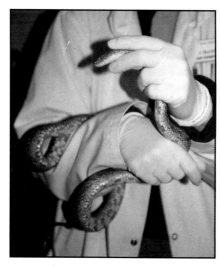

4.36 Holding the head of a snake. (Courtesy of Anna Meredith.)

Breeding

Most commonly kept snake species (e.g. cornsnakes) can be bred relatively easily in captivity.

Snake species can be divided into:

- Viviparous or live-bearing (e.g. boas, garter snakes)
- Oviparous or egg-laying (e.g. pythons).

Incubation facilities will be required for reptile eggs. The eggs have soft shells and require a high humidity. Incubation temperature can affect the sex of the hatchling in some species.

Lizards

Anatomy and physiology

The lizard skeleton follows the basic vertebrate pattern, with four limbs in most species and a tail.

- Some lizards are able to shed their tail (autotomy) as an escape mechanism, and can grow a new one. The replacement does not contain bony vertebrae, only cartilage, and will be dull in colour and have smaller scales than the rest of the body.

- Lizards shed their skin in large pieces and will often eat the dead skin.
- The structure of the digestive system varies depending on the diet. For example, herbivorous lizards such as the green iguana have a large caecum.
- Lizards have simple teeth.

Sexing

Lizards can be sexed in several ways:

- Femoral pores on the medial aspects of the hindlimbs are more obvious in males than in females (Figure 4.37)
- Some males have head ornamentation
- Hemipenes can be seen as bulges at the base of the tail in sexually mature males
- Radiography of certain monitor species will reveal the os penis.

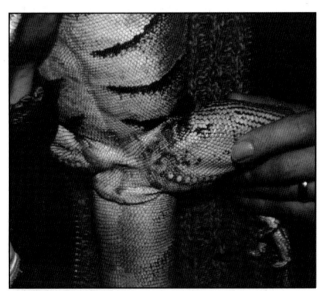

4.37 Femoral pores in a male green iguana. (Courtesy of Sharon Redrobe.)

Nutrition

- A calcium:phosphorus ratio of 1.5:1 plus vitamin D3 is essential for all species.
- Insectivores (e.g. bearded dragons, geckos) may be offered live crickets, waxworms, etc. coated with a reptile mineral/vitamin supplement. Ensure that the insects themselves have been fed (nutrient-loaded) before being offered to the reptile.
- Herbivores (e.g. iguanas) should be offered a wide variety of leafy greens, other vegetables and fruit, dusted with a proprietary reptile vitamin/mineral supplement.
- Lizards are generally fed daily.

Handling

- Lizards should be held around the neck and pelvic girdle with one hand, with the other around the pelvis and hindlimbs (Figure 4.38).

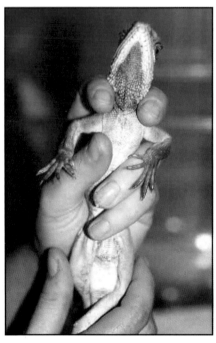

4.38 Holding a Chinese water dragon. (Courtesy of Anna Meredith.)

- For further restraint and to prevent being scratched, the limbs can be held down against the body. The limbs should be held near the top: if held down by the feet, violent struggling could result in a fracture, especially if the lizard has metabolic bone disease.
- A soft cloth may be used to catch the delicate-skinned geckos.
- Never handle a lizard by the tail – some species shed them.

Breeding

Some species of lizard are still wild-caught or imported from a farmed situation (e.g. iguanas) but many species are now captive-bred (as for snakes, see above).

Chelonians

Anatomy and physiology

The body of the chelonian consists of a bony box or shell. The upper shell is the carapace; the lower shell is the plastron.

- All chelonians shed the skin on the limbs, neck and head, in small pieces.
- Only terrapins shed scales (scutes) from their shell.
- Chelonians possess a hard horny beak and do not have teeth.

Contrary to popular belief, it is not possible to age a tortoise from the rings on its shell. These rings correspond to periods of rapid growth, which are not necessarily annual.

Sexing

- The single hemipenis in the male makes the tail larger and longer, and the cloaca is further away from the plastron than in the female (Figure 4.39).

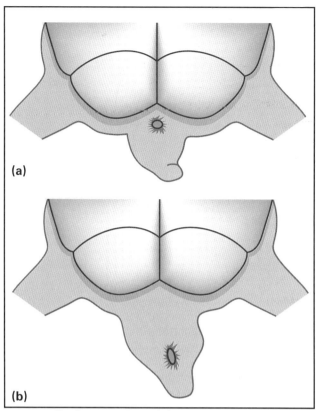

Nutrition

- Most commonly kept tortoises are herbivores and require high-fibre foods. A wide selection of leafy green vegetables is required, and natural foraging on wild plants in the garden is beneficial.
- Omnivorous species (e.g. box turtles) should be offered vegetable matter but will also take animal protein, such as crickets and other insects, mealworms, pinky mice, fish and small amounts of low-fat dog food.
- Aquatic species (which feed in water) should be fed in a separate feeding tank to prevent water fouling.
- All food (except complete pelleted commercial diets) should be dusted with a reptile vitamin/mineral supplement.

Handling

Chelonians are easily handled by holding the shell between the fore- and hindlimbs or around the back of the shell between the hindlimbs (Figure 4.40).

Breeding

As for snakes (see above).

4.39 Sexing tortoises. **(a)** Female: short tail; cloaca close to plastron. **(b)** Male: larger tail; cloaca further from plastron.

- In some species the plastron is concave in the male, but this is not always reliable as some older female tortoises can develop a concavity also.
- In the terrapin, the male has longer forelimb claws (used in courtship).

Veterinary care of reptiles

Administration of medicines

Reptiles have a renal portal venous circulation, which means that injections into the hindlimb musculature may be eliminated via the kidneys before reaching the rest of the body. There is still debate as to whether this system significantly affects drug distribution.

Suggested routes of administration of medicines in reptiles are given in Figure 4.41.

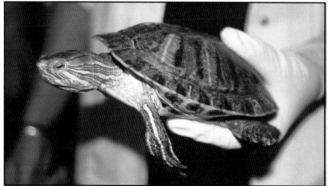 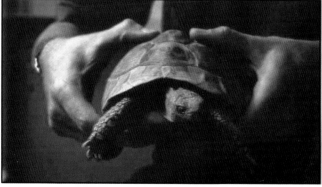

4.40 Alternative methods of handling chelonians. (Courtesy of Anna Meredith.)

Route	Reptile	Site
Subcutaneous	Snake/lizard	Loose skin over ribs
Intramuscular	Snake	Intercostal muscles of body
	Lizard	Fore/hindleg, tail muscles (with care)
	Chelonian	As lizard, plus pectoral muscle mass at angle of forelimb and neck
	In patients weighing less than 100 g, no more than 0.2 ml should be given at any one site	

4.41 Routes of administration of medicines in reptiles. (continues) ▶

Route	Reptile	Site
Intracoelomic	Snake	Off midline, cranial to cloaca
	Lizard	Off midline caudal to ribs, cranial to pelvis
	Chelonian	Cranial to hindlimb in fossa
	Large volumes should not be given by this route as respiration may be impaired	
Intravenous	Snake	Ventral tail vein, jugular vein, intracardiac
	Lizard	Ventral tail vein
	Chelonian	Dorsal tail vein, jugular vein
Intraosseous	Lizard/chelonian	Femur, tibia

4.41 (continued) Routes of administration of medicines in reptiles.

Force-feeding

- Stomach volume in reptiles is 10 ml/kg bodyweight.
- Some reptiles will accept liquid food being placed in the mouth via syringe.
- Carnivorous and insectivorous species should be given a meat-based liquid diet.
- Herbivorous species should be given a vegetable-based diet.
- Commercial critical care formulae are available.
- Placement of a pharyngostomy tube is the preferred method for force-feeding in the longer term.

Methods of tube-feeding reptiles are given in Figure 4.42.

Snakes

1. Manually restrain animal, open mouth and insert gag.
2. Hold anterior of snake vertically.
3. Insert well lubricated end of feeding tube into oesophagus to level of stomach (approximately one-third down length of snake).
4. Syringe in fluids/food slowly.
5. Hold snake vertically for 2–3 minutes to avoid regurgitation.
6. After several feedings of liquid died with no regurgitation, the snake can be force-fed whole animals or given liquidized whole animals by tube-feeding.

Lizards

1. Locate the stomach – it is positioned just behind the caudal edge of the ribs.
2. Proceed as above.

Chelonians

1. Locate the stomach – it is positioned midway down the plastron.
2. Measure stomach tube from mouth to caudal end of abdominal shield just beyond gular notch.
3. Hold chelonian upright.
4. Extend neck and hold head behind mandible.
5. Prise open mouth and hold open with a gag.
6. Proceed as above.

4.42 How to tube-feed reptiles.

Fluid therapy

- Most sick reptiles will present at least 10–15% dehydrated, requiring fluid therapy.
- Oral fluids (e.g. lactated Ringer's solution) should be given daily equal to 4–10% bodyweight if the reptile is not drinking.
- Oral fluids are given by stomach tube (see Figure 4.42).
- Fluids should be warmed to the reptile's preferred body temperature before administration.
- Fluids can be given by the subcutaneous, intracoelomic, intravenous or intraosseous route.

Amphibians

Frogs, toads, salamanders, newts and axolotls are all kept as pets.

Points to consider when choosing amphibians

- Amphibians have delicate moist permeable skin that is easily damaged, so these animals should not be handled on a regular basis.
- They need a vivarium tank and some species will need special heating and lighting and water filtration arrangements.

Anatomy and physiology

Amphibians have a basic vertebrate skeleton.

- Frogs and toads are tailless and have long hindlegs, whereas newts and salamanders have tails.
- All have moist permeable skin across which oxygen is absorbed.
- Some species (e.g. toads) have skin glands that secrete toxins.
- All amphibians require water to breed. Their life cycle involves a larval tadpole stage with gills,

which undergoes metamorphosis into the adult form. Axolotls are unique in that they remain and can become sexually mature in the larval stage, although they can metamorphose under certain conditions.

Sexing

Sexing of newts and salamanders involves looking at the cloaca, which has more swollen edges in the male. In the breeding season, the males of these species often become more brightly coloured and develop crests, and the females swell with eggs. Male frogs and toads develop swellings called nuptial pads on their forelegs and are more vocal than the female during the breeding season.

Housing

Vivaria or fish tanks are suitable for housing amphibians.

- High humidity (75–95%) is required.
- Some species will live in water all the time (e.g. newts, xenopus toads).
- Additional heating is required for tropical species (21–29°C).
- Temperatures are generally lower than those for reptiles.
- Moist bark chippings and moss make a suitable substrate.
- An ultraviolet light should be provided, as for reptiles.

Nutrition

All invertebrate food items should be nutrient-loaded or dusted with a vitamin/mineral supplement.

- Frogs and toads: crickets, mealworms, waxworms, pinkies.
- Salamanders: earthworms, mealworms, waxworms, crickets.

Handling

Because of their delicate skin, amphibians should only be handled if absolutely necessary. Hands should be wet before handling, or wet surgical gloves can be worn.

- Aquatic species, such as newts, should be picked up using a soft fine-meshed net.
- Amphibians can be coaxed into a small clear plastic box or bag, which will allow close inspection without the need to handle them directly.
- When handling frogs and toads, care should be taken to ensure that they do not leap out of the hand. Placing the animal's head between the first two fingers, with its back lying against the palm of the hand, will restrain them.

Veterinary care

Administration of medicines

Drugs for amphibians can be administered:

- Orally, by syringe into the mouth
- Topically – but beware toxicity, as the drug will be systemically absorbed
- In water, as for fish (see below).

Force-feeding and fluid therapy

Small rubber tubes or catheters can be used as feeding tubes for amphibians. Great care must be taken when opening the mouth, to avoid damage to the delicate mandible. Some animals will swallow food items placed directly in the mouth.

Fish

Points to consider when choosing fish

- Fish are not very interactive pets, but many people find them soothing and therapeutic to watch.
- Fish are low-maintenance pets and relatively easy to keep, as long as the water quality is good.
- Freshwater species, such as goldfish, and many species of tropical fish are widely available.

Anatomy and physiology

- Fish are ectothermic. They possess gills, which extract oxygen from the water as it flows over them.
- The skin is covered with scales.
- Fish have no eyelids.
- The digestive system is simple and has intestinal (pyloric) caecae.
- The swim bladder connects to the digestive tract in most species (Figure 4.43).

Housing

- The aquarium tank should be sited away from heaters, draughts and direct sunlight, and near sources of water and power.
- A firm level base must be provided.
- Consideration should be given to the weight of the tank when full (1 litre of water weighs 1 kg).
- Exposure to tobacco smoke and paint fumes must be avoided: these can dissolve in the water and harm the fish.

The larger the tank, the better, but the most important factor is to provide a large surface area for good oxygenation. For this reason, the traditional goldfish bowl is completely unsuitable. The best type of tank is all-plastic or stainless steel with glass sides.

For tanks that are not artificially aerated, the stocking density should be 75 cm^2 surface area for each 2.5 cm body length of fish. This can be increased up to a point if aeration is provided. Cold-water tanks can be stocked more densely than a tropical tank of similar size, due to the higher oxygen content of the colder water.

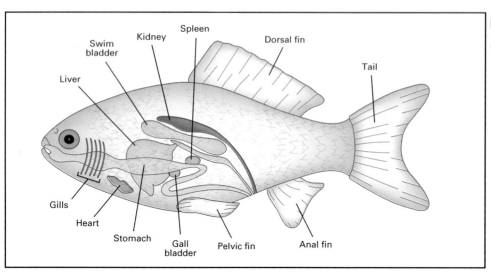

4.43 External features and internal organs of a fish.

Labels: Swim bladder, Kidney, Spleen, Dorsal fin, Liver, Tail, Gills, Heart, Stomach, Gall bladder, Pelvic fin, Anal fin

- Cold-water fish require an average temperature of 15°C.
- Tropical fish will require a heater and thermostat. These are generally sold as a combined unit, plugging directly into the mains electricity supply.

There are three main types of mechanical filtration available, and these systems aerate the water as well as removing particulate matter from it:

- Bottom filter – hidden below the gravel; this works as a simple slit system
- Inside filter box – suspended in the water, usually in a corner of the tank; it contains nylon or gravel plus activated charcoal, which need to be changed regularly
- Outside filter box – similar to the inside box but situated outside the tank
- Biological filters are also available; these contain bacteria that breakdown metabolic waste products.

Extra aeration is seldom required in a good tank (i.e. one that is not overcrowded and is well filtered, with a good surface area) but is often needed to stock smaller tanks at densities that aquarists find aesthetically pleasing.

- Aeration (diffuser) blocks are often used, but some fish dislike violent aeration.
- Excessive aeration can lead to 'gas bubble disease', seen on the skin and fins.

Light is essential for a healthy aquarium: it ensures plant survival, and is necessary to display the fish well. In the wild, light enters from the surface only. It is unnatural for fish to receive light from all sides, as they do in a tank.

- Fish have no eyelids and need shelter (e.g. plants) to avoid too much light.
- Fish need dark periods in order to rest. A 12 h light/dark cycle is adequate (at least 9 h light is necessary).
- Artificial light is essential, as sunlight is unpredictable, warms the water and promotes algal growth.
- White fluorescent strip lighting is best.

Other aquarium equipment might include:

- Gravel and rocks
- Plants for oxygenation, decoration, shelter and food
- Dipping nets for catching fish
- Scraper for removing algae.

Setting up an aquarium is detailed in Figure 4.44. The aquarium must be set up for at least 5 days before fish are added.

1. Clean the tank and all fittings thoroughly with dilute detergent and rinse thoroughly.
2. Place in a suitable position. Once in place, the tank should not be moved.
3. Wash the gravel and rocks several times in running water and lay them at the bottom of the tank to a depth of 5 cm, sloping up towards the back of the tank. Position any rocks. (If a bottom filter is being used, this will have to be in place first and gravel should be level.)
4. To minimize gravel disturbance during water-pouring, place brown paper or a plastic sheet over the gravel. Fill the tank with conditioned water (water can be conditioned artificially by adding a conditioning solution, or by allowing it to stand for a few days to allow for the chlorine gas to evaporate). Remove the paper or plastic sheet.
5. Plant the plants in the gravel, with the tallest at the rear and sides.
6. Place the thermometer in position.
7. Set up lighting, heater and thermostat, pump, aerators and filters.
8. Put on top cover or, if not available, a sheet of glass supported by four corks or pads. This keeps dust out but allows free entry of air.
9. Run the tank with no fish for a few days, checking that the thermostat and heater are working.
10. Add the fish, contained in the plastic bag in which they were purchased, to the tank. After 15 minutes, when the temperatures of the bag water and the tank water have equilibrated, gently tip the fish into the tank. Allow them to settle for a day before feeding.

4.44 Setting up an aquarium.

Nutrition

Commercial fish diets are often fed to exclusion, but fish require a varied diet and live food is essential, especially for tropical fish.

- Dried diets are made of meat and cereal, with added vitamins and minerals.
- Dried *Daphnia* (water fleas) and tubifex worms are also available. Homemade additions include brown bread crumbs and grated cheese. Ant eggs should only be given occasionally.
- Live food should be fed regularly. *Daphnia* can be added direct to the tank but tubifex worms should be thoroughly washed first in running water, as they are reared in detritus.
- Overfeeding and giving too much dry food are common mistakes. They result in fouling of the water and constipation of the fish (trailing faeces).
- Fish should be fed *once daily* at a regular time and place. Food should either be sprinkled on the surface or given via a plastic floating feeding ring.
- A pinch as large as the eye of the fish is a good rule for the amount to feed per fish.
- After 10 minutes, or when the fish show no interest, remove the excess with a siphon or pipette.
- Outdoor fish eat less in the winter than in the summer.

Handling

Fish can be moved from tank to tank by using a soft fine-meshed net. Time spent out of the water must be kept to an absolute minimum.

Veterinary care

If a fish is thought to be ill it should be isolated immediately, in a separate tank filled with water from the main tank to avoid further stressing the fish. The rest of the original tank should be quarantined and the advice of an experienced aquarist or veterinary surgeon should be sought.

Administration of medicines

Fish are not covered by the Veterinary Surgeons Act; therefore owners are able to diagnose disease, obtain non-prescription drugs and administer them. Unfortunately, the diagnosis is often inaccurate and fish may have been treated with numerous over-the-counter preparations before presentation to a veterinary surgeon.

In-feed medication

Medicated feed is commercially available for farmed fish and may be used where large numbers are kept (e.g. Koi carp). Medicated pellets can be made at home by mixing the drug with softened diet pellets and allowing them to dry.

Intramuscular injection

This is possible with larger individual fish. Commonly used sites are the base of the tail or in front of the dorsal fin.

In-water medication

Liquids or soluble powders may be added to the water. Calculation of the water volume is essential for accurate dosing. A separate treatment tank should be used.

Invertebrates

Spiders and other invertebrates such as giant African land snails, scorpions, millipedes and stick insects may be kept as pets.

Anatomy and physiology

Many invertebrate species have exoskeletons that may be shed (moulted). Invertebrates are ectothermic.

Housing

Most are kept in a vivarium. It should be of sufficient size to allow the animal full movement, including that required when moulting. Long insects such as stick insects require a height of at least twice their length. Vivaria should have a close-fitting lid that allows ventilation but is secure to prevent escape.

- Heat should be provided via a heat mat covering two-thirds of the vivarium floor. For example, tarantulas can be maintained at 25–26°C.
- Different species have different requirements for humidity – molluscs (slugs and snails) need damp environments and most arthropods require drier environments.
- Vermiculite is recommended as substrate for many species, as it retains moisture and remains relatively sterile. Moist peat may be used for molluscs.
- Vivarium hygiene is very important, especially in humid environments.

Nutrition

Dietary requirements vary widely, depending on the species.

- Herbivorous species should receive fresh food, with foliage kept in water to prevent wilting but protected so the animal does not fall in and drown.
- Spiders are carnivores and require live prey – usually insects. Live food should be fed with care, as they may damage the invertebrate predator.
- Molluscs have a high calcium requirement and should be given cuttlefish.

Handling

Invertebrates should be handled over a table, because if they are dropped they may rupture the exoskeleton.

- Tarantulas should be handled with care as they can flick abdominal hairs that are highly irritant to eyes.
- Aquarium nets can be used to encourage animals into a clear plastic box for examination. If there is any doubt about whether handling is safe for either animal or handler, it should be viewed within a clear plastic container or by restraining it with clear plastic wrap on a sheet of glass.

- Long-handled forceps are useful for encouraging invertebrates into containers.
- Scorpions can be grasped with padded forceps at the end of the tail just in front of the stinger (telson).
- Some species, such as snails and millipedes, will tolerate grasping with the hand.
- Hypothermia can be used to facilitate handling – 30 minutes in a fridge at 4°C is usually sufficient but has no analgesic effect.

General care of wildlife casualties

Although they are included in this section of the manual, wild animals and birds differ a great deal from domesticated species and should not be considered as exotic pets. Wildlife may require care and treatment as a result of becoming injured, trapped, weakened through exhaustion or starvation, diseased or orphaned. Some animals and birds may simply have reached the end of their normal lifespan. Wild animals can be difficult to treat and care for successfully, and for many casualties euthanasia may be the kindest course of action.

There can, however, be some good reasons for treating wildlife. The treatment of wildlife casualties can be an important part of conservation in some countries. Treatment of wildlife can help to prevent suffering of individuals and heal creatures that have been damaged by human actions (trapping, shooting, road traffic accidents). Additionally, monitoring disease in wildlife can be an important part of disease prevention in humans and livestock and assist in the assessment of environmental factors such as pollution and global warming.

The aim of treating any wildlife casualty is to be able to release it successfully back to the wild. Any released animal or bird must be able to run or fly, feed, defend itself, reproduce, and behave in a normal manner towards its own and other species. As few British wildlife species are endangered, life in captivity is not considered a humane alternative to release, with euthanasia being a kinder option. The process of treatment, rehabilitation (preparation for eventual release back into the wild) and release of a wild animal into its own environment can be a long and involved process. Often the skills of several professionals are needed, such as veterinary surgeons, specialist wildlife carers and ecologists. Suitable facilities are also required for treatment and rehabilitation and a suitable site for eventual release. There are many specialist organizations in the UK that are happy to assist with this care.

The treatment of wildlife casualties is covered by the same legislation as for other species. Additionally specific legislation applies to keeping and release of some species. Those not qualified as veterinary surgeons or veterinary nurses can provide first aid to wildlife until professional help can be obtained. Professional assessment should be sought as soon as possible so as to provide the best possible care, avoid unnecessary time in captivity and carry out euthanasia if the casualty is felt to be unfit for eventual release.

Capture and handling of wildlife

All wildlife species must be handled with great care so as to prevent further injury to themselves or to the handler (Figure 4.45ab). All birds and mammals can cause injury through pecks, scratches and bites. Infections (zoonoses) can be contracted from wildlife as a result of lack of personal safety and hygiene.

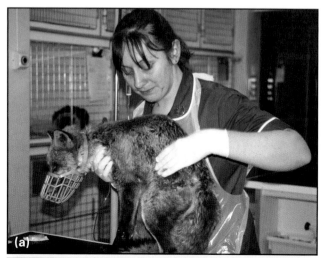

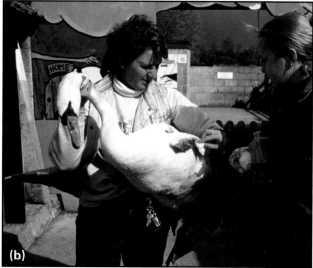

4.45 **(a)** Wildlife casualties must be handled with great care to prevent further injury to themselves or the handler. **(b)** First aid techniques, such as cleaning a wing wound in this swan, are similar to those performed in domestic species. (Courtesy of the Secret World Wildlife Rescue.)

Figure 4.46 illustrates suitable capture and handling techniques for the common groups of British wildlife casualties, together with some of the dangers associated with them. Special equipment together with help from specialist organizations may be needed. Wildlife should be handled with minimal human contact and all noise, such as talking and the sounds of other animals, must be kept to a minimum to avoid unnecessary distress.

It is important to record as much detail about the casualty as possible, including how and where it was found and what condition it appeared to be in when it was recovered. As many animals and birds are territorial, it is necessary to record exactly where

Species	Capture techniques	Transportation methods	Dangers of handling
Small and medium-sized birds	Cover with cloth, coat or blanket Catching net	Short journeys: hand-hold in covering cloth Dark box or pet carrier with air holes and non-slip floor covering Pillowcase or hessian sack	Bites and scratches Zoonotic infections
Seabirds (e.g. gulls, gannets)	Prevent re-entry to water Cover with blanket or coat Angler's landing net Immobilize head	Short journeys: hand-hold in covering material Dark box or pet carrier with air holes and non-slip floor covering Hessian sack	Painful bites Stabs at face and eyes Zoonotic infections
Large water birds (e.g. swans, geese, herons)	Prevent re-entry to water If on water, seek expert assistance Immobilize head	Restrain body in blanket or sack 'Swan bag'	Painful bites Stabs at face Strikes with wings Zoonotic infections
Raptors (e.g. falcons, hawks, owls)	Cover with cloth, coat or blanket Angler's landing net Allow to grip material with talons Restrain legs	Short journeys: hand-hold in covering material Dark box or pet carrier with air holes and non-slip floor covering	Painful bites Injuries from talons Zoonotic infections
Small rodents and bats	Leather gloves or cover with cloth	Escape-proof box with air holes Pillowcase or cash bag	Bites Zoonotic infections (including rabies in bats)
Rabbits, hares and hedgehogs	Cover with cloth or towel Thick leather gloves Angler's landing net	Dark box or pet carrier with air holes and non-slip floor covering or soft bedding	Bites, scratches Zoonotic infections
Stoats, weasels and squirrels	Thick leather gloves Angler's landing net	Plastic box or dustbin with well fitting lid Plastic or fine-meshed wire carrier (covered)	Bites, scratches Zoonotic infections
Foxes and badgers	Approach with caution: shocked animals appear tame Prevent escape (with loop around animal's neck) Seek expert assistance	Once restrained, lift with care into plastic dustbin with well fitting lid or stout hessian sack Wire crush cage	Serious bites Zoonotic infections
Deer	Approach with caution: shocked animals appear tame Cover animal's head, legs and feet Seek expert assistance	Do not attempt to move without expert assistance or advice	Serious injury from antlers and feet Zoonotic infections

4.46   Capture and transport of common wildlife casualties (adapted from *BSAVA Manual of Wildlife Casualties*).

they were found (OS map grid reference if possible) in order for them to be safely released in the same area at a later date.

Rapid identification of the species concerned will help with decisions about its care and prognosis. Field guides and the knowledge of others may be required to assist with identification.

Basic first aid

Like all species, wildlife cases may require first aid to stop deterioration before professional help can be obtained. Handling should be kept to a minimum to prevent unnecessary stress, but some handling may be needed to stop profuse haemorrhage or support damaged wings. The techniques for such first aid are technically the same as for domestic species, but extra care must be taken to avoid unnecessary stress to the casualty or injury to the handler.

Many wildlife casualties will be cold (hypothermic) and dehydrated on admission.

- Heat should be provided through the use of appropriate bedding together with lamps, heat pads or bags and incubators as available. The aim of these is to prevent further heat loss rather than warm the patient up quickly.
- Oral fluids should be given with care, but otherwise in the same ways and in the same volumes as for domestic species (birds by gavaging and mammals by syringe or stomach tube, as appropriate).
- If the patient is collapsed or very dehydrated, fluid therapy by other routes (intravenous, intraperitoneal, intraosseous) will need to be carried out by a veterinary surgeon or veterinary nurse.
- Suitable pain relief (analgesia) should be given.

Care in captivity

Figure 4.47 gives requirements for the short-term housing and feeding of common wildlife species.

For longer-term captivity (over 5 days) all species benefit from specialist care in purpose-built accommodation. Wildlife should be kept away from domestic species to avoid the smell and noise of predators and reduce disease transmission. Covering of cages, provision of bedding or nest boxes and dim lighting all help to provide visual seclusion and further reduce stress. Good general hygiene of cages, bowls and bedding should be carried out as for domestic species but in such a way as to minimize handling of the patient.

Feeding should mimic a natural diet as far as possible. Water in suitable spill-proof containers should also be provided.

Orphans of wildlife species

Many young birds and mammals are brought into captivity unnecessarily, having been assumed to be orphaned. The prognosis for these juveniles is extremely poor, as hand-reared animals adapt poorly when released back into the wild. It is perfectly normal for the adults of many species (e.g. hare, fox, deer, nest-rearing birds) to leave their young unattended for periods of time, returning only intermittently to feed them.

- If such juveniles are found, they should be left untouched exactly where they are unless they are obviously injured.
- If they are at real risk of injury from predators (e.g. cats), they should be placed under cover of vegetation.

Where it is genuinely necessary to bring a juvenile bird or mammal into captivity, handling and basic first aid are the same as for adult casualties. Veterinary attention and specialist rearing care should be sought immediately (Figure 4.48).

Species	Short-term housing	Short-term feeding
Small birds	Escape-proof cage For perching species: a suitably sized natural or plastic perch Newspaper on floor	Insectivores: commercial diets, mealworms, waxworms, maggots Granivores: commercial diets, small seed mixtures Fish eaters: small fish Omnivores: commercial diets, commercial dog/cat food
Sea and water birds	Hospital cage Newspaper or sheet bedding (moisten bedding for seabirds and waders)	Fish eaters: small fish Omnivores: commercial diets, commercial dog/cat food
Raptors	Solid-walled cages or boxes Carpet on floor Suitable perch Care to prevent tail damage (guard)	Convalescence diets (gavaged) Day-old chicks or mice (skinned)
Rodents	Escape-proof weld-mesh or stainless steel cages (squirrels); plastic or glass vivarium with lid (other species) Hide-tubes or boxes of wood or cardboard Hessian or paper bedding or natural substrates (hay, moss, leaves) Tree or shrub branches	Pelleted rodent food Seeds, fruit, nuts
Bats	Plastic tank with lid Paper towel or thin cloth, some of which hangs vertically in the tank	Commercial tinned cat food or convalescence diets Mealworms
Rabbits and hares	Escape-proof weld-mesh or stainless steel cages Hide-tubes or boxes of wood or cardboard Hay or straw bedding	Hay, vegetables, commercial rabbit food
Hedgehogs	Secure cardboard or plastic boxes Newspaper or shavings for bedding	Commercial tinned or dried dog food
Badgers	Stainless steel kennel with shredded paper, straw or blankets – enough for the animal to bury itself in	Commercial tinned or dried dog food Meat, fruit, seeds, day-old chicks
Foxes	Stainless steel kennel with shredded paper, straw or blankets Wooden or cardboard nest box	Commercial tinned or dried dog food Rodents, rabbits, day-old chicks

4.47   Short-term housing and feeding of common wildlife species.

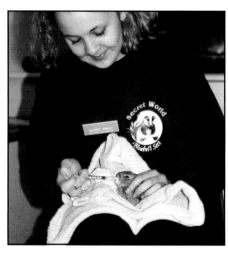

4.48

Hand-rearing of wildlife orphans, such as this wild rabbit, is time-consuming and requires specialist skills, but can be very rewarding. (Courtesy of the Secret World Wildlife Rescue.)

References and further reading

Girling S and Raiti P (2004) *BSAVA Manual of Reptiles, 2nd edn.* BSAVA Publications, Gloucester

Harcourt-Brown N and Chitty J (2005) *BSAVA Manual of Psittacine Birds, 2nd edn.* BSAVA Publications, Gloucester

Meredith A and Flecknell P (2006) *BSAVA Manual of Rabbit Medicine and Surgery, 2nd edn.* BSAVA Publications, Gloucester

Meredith A and Redrobe S (2002) *BSAVA Manual of Exotic Pets, 4th edn.* BSAVA Publications, Gloucester

Mullineaux E, Best D and Cooper JE (2003) *BSAVA Manual of Wildlife Casualties.* BSAVA Publications, Gloucester

Wildgoose W (2001) *BSAVA Manual of Ornamental Fish, 2nd edn.* BSAVA Publications, Gloucester

5

Management of an animal ward

Dawn Platten

This chapter is designed to give information on:

- Types of animal ward
- Preparation of accommodation
- Restraint of patients
- Cleaning animal accommodation
- Health and safety in the animal ward
- Design and nursing in the isolation ward

Introduction

The basic requirements of the ward accommodation are:

- To provide accommodation for animals to be housed for both short and longer periods of time
- To enable ease of handling, examining and treating as required
- To protect the patient from fear and distress
- To provide warmth and comfort for the patient
- To enable varying feeding protocols to be undertaken
- To be secure, with no possibility of escape
- To provide an area for exercise and toileting as appropriate
- To protect the patient from injury
- To minimize risk of the patient contracting a disease
- To provide a caring environment where the patient receives companionship, mental stimulation and the opportunity to express normal behaviour.

Ward design and equipment

Animal wards can take many different forms. This is dependent on a number of issues. Considerations include:

- The amount of space available for the ward
- The number of animals to be housed
- The type of animal to be housed in the ward
- The expected length of stay of the animals
- The expected medical and surgical conditions
- The number of staff members who will work on the ward
- Any additional equipment that will need to be stored (of particular importance for intensive care units).

Types of animal ward

Run access

This is an outdoor cage for dogs or cats. Access is gained to the cage through a gate in the exercise run. This type of accommodation is commonly used in boarding or breeding situations. It is not suitable for hospitalized patients.

Parasol or circular

This is a fairly recent design that may be used for larger hospitals or treatment wards in rescue centres. It consists of a circular design with the animal cages placed around the outside of the circle, facing inwards. The centre of the circle contains the working area for staff. Patients have access to individual exercise areas via a hatch, which the staff operate as required.

Corridor

This is a common design consisting of a building with kennels running along each side (Figure 5.1). Access to the exercise areas is often via a hatch, which is operated on a pulley system from the corridor.

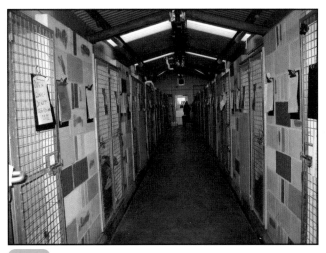

5.1   Corridor kennels.

H block

This design consists of four separate wards forming an H shape where the working area for staff forms the crossbar of the H. It is used where large numbers of animals are to be housed under one roof.

Tiered

This is probably the most common type of ward seen in veterinary practice (Figure 5.2). It consists of a bank of cages on one side of the ward. The cages are relatively small, allowing many patients to be housed in one area. The small cage size is also suitable as most patients will either require rest or only stay for a short time.

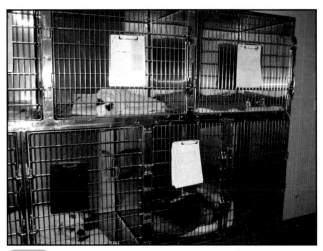

5.2   Tiered kennels.

The lower cages are usually larger, for dogs, and the higher cages are of a smaller size, for small dogs or cats. Large or long-stay dogs will need bigger, preferably walk-in, kennelling (Figure 5.3).

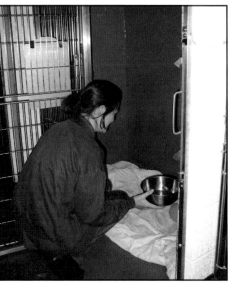

5.3 Preparing a walk-in kennel for a large dog.

Care should be taken with the type and temperament of animals placed in the higher cages. Large, timid or aggressive patients should not be put in these cages.

A food preparation area is usually incorporated in the ward.

Sneeze barriers

Sneezing results in aerosol droplets flying into the air at high speed. This has an important role in the spread of respiratory disease. Nasal discharge from an animal can travel up to half a metre during a sneeze. Cages should be arranged so that it is not possible for one patient to sneeze at another. This is achieved by:

- Ensuring that all cages face the same direction
- Separating cages that do face each other in a ward by a distance of at least 0.6 metres
- Using cages with a solid front to the cage (e.g. glass) (Figure 5.4).

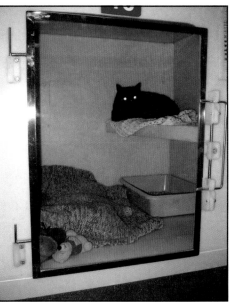

5.4 Glass-fronted cage.

Kitchen or food preparation area

If there is only one ward in a clinic, the food preparation area is usually close to or part of the ward. If a clinic has more than one ward, each can have a food preparation area or it may be more suitable to have a separate kitchen area. This limits the likelihood of cross-infection from one ward to another.

- The kitchen should have vermin-proof bins for food storage, a sink with hot and cold water, a refrigerator, scales to weigh food and a microwave (or similar) to warm food.
- A separate sink for washing of hands should be provided.
- Food storage areas should be cool and dry.
- Expiry dates of food should be checked regularly.
- Sacks of food should be stored raised from the ground.
- Stock rotation should be in place to ensure that food used is fresh.
- A range of food and water bowls should be stored to allow choice of the most appropriate type for each patient.

Grooming room

The size and facilities in this area will depend on the level of use. A grooming room that is used frequently should ideally contain:

- Raised bath with mixer hose for hot and cold water
- Table with non-slip mat
- Hair dryer
- Storage and disinfection facilities for brushes, combs and scissors.

Ventilation

Ventilation in the animal ward is necessary to:

- Ensure that there is an adequate supply of clean air for the animals and staff
- Remove stale air (which contains carbon dioxide from exhalation and ammonia and methane from excretions)
- Remove unpleasant odours
- Reduce the spread of airborne infections.

The degree of ventilation taking place within a building is normally expressed in terms of air changes per hour, i.e. how many times all the air is replaced in an hour.

Types of ventilation

Passive ventilation

Passive ventilation relies on the opening and closing of doors, windows and vents.

There are some obvious drawbacks:

- It can be draughty and lead to cold areas in the ward
- Heat loss can be a problem
- Frequent adjustments of the vents and windows are required
- In hot, still weather it can be difficult to maintain adequate ventilation.

Active ventilation

Active ventilation involves air being forced into or out of the building, usually by the use of extractor fans or an air-conditioning system.

- In the animal ward, it is advantageous for the ventilation system to provide fresh air to each kennel and then remove it before other animals in the ward inhale it.
- Where there is more than one animal ward, separate ventilation systems reduce the likelihood of cross-infection of airborne disease.

Heating

Animal wards require heating to:

- Provide a warm and comfortable environment for the animals
- Reduce the time taken for cages to dry after cleaning and disinfecting
- Reduce condensation and humidity, thus in turn reducing the incidence of respiratory disease
- Improve the working environment for the staff.

The ward should be maintained at a constant temperature of approximately 18–23°C.

Animal wards are commonly heated by environmental heating systems, but there will be instances when additional heating may be required for patients. There are many different methods to provide this, some of which are compared in Figure 5.5.

System	Advantages	Potential problems	Safety considerations
Electric fan heater	Can be controlled individually Heat can be directed towards animals	Noisy Increased risk of spreading airborne disease Can cause overheating of individual animals	Small fire risk Cables must be protected from interference by animals Switches and sockets should be waterproof
Infra-red dull emitter lamp	Good source of local heat Can be controlled by adjusting distance of lamp from the animal	Can cause overheating and burning if too close to animal or not thermostatically controlled	Cables must be protected from interference by animals Switches and sockets should be waterproof

5.5   Comparison of heating devices. (continues)   ▶

System	Advantages	Potential problems	Safety considerations
Heated bed or pad	Animal is directly heated by low constant heat from below	Difficult to clean	Risk of electrocution of animal if chews wires Circuit breaker must be used to minimize risk
Hot-water bottle or 'hot hands' (latex gloves filled with warm water and tied up)	Direct heat to individual	Scalding can occur if leaks or chewed Requires regular replacing	Never use boiling water Cover with blanket or towel
Incubator	Useful for neonates and small intensive care patients Thermostatically controlled		Cables must be protected from interference by animals Switches and sockets should be waterproof
Tin foil (shiny side towards patient) or bubble wrap	Retains patient's own body heat	Could cause blockage or choking if chewed	

5.5   (continued) Comparison of heating devices.

Lighting

Good lighting is necessary in order to:

- Create a safe working environment for the staff
- Allow the animals to be observed properly.

Natural light

Natural daylight is beneficial for animals. The ward should have a window for natural light to enter, but in warm sunny weather it may be necessary to use a screen at the window to prevent overheating. Windows in the ward that may be opened must be protected by wire to avoid patient escape.

Artificial lighting

The most commonly used form of artificial lighting is fluorescent strip lighting with a diffuser. These lights produce little shadow and are therefore helpful when cleaning and examining patients. Spotlights may be of use if additional lighting is required when dealing with individual patients.

Light switches within the ward area should be waterproof, as they may become wet due to either the cleaning process or staff using them with wet hands.

Preparing accommodation for a patient

- Ensure that the cage to be used is of suitable size and is appropriate for the species it will house.
- Check whether there are any special requirements for the animal (e.g. provision of additional heat or certain types of bedding).
- Ensure that there are suitable facilities for toileting (litter trays for cats, regular trips outside for dogs, if condition allows).
- Choose appropriate bedding.
- Choose suitable food and water bowls.

- If appropriate, provide a form of mental stimulation (i.e. toys).
- If possible, dogs and cats should be housed in separate wards to reduce stress.
- Consider pheromone treatment. There are a number of pheromone treatments on the market that claim to reduce stress for animals in unfamiliar environments (e.g. Feliway diffuser for cats).

> **CAUTION**
> When preparing a cage for a very small patient, it is important to check that the distance between the bars on the front of the cage is small enough to avoid the animal escaping or getting its head stuck.
> This precaution is often overlooked when a queen or dam has undergone a Caesarean section: the animal is placed back in the original cage (with wide spaces between the bars), which is no longer suitable due to the presence of her newborn offspring.

Beds and bedding

All animals should be provided with some form of bed. This indicates their sleeping area and is used for comfort, warmth and security. There are many types of bed available commercially, with varying degrees of usefulness within the veterinary practice. There may be limited space for bedding due to the cage size, but it is extremely important that the patient should be able to lie fully stretched out.

Selecting bedding material

Bedding may be divided into disposable (Figure 5.6) or non-disposable (Figure 5.7). When considering an appropriate choice of bedding for an animal, account must be taken of species, size, weight and health status (Figure 5.8).

Bedding	Advantages	Disadvantages	Comments
Newspaper	Good lining for cages Helps prevent top bedding layer from slipping around cage Absorbs any liquid on floor of cage	Not suitable for use alone Provides little comfort or insulation Can stain coat of light-coloured animals	Most common form of disposable bedding used in veterinary practice Free and easily available Recyclable if unused
Shredded paper	Good padding and insulating properties Enables animals to make 'nest' (natural behaviour)	Can be messy to deal with in practice Can stain coat of light-coloured animals	Free and easily available
Incontinence pads	Good absorbency Provides some warmth and padding	Plastic backing could cause blockages if chewed and swallowed	

5.6 Disposable bedding.

Bedding	Advantages	Disadvantages	Comments
Plastic moulded beds	Raised sides protect animal from draughts Low entrance allows easy access for patient Easy to clean Strong and durable Cheap to purchase	Rigid with hard base Need additional soft bedding inside	
Wicker basket/bed	Warm	Hard uneven floor Needs additional soft bedding inside Difficult to clean Broken ends of wicker are sharp and could cause injury	Not recommended for use in veterinary practice due to inability to clean effectively
Acrylic (e.g. Vetbed, Drybed)	Allows fluids to soak through, leaving top layer dry Good insulating and padding properties More durable than most bedding material Easy to wash and quick to dry	Expensive to purchase	Cheaper if bulk purchased on roll and cut to required size
Beanbags	Good insulating and padding properties Conform to body shape	Difficult to launder Easily destroyed by dogs Expensive to purchase Animals with limited movement can find them difficult to get into	
Covered foam pads	Good insulating and padding properties Relatively cheap to purchase	Difficult to launder and dry Can be destroyed by dogs	Nervous animals enjoy security of enclosed igloo types
Blankets	Good insulating and padding properties if several layers used Easy to launder but slow drying	Easily destroyed by dogs Expensive to purchase	Often donated
Duvets	Excellent insulating and padding properties Easy to machine wash	Can be destroyed by dogs Slow drying Expensive to purchase	Often donated

5.7 Non-disposable bedding.

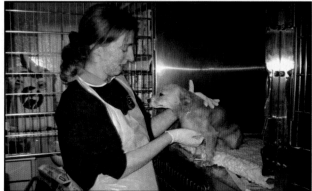

5.8 The bedding should meet the needs and size of the patient.

In veterinary practice the most common arrangement is to line the cage with newspaper and then place non-disposable bedding, such as acrylic bedding, on top. The type of bedding chosen for a patient may depend on how long they are expected to be using it:

- A day surgery case (e.g. a cat for routine spaying) must be provided with bedding primarily for warmth and comfort. This bedding will be used for one day only, so ease of washing and drying is important. There is little need for bedding to prevent pressure sores – this patient should be home long before that is a risk factor

■ Patients that may be staying for longer or that have limited movement have different bedding needs from the very beginning. It is important to try to avoid using bedding that allows the patient to put pressure on any one area of the body for long periods. The bedding used should be warm and soft with sufficient padding to prevent any pressure sores.

As soon as a patient becomes soiled with urine, faeces or other bodily fluids, there is an increased risk of contaminated wounds, irritating the underlying skin and ingestion of the offending substance if the patient attempts to lick itself clean. The type of bedding used can be an important factor in limiting patient soiling. Acrylic bedding, which allows fluid to soak through, leaving the top surface dry, is of great use for these patients.

When considering soiling, it should also be noted that if a patient urinates on the bedding, it is not always obvious that this has happened. This is particularly true with some bedding types. For example, beanbags and covered foam pads may be sodden with urine but do not look any different from when they were clean and dry. It is important to feel the bedding to ensure its cleanliness.

The bedding needs of different categories of patient are outlined in Figure 5.9.

Management of patients

Staff

The number and type of staff working on the animal ward will vary according to the number of patients, the degree of care required and often the pressure of workload in other areas of the clinic. There should, however, be one member of the nursing staff who is responsible for overseeing the care of ward patients.

Ward staff must be in control of various aspects of their patient's care, taking instruction from senior nursing staff and ultimately the veterinary surgeon.

Daily routine

On arrival in the ward the duty nurse should quickly check the hospitalized patients to ensure that no animal requires urgent attention. If taking over from another staff member, a thorough handover procedure should take place to discuss the patients and their care.

The following routine need not be carried out in exactly the order listed here, but provides a guide for best practice patient management:

■ Clean and disinfect the cage
■ Feed as directed by veterinary surgeon
■ Medicate as directed by veterinary surgeon
■ Temperature, pulse and respiration monitoring
■ Brief physical assessment of the patient (e.g. recumbent, bright and alert).

It can be difficult to decide what should be done first when faced with a ward full of animals that all need cleaning, treating and feeding. The following guidelines will assist in making these decisions.

Disease status

Patients with compromised or immature immune systems are at high risk of developing infection from other inhabitants of the ward (so-called cross-infection). These patients should take priority in the ward routine.

Patient category	Bedding needs	Reasons
Recumbent	Warm	Inactive patient often requiring additional warmth
	Soft	Patient remaining in one position for increased time
	Well padded	To avoid pressure sores
	Absorbent	Patient likely to urinate and defecate on bedding
	Not high-sided	Easy access for nursing staff
	Easy to launder	Bedding likely to be soiled
Vomiting and/or diarrhoeic	Absorbent	Patient likely to urinate, defecate and vomit on bedding
	Easy to launder	Bedding likely to be soiled
	Disposable (in some cases)	Infectious pathogens may be present
Patients with wounds	Absorbent	To soak up any discharge from wounds
	Disposable (in some cases)	Infectious pathogens may be present
	Non-adherent	To avoid fabric or fibres sticking to wounds
Patients requiring movement restriction	No high-sided beds	Easy access for animal without need for jumping
	Non-rigid bedding	To avoid patient knocking injured area
	Durable	Bored patient more likely to damage or chew bedding
	Easy to launder	Bedding likely to be soiled

5.9 Bedding needs of different patients.

Isolation patients suffering from a contagious disease, even though they may well have weakened immune systems, should be dealt with *after* other patients have been cared for, or by a separate dedicated member of staff. (See section on isolation nursing, below.)

Medication

The timing, duration and type of treatment required may dictate that certain patients are seen at highly specific times.

Number of meals

Feeding at correct times is important, particularly for young or debilitated patients. Therefore the number of feeds a patient requires and the timing of these meals will guide the nursing staff to the order in which patients are seen.

Soiled cages

Cages that are badly soiled will need to be cleaned quickly to reduce the likelihood of the patient itself becoming soiled.

Exercise or outdoor toileting

Most dogs are housetrained and so require regular access to an outdoor area to relieve themselves. It would be inappropriate to expect a dog to wait to use the outdoor area, particularly after it has been caged for a considerable time (e.g. overnight).

Dealing with aggressive patients

When a patient is uncooperative or aggressive, the situation must be dealt with professionally and calmly. However aggressive a patient may be, it is the nurse's duty to deal with the situation in an ethical, ordered manner:

- If the situation is escalating out of control: *stop*! Consider other ways of working through it.

Animals become stressed in situations that are new to them and respond in a variety of ways. For example, they may freeze; they may show differing levels of aggression; or they may simply demand attention.

'Freezing'

This reaction applies particularly to cats. They come out of their cage on to an examination table and allow anything to be done to them, because they stand absolutely still, immobilized by fear.

Aggression

Response aggression

These patients react when whatever is being done to them exceeds their threshold of pain, or their perceived acceptable intrusion. For instance, some animals may allow an examination, but having their temperature taken is too intrusive.

Fear-induced aggression

This is the 'I'll get you before you do anything unpleasant to me' approach. It often applies to dogs that have tried such a behaviour in the home and seen that it can work. Success reinforces the behaviour.

Territorial aggression

This might also be termed cage guarding. A normally well behaved pet may see its cage as a safe haven and therefore be aggressive to anyone trying to remove them from it.

Attention seeking

Attention seeking may be expressed by making a noise (bark or miaow) or by displaying a high level of excitability, commonly resulting in a pet becoming overly friendly in an attempt to make the staff member stay with them.

Restraint

Restraining aids (Figure 5.10) are used when it is not possible to guarantee reasonable safety of the handler or persons treating the animal.

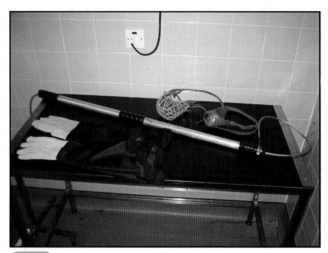

 An assortment of restraining aids.

> ⚠️ **WARNING**
> - **Only personnel who have received *training in their use* should use restraining aids.**
> - **Restraining aids must only be used on patients under *constant supervision*.**
> - **Restraining aids should be used for the *minimum time period* possible.**

Full details of restraint equipment and use are given in Chapter 6.

Dog restraining aids

Collar and lead

A well fitting collar with a lead attached is adequate restraint for most dogs.

Muzzle

The aim of this device is to stop a dog from opening its mouth, thereby preventing it from biting. It can be of the simplest form (a woven bandage tied around the dog's muzzle) or a more substantial box-type muzzle made from leather, fabric or plastic (see Chapter 6).

Dog grasper

This is a pole with an adjustable loop at one end (see Chapter 6). It can be used for dogs that are too dangerous for staff to get close to. The loop of the catcher is placed around the dog's neck and holds the dog still while the procedure or further restraint procedures take place (muzzling or sedation).

Cat restraining aids

Towel

The fractious cat is wrapped in a towel with just the parts of the body needing to be examined remaining outside the towel (e.g. head and forelimb for induction of general anaesthesia). This technique provides security for the cat and prevents the handler from being scratched.

Cat gloves

These gloves are made of heavy-duty leather, offering the user protection from scratches and, to a lesser extent, bites from cats.

Cat grasper

This is a similar device to the dog grasper. It has a 'grasping' section, which holds the cat around the neck to restrain it for short periods of time (see Chapter 6).

Cat muzzle

The cat muzzle fits over the cat's head, preventing it from biting. The muzzle also covers the eyes and this can help to calm a fractious cat.

As this device does not affect use of the limbs, care must be taken to prevent the cat from scratching either the handler or its own face if it attempts to remove the muzzle.

Cat bag

The cat's body is placed inside the restraining bag, which prevents scratching.

Crush cage

This is an adapted wire basket. It has a movable internal wall that can be used to hold the cat against one side of the basket. It is often used to assist in administering injectable sedation, particularly in feral cats.

Mental stimulation

Mental stimulation is an important part of helping patients to be happy in the ward and in turn can assist in their recovery.

Most animals will be feeling isolated and missing their owners' company. A stressed animal will have a depressed immune response, leaving them open to contracting further disease. They are also less likely to eat, which is an important factor in their general welfare and recovery from disease or surgery.

Company and environmental enrichment play an important role in keeping a patient 'happy', ensuring that they eat and encouraging wellbeing (Figure 5.11). In turn this may reduce the length of stay for the patient.

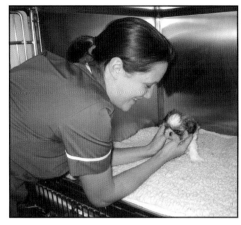

5.11
Reassurance for an inpatient.

Dogs

Grooming

A grooming session is useful as a time for the ward staff to build up a bond with a patient, as well as assisting with general coat care (see Chapter 6 for detailed information on grooming procedures).

Exercise

Most dogs are housetrained and are reluctant to defecate or urinate in their cage. If the condition allows, a dog should have access to a secure run or be taken for a short walk outside to relieve itself. Some dogs will only urinate on grassed areas. Disease spread must be considered if many animals use a small area of grass for this purpose.

Dogs usually return from a trip outdoors brighter and happier. This is a good time to try to encourage inappetent patients to eat.

Food

Many dogs are stimulated by food. This can be a useful tool in keeping a dog busy while it is in the practice. For example:

- Scattering dry kibble food around the cage encourages the dog to search for its meal
- Food-containing toys, filled with dry food kibble, have a hole on one side allowing the food to drop out as the dog moves the toy around
- Tinned food stuffed into the cavity of a toy can keep a dog well occupied as it tries to lick the food out.

Cats

Cats are particularly sensitive to being hospitalized. A stressed cat will be less likely to respond positively to medical or surgical intervention. By making attempts to reduce the stress for these patients on the hospital ward, staff can play an important role in the eventual outcome of the hospitalization. Cat-only wards are now viewed as very useful in reducing cat stress.

Grooming

The majority of cats enjoy being groomed and petted. Cats are usually fastidious about keeping themselves clean. If the cat is unable or unwilling to clean itself, it can be assisted with a twice-daily grooming session.

This involves brushing the coat with a comb or soft brush to remove dead hair. Moistened cotton wool can be used to wipe the coat clean (this emulates the mother cat cleaning her kittens and can make patients feel calm and secure). Wet cotton wool is also used to clean around the eyes, nose and anal area.

Toys

Toys are a good way to encourage interaction with a hospitalized cat (Figure 5.12). These may be of the simplest form – a scrunched-up piece of newspaper is often a favourite, especially for kittens. Balls, toys with bells inside and pretend mice are usually successful.

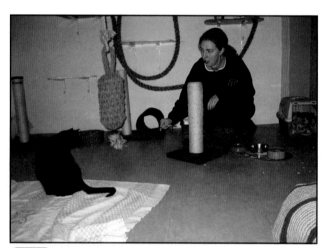

5.12 An enriched environment for a cat.

Catnip is a plant that can cause a 'trance-like' reaction in some adult cats. It is often used to impregnate cat toys to make them more appealing. The effect is short lived but if the toy is removed for an hour or so then it will be effective again when returned.

'Room with a view'

Cats enjoy being able to see the outside world. Some cats will benefit from being able to look out through a window. If there is not a suitable cage for this, the cat can be placed in a secure basket and put somewhere that they can see out, for a short time.

Cats feel more secure if they are above ground level. They should be placed on an elevated surface or cage.

Meals without litter trays

Due to the smaller size of cages in veterinary practice, it is common that the cat's litter tray and food bowl are in close proximity to one another. Cats have a very sensitive sense of smell and will often not eat if the litter tray is close by. It is good practice to remove the tray while a cat is eating. Eating often results in the need to pass a motion, so the tray should be returned immediately the food has been finished.

Scratching post

Cats that remain hospitalized for lengthy periods often make use of scratching posts. These help the cat to keep its claws in good condition and may act as a distraction for a stressed animal.

Owner visits

The use of visits by the owner will depend on the individual patient, their condition and the practicalities of ward care routines.

Most animals, especially those hospitalized for lengthy periods, appear to enjoy being visited by their owner. Visits seem to be of particular use when a patient is inappetent, stressed or just depressed. The owner can be encouraged to supply the patient's favourite food (if no feeding restrictions are in force) and may be able to offer more comfort and contact than the ward staff can provide.

A disadvantage arising from owner visits is that the patient may become stressed when the owner leaves.

Antiseptics and disinfectants

Terminology

Before the most effective cleaning method can be chosen, the relevant terminology must be understood.

Sterilization

Sterilization is defined as the destruction of *all* microorganisms, including the most resilient form of some bacteria: the bacterial spores.

In veterinary practice, sterilization is usually carried out by:

- Moist heat, under pressure (autoclaving) – the most widely used for drapes and surgical instruments
- Chemical methods (ethylene oxide, formaldehyde gas or glutaraldehyde solution) – generally restricted to use for fragile specialist instruments that will not withstand heat
- High temperatures at atmospheric pressure (hot air oven) – declining in use, as can cause damage to instruments.

Disinfection

Disinfection is defined as the destruction or reduction of microorganisms that cause disease (pathogenic organisms). Less harmful bacteria are also reduced in number, or removed. Bacterial spores are not usually destroyed.

Methods of disinfection include:

- Chemical disinfection (to be effective, recommended contact times must be adhered to)
- Mechanical removal (e.g. scrubbing, mopping, wiping).

Antisepsis

Antisepsis is the opposite of sepsis. It is the destruction of microorganisms *on living tissue*. The delicate nature of tissue means that methods used for antisepsis cannot destroy bacterial spores.

Antisepsis is achieved with the use of antiseptics. Many antiseptics are a weak solution of the disinfectants used on non-living objects, and when used as an antiseptic they can be referred to as skin disinfectants.

Not all disinfectants are safe to use on tissue; and even at a very low concentration some disinfectants can destroy living tissue.

Bactericides and bacteriostats

■ Bactericides destroy or kill bacteria – the suffix '-cide' indicates killing, rather than simply preventing an increase in the numbers of bacteria.
■ Bacteriostats slow down or stop bacterial growth (multiplication of their numbers). The suffix '-stat' indicates no growth or increase in numbers of bacteria.

An ideal disinfectant or antiseptic should clearly be a bactericide.

Virucides

Virucides are disinfectants that are effective in the destruction of viruses.

Disinfectant effectiveness

Viruses (and to a lesser extent bacteria) vary widely in their susceptibility to various disinfectants. The ability to eliminate parvovirus is often used to test the effectiveness of a disinfectant.

Various brand names are marketed with emphasis on their effectiveness against a particular agent or agents, according to the current diseases of concern in veterinary practice. At the time of writing, efficacy against methicillin-resistant *Staphylococcus aureus* (MRSA) (see below) is receiving much attention.

Fungicides

Fungicides are disinfectants used to destroy fungi and their spores. Most disinfectants will destroy these. One exception is the quaternary ammonium compound group.

Principles of cleaning

A hygienic environment is important in maintaining good health for animals. This is particularly so when dealing with situations where many animals are being accommodated in a ward. It is also important in the veterinary situation, as patients are staying for many different reasons. Due to space limitation, it is not unusual for a day surgery patient to be caged in the same ward as an inpatient. In these situations good hygiene and effective cleaning routines must be in place to minimize the risk of cross-infection.

Disinfection can only be achieved if the product is in direct contact with the target organism and remains so for the specified contact time. This means that any trace of debris left in the kennel affects the process, by inactivation, by absorption or by acting as a physical barrier. For this reason it is vital to remove all grease, dirt, urine, vomit, faeces and other bodily secretions *before* the disinfectant is applied. This is achieved by scrubbing with a brush or cloth, using warm water and detergent. Once the cage is visually clean it is rinsed out with clean water. Then the disinfecting agent can be applied.

Routine cleaning of cages

One thorough cleaning of a cage should be carried out daily (Figure 5.13). This is usually performed in the morning. Localized cleaning during the day deals with further soiling. If gross soiling of the kennel occurs, it may be necessary to perform the thorough clean-out more often. Care should be taken to maintain the kennel in as dry a condition as possible between cleanings, as this reduces humid conditions in which microorganisms thrive.

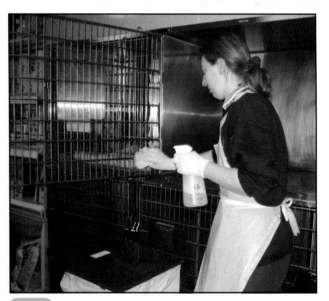

5.13 Cleaning a cage.

To summarize cage cleaning:

1. Remove animal from cage and place it in a secure holding area or exercise run.
2. Remove bedding, bowls, toys, etc. for separate cleaning.
3. Pick up and dispose of any solid waste.
4. Scrub the cage with detergent to remove grease, hair and other debris.
5. Rinse with water if using separate disinfectant.
6. Cover all surfaces of the cage with disinfectant.
7. Leave for recommended contact time.
8. Rinse out thoroughly.
9. Dry, using clean cloth.
10. Leave to air dry.
11. Replace bedding, bowls, toys, etc.
12. Return animal to cage.

Although many modern disinfectants include a detergent agent, it is still important to scrub using the detergent/disinfectant mix to remove debris before applying the same mix to act as a disinfectant.

Cleaning of toys, food bowls and bedding

Toys

Toys should be cleaned on a daily basis. They should be cleaned with detergent, rinsed with water and then soaked in disinfectant for the recommended contact time. Toys that cannot be easily or effectively cleaned should not be used in the practice or should be disposed of after use. If a toy is chewed or scratched by a patient, the cleaning process is less likely to be effective and the toy should be discarded.

Bowls

Food and water bowls should be washed and disinfected in a designated kitchen area. This must be in a separate sink to that which is used for cage cleaning. Bowls should be allowed to dry naturally or by using disposable paper towels.

Certain types of feeding bowls may be sterilized in an autoclave or using chemical sterilization. It is important to check that the chosen method will not damage the bowl.

Bedding

Soiled bedding should be cleared of any solid waste and then rinsed in water to remove loose particles of organic matter.

Non-disposable bedding is usually washed in a washing machine. Some detergent/disinfectant mixes are suitable for use in a washing machine, or the bedding may be pre-soaked in a bucket and rinsed before being placed in the washing machine.

A separate washing machine should be used to wash drapes and theatre clothing.

Cleaning the cleaning equipment

Equipment used to clean kennels must itself be kept clean and regularly disinfected. This point is all too often overlooked. Dirty or contaminated equipment can play an important role in cross-infection.

Cloths, brushes, mops, squeegees and buckets should be cleaned in detergent and then soaked in disinfectant at the recommended strength, observing contact times. They then are rinsed carefully and allowed to dry.

Cleaning the working environment

The ward itself must be kept clean. The floor should be washed with detergent and disinfectant at least once daily. Buckets of water must be emptied after use: fresh disinfectant and water are required for each clean.

Many areas of the ward, including surfaces, examination tables and food preparation areas, will be wiped down after each use. In addition to this, these areas should be *thoroughly* cleaned once a day, ensuring that all visible traces of dirt are removed. The cupboards, walls (to a height of approximately 1 metre) and waste bins should be wiped down on a regular basis, preferably daily.

Misting

Misting is a powerful technique to remove microorganisms that are spread through the air. The technique is typically appropriate for isolation units or large multi-occupant units (e.g. rescue kennels) faced with an outbreak of disease.

1. The ward is cleared of all patients and staff before misting takes place.
2. The operator wears protective clothing, including goggles and a facemask or ventilator (the degree of personal protective equipment required varies according to the disinfectant used).
3. Correctly diluted disinfectant is placed in a knapsack sprayer or in a pressure washer set at the finest spray. (A trigger sprayer on a mist setting would produce the same effect, but it will take much longer to apply to large areas.)
4. The disinfectant is then sprayed into the air of the ward to destroy pathogenic aerosol particles.

Standard sanitary operating procedures

Standard sanitary operating procedures (SSOPs) are sets of procedures to be carried out as an area is cleaned. The objective is to achieve a standard cleaning system, which all staff will follow, and one that can be checked once completed to ensure that it reaches the required standard.

This technique is widely used in human healthcare and indicates best practice standards. It ensures that all areas are cleaned, for example light switches, not just those that are obviously contaminated, e.g. floors.

The implementation of the technique is recommended for the veterinary world.

The SSOP for the animal ward would detail:

- Areas that should be cleaned on a daily basis (this would probably include the floor, the work surfaces and the sink)
- Areas that should be cleaned every other day (e.g. walls and cupboards)
- Areas that are cleaned weekly (e.g. door handles, light switches, telephones)
- Which chemical is used for each item, at what strength and for how long it must be in contact.

Staff should sign a chart when the cleaning has been completed (Figure 5.14). In this way no area will be overlooked or forgotten. If an area has been cleaned but fails to reach the required standard, it is easy to tell from the chart which staff member undertook the cleaning. They can then receive further training as deemed necessary.

Daily Ward Cleaning.			Week commencing:		DD/MM/YYYY		
Task	**Mon**	**Tue**	**Wed**	**Thu**	**Fri**	**Sat**	**Sun**
Empty waste bins (am)	✓ DP	✓ DP	✓ KE				
Empty waste bins (pm)	✓ DP	✓ DP	✓ KE				
Vacuum and mop floors	✓ DP	✓ DP	✓ KE				
Clean work surfaces	✓ DP	✓ DP	✓ KE				
Clean sink, including taps	✓ DP	✓ DP	✓ KE				
Clean cupboard fronts	✓ DP	✓ DP	✓ KE				
Clean walls to height of 3 ft	✓ DP	✓ DP	✓ KE				
Clean door handles	X	X	X	X		X	X
Sanitize telephones	X	X	X	X		X	X
Clean light switches	X	X	X	X		X	X

5.14 Example SSOP chart.

Effectiveness of disinfectants

The effectiveness of all agents and methods is dependent upon:

- Freedom from organic debris (principles of removal discussed above)
- Correct dilution
- Correct contact time with agent
- Correct temperature.

All modern proprietary disinfectant mixtures are supplied with a data sheet, clearly setting out the correct dilutions, contact times and optimum temperatures if appropriate. Many disinfectants have two or more dilutions listed for use with differing levels of soiling and with different pathogens that may be present.

- A solution of inadequate strength will be ineffective.
- Too strong a solution is not only wasteful but also works no more effectively and may be irritant to both patient and operator.

It is extremely important to refer to the data sheets and to adhere to the manufacturer's recommendations for the product that is being used. When a different disinfectant is used, or alterations are made to cleaning routines/SSOPs, or in the event of a suspected breakdown of disinfection, the data sheets must be reviewed and changes to the regime made as required.

The data sheet will also contain all relevant operator safety precautions and storage requirements for the product. All disinfectants should be stored in their original containers so that this information is clearly visible to those using the products.

Disinfectants have traditionally been classified into groups according to the agent that actually effects the killing of microorganisms, or to the class of chemical to which they belong to (Figure 5.15). Details of some commonly used disinfectants are set out in Figure 5.16, which is not intended to be an exhaustive list. Inclusion or otherwise in the list does not imply any particular recommendation.

Chemical group	**Examples**	**Trade names**	**Comments**
Halogens: chlorine-releasing	Hypochlorites (bleach)	Domestos Milton	Release corrosive, toxic, irritant chlorine gas
	Chlorine dioxide	Viruchem V26	New very broad-spectrum agent Use for 'high risk', not daily use
	Sodium dichloroisocyanurate [a]	Presept Vetaclean Parvo tablets	See Figure 5.16 and text
Halogens: iodine-releasing	Povidone–iodine [a]	Vetasept–povidone–iodine Medine Betadine	See text

5.15 Disinfectants and antiseptics. [a] Denotes those of particular importance in current veterinary practice. (continues) ▶

Chemical group	Examples	Trade names	Comments
Peroxides: oxygen-releasing	Peroxygen compounds [a]	Vetaclean Parvo liquid Virkon	See Figure 5.16 and text
	Hydrogen peroxide		Very irritant to tissues Superseded
Quaternary ammonium compounds [a]		Vetaclean liquid	See Figure 5.16 and text
		Savlon	Limited veterinary use nowadays
Halogenated tertiary amine with quaternary ammonium compounds		Trigene [a]	See Figure 5.16 and text
Biguanides	Chlorhexidine [a]	Hibiscrub Hibitane Vetasept–chlorhexidine Medihex 4	See text
Alcohols	Surgical spirit [a]	Surgical spirit	See text
	In many mixtures	Trigel Vetasept–chlorhexidine hand rub	See text
Aldehydes	Glutaraldehyde	Cidex	Toxic, very limited use
Phenolics	Chlorophenol (Triclosan) [a]	Mediscrub	See text
	Clear and black/white phenols	Jeyes	Highly toxic to cats, unpleasant smell and residue Superseded

5.15 (continued) Disinfectants and antiseptics. [a] Denotes those of particular importance in current veterinary practice.

Agent	Effective against	Oxidizing or non-oxidizing	Dilution rates	Notes
Trigene	Bacterial spores, bacteria, viruses and fungi	Non-oxidizing, so does not damage surfaces	Many, varying with level of risk	Contact time 1–2 minutes Long shelf-life once made up
Vetaclean Parvo	Viruses, bacteria, bacterial spores and fungi	Oxidizing (but manufacturers claim will not damage surfaces if used at correct dilution)	1:100 as general cleaner, to 1:25 to eliminate parvovirus	Available as liquid format (peroxy compound) or as soluble tablet (sodium dichloroisocyanurate)
Vetaclean liquid	Bacteria, fungi and some viruses	Non-oxidizing	1:200	
Virkon	Viruses, bacteria and fungi	Oxidizing (but manufacturers claim will not damage surfaces if used at correct dilution)	1:100 for high-risk areas	Short shelf-life once made up

5.16 Commonly used disinfectants.

Inactivation of disinfectants

Generally the presence of organic matter will reduce the activity of disinfectants and of antiseptics. However, with most of the newer agents now in common use, inactivation is far less common. Good cleaning habits are obviously still of great importance and manufacturers will still confirm that the less organic material present when using these products, the more effective and faster acting the agent will be.

Antiseptics

Antiseptics are used to destroy or reduce growth of microorganisms on the skin. They may be used as pre-surgical scrubbing agents for both the patient and for theatre staff. Some are suitable for cleaning wounds. They are often referred to as skin disinfectants.

There are four groups of antiseptic commonly used in veterinary practice:

- Chlorhexidine
- Iodine
- Alcohol
- Triclosan.

Chlorhexidine

Chlorhexidine is a rapidly acting antiseptic that is effective against fungi and a wide range of bacteria. It is not active against bacterial spores and has limited activity against viruses.

It is available with or without added detergent and with or without alcohol, and is widely used in veterinary practice for surgical preparation of both the patient and theatre staff. It is of particular use when the surgical procedure will take place quickly after scrubbing up, as it has been shown to produce a 99% bacterial kill rate 30 seconds after application. After a 3-minute scrub, 99.9% of surface bacteria will be destroyed.

Disadvantages include the following:

- It is inactivated by organic material (and soap), and so may not be the scrub of choice for surgical sites that cannot be cleaned thoroughly (e.g. surgery involving the anus or an infected wound)
- It may cause drying and irritation of the skin
- It is a corneal irritant and must not be used around the eyes.

Dilutions for chlorhexidine, based on a standard 4% presentation, are:

- Surgeon's hands: undiluted
- Operation site, unbroken skin: undiluted
- Wound cleansing: 0.5%, without detergent or alcohol (i.e. 1:7 parts with water).

Iodine/iodophors

Povidone–iodine is the most common iodine antiseptic used in veterinary practice. It is generally recognized to be more powerful than chlorhexidine. It is effective against a wide range of bacteria and fungi; it will also destroy bacterial spores, but this only occurs 15 minutes after application. After a 2–3-minute scrub 99.9% of bacteria will be destroyed.

Povidone–iodine continues its bacterial activity by the release of free iodine as it dries and the colour fades; therefore this antiseptic is especially useful in surgical cases where there may be some time delay between scrub and first incision. This may occur in cases where a complicated draping technique or preparation of specialized equipment is required.

Disadvantages include the following:

- Its effectiveness is reduced by the presence of organic material
- It can cause skin irritation and staining
- It should not be used on or by those with a thyroid condition.

Dilutions for povidone–iodine are:

- Surgeon's hands: undiluted proprietary 7.5% solution

- Operation site, unbroken skin: undiluted proprietary 10% solution
- Wound cleansing: 1:10 parts with water of non-detergent or alcohol-containing 10% solution
- Conjunctival area: 1:50 parts with water of non-detergent or alcohol-containing 10% solution.

> ⚠️ **WARNING**
> - **In veterinary practice it is common to prepare, and leave on the side ready, a kidney dish containing diluted chlorhexidine or povidone–iodine and cotton wool for scrubbing up surgical sites. This practice should be discouraged.**
> - **Chlorhexidine and povidone–iodine should be used undiluted.**
> - **Chlorhexidine, which is inactivated by cotton wool, should only come into contact with cotton wool as it is being used on the patient.**

Alcohol

Alcohols are used either as a stand-alone antiseptic (surgical spirit) or as a constituent of many proprietary antiseptic mixtures, especially in combination with chlorhexidine, povidone–iodine or triclosan. The combination products are fast acting and effective against bacteria and fungi.

Surgical spirit is relatively slow acting and must not be used in open wounds or anywhere near the eye. The value of its use as a skin swab prior to intravenous injection or as a final rinsing after preoperative skin scrubbing is debatable.

Alcohols as the solvent base for other disinfectants are commonly used in veterinary practice for quick hand disinfection between patients and when away from the practice (e.g. on a house visit). Drying of the skin is a disadvantage, but many products include other ingredients to counteract this.

Triclosan

Triclosan is a chlorophenol. It is deemed to be a very effective hand scrub for operating theatre staff, and is effective against bacteria, fungi and viruses. There has been some debate regarding potential health risks of using chlorophenols on a daily basis.

Methicillin-resistant *Staphylococcus aureus* (MRSA)

The bacterium *Staphylococcus aureus* is found in the nose and on the skin of up to 50% of healthy people. For the majority of the population it causes no ill effects. It can cause illness if it is able to enter the body of a susceptible individual. The bacterium is easily treated with antibiotics such as penicillin and erythromycin.

Methicillin is a type of penicillin. Methicillin-resistant *S. aureus* was first identified in the 1960s. This variety is often also resistant to other antibiotics, complicating treatment.

MRSA infection is of importance in human health as it is commonly acquired in hospital, usually affecting debilitated individuals.

MRSA in veterinary practice

MRSA is becoming an issue of some concern in veterinary practices. Although it primarily infects humans, it has the ability to colonize other species and has been reported in dogs, cats, rabbits and horses. Other strains of *Staphylococcus* that are more commonly isolated from dogs and cats also have resistance to methicillin.

MRSAs are most commonly associated with wound infections, including postoperative infections. Humans are the main source of infection and most transmission is human to human. The source of animal infection is being researched, but it seems likely that a pet infected with MRSA will have contracted the bacterium from an infected human, commonly their owner.

Animals infected with MRSA can pass the infection back to humans, though it appears that this happens relatively infrequently. Therefore, according to current advice, animal patients infected with MRSA should not pose significant risk to the staff caring for them as long as the staff members themselves are not debilitated.

Preventing the spread of these organisms is of the utmost importance. A good cleaning protocol for both the environment and the staff working within the practice is the key to limiting disease spread. Practices should implement an infectious disease control policy to monitor and control MRSA. It is important to note that MRSA is no more difficult to eradicate from the environment than most other bacteria.

For nursing staff, risk of contracting MRSA can be reduced by:

- Good personal hygiene, particularly hand washing
- Use of skin-disinfecting hand rubs between patients
- Use of disposable gloves to handle suspect patients
- Use of disposable gloves when dealing with body fluids or wounds, particularly infected wounds
- Isolation and barrier nursing of suspected cases
- Effective environmental cleaning procedure
- Careful handling of hazardous waste.

At the time of writing, MRSA in veterinary practice is a 'hot topic' and is being further investigated.

Health and Safety legislation

The following section gives a summary of relevant legislation.

Health and Safety at Work etc. Act 1974

The Health and Safety at Work etc. Act is designed to make everyone in the workplace responsible for safety standards. This includes not only their own health but also the health of their colleagues and of visitors and clients using the premises. The duty of the employer is to ensure that adequate training has been given to all staff in areas of health and safety and that appropriate measures have been taken to minimize risks in the workplace.

Control of Substances Hazardous to Health (COSHH) Regulations 2002

COSHH is concerned with the safe use of chemicals or any other potentially hazardous substance within the workplace. A risk assessment must be undertaken for each hazardous substance used in the workplace. This examines whether exposure to each substance can be prevented or limited and what precautions should be taken when using these substances. It also details what actions should be taken in the case of accident or spillage.

For each chemical used, a COSHH data sheet should be kept in the practice's health and safety records.

Personal Protective Equipment at Work Regulations 1992

These regulations cover the use of protective equipment for staff in the workplace. The use of personal protective equipment (PPE) is based upon a risk assessment carried out at the workplace. The employer must provide suitable equipment, ensure that instruction and training on its use have been given and ensure that staff use the equipment as detailed. The risk assessment must also record how to store and maintain the equipment and what action to take if it becomes damaged or lost.

Manual Handling Operations Regulations 1992

Manual handling is transporting or supporting loads by hand or using bodily force. The regulations state that the employer is responsible for ensuring that employees are aware of the risks involved when handling loads and for providing instruction on how these risks can be minimized.

Social Security (Claims and Payments) Regulations 1979

These regulations state that an employer must provide an accident book for the reporting of injuries that occur in the workplace. The book must be of an approved format and is retained for at least 3 years after the last entry.

Health and Safety (First Aid) Regulations 1981

These regulations require the employer to provide adequate and appropriate equipment, facilities and personnel to enable first aid to be given to employees if they are injured or become ill at work. The employer is also responsible for making all employees aware of the cover provided.

The minimum first aid provision for any workplace is a suitably stocked first aid box and an appointed person to take charge of first aid arrangements.

In veterinary practice it is advantageous for at least one member of staff to be trained as a first aider. This involves attending an approved training course in administering first aid at work.

Reporting of Injuries, Disease and Dangerous Occurrences Regulations (RIDDOR) 1995

This piece of legislation states that certain injuries, accidents and diseases have to be reported to the Health and Safety Executive. Incidents that require a report are:

- An accident connected with work resulting in death or major injury of a staff member or a member of the public
- An accident connected with work resulting in the employee suffering an injury that keeps them from working for over three days
- Notification by a doctor that an employee suffers from a reportable workplace disease
- Any dangerous occurrences as outlined by the regulations.

Waste disposal

New regulations

The regulations relating to waste disposal underwent substantial changes in July 2005, with a complete overhaul of waste categorization. The way in which these changes are being implemented is currently under review; therefore some further changes are possible. The following recommendations are made using current advice.

Duty of care

Since the introduction of the Environmental Protection Act 1990, a 'duty of care' has been placed on any business generating waste to dispose correctly of the waste it produces. It is the legal responsibility of the practice owner to develop a system for waste segregation, packaging and disposal, and to ensure that all employees are familiar with it. Any establishments that are found not to be complying with current regulations are subject to prosecution.

Segregation of waste

Waste produced must be sorted and placed in the correct receptacle for suitable disposal (Figure 5.17). Colour-coded containers are used to assist good segregation practice. Staff should expect to receive full training in practice policy for waste sorting.

Storage and collection

Full waste containers will need to be stored at the practice prior to collection. They should not be allowed to accumulate in corridors, wards or public areas. A refrigerated room or freezer is an ideal place to store waste, especially in hot weather.

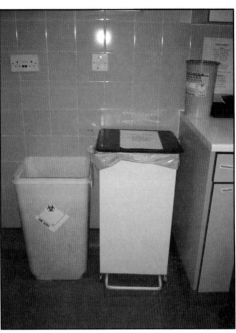

5.17
Disposing of waste.

Waste should be collected at least weekly. Sharps containers should be collected at least every three months.

Transportation of waste is regulated carefully. All sacks must be placed in UN-approved containers on the transporting vehicle to guard against leak or spillage.

All infectious waste produced must be labelled with the name and address of the practice.

Infectious waste

Infectious waste is defined as: 'Substances containing viable micro-organisms or their toxins which are known or reliably believed to cause disease in man or other living organisms.' Waste from animals that are deemed (on clinical examination or by laboratory determination) to be suffering from a disease that may infect humans is deemed as infectious. At present, regulations are not clear on disposal of waste from animals with diseases that affect other animals (e.g. cat 'flu).

Most of what would have previously been classed as clinical waste will, in fact, not be infectious waste.

Infectious waste is disposed of by incineration at a licensed plant. Anatomical waste must also be incinerated.

'Sharps'

Sharps are items that could cause cuts or puncture wounds. This includes needles, scalpel blades, the sharp section of infusion sets and broken glass ampoules. Sharps must be fully discharged. They are disposed of in a UN-approved sharps container, which is collected with other hazardous waste and incinerated.

Pharmaceutical waste

Out-of-date drugs, used vials or syringes not fully discharged of pharmaceutical drugs are classed as hazardous waste. They are placed in puncture- and leak-proof containers for collection and incineration.

Radiographic waste

X-ray fixer and developer are classified as hazardous waste. The disposal company employed will provide large leak-proof containers to drain the chemicals into. Once filled, they are sealed and collected.

Cytotoxic and cytostatic waste

Waste containing cytotoxic and cytostatic drugs is treated as a separate class of hazardous waste and must be placed in a correctly colour-coded container, which is incinerated at suitable licensed facilities. Where a sharps box contains sharps used with these products, the whole box must be treated as cytotoxic waste.

Cadavers

Veterinary surgeons have no legal obligation to dispose of cadavers. The body of an animal is still the property of the owner. An owner who wishes to bury their pet's body in their own garden is allowed to do so: it is not illegal, as often believed. Individuals are not subject to the same waste disposal legislation as veterinary practices or other businesses.

In practice, however, most cadavers are disposed of by the surgery. The local authority or a commercial disposal company for mass incineration may collect cadavers. They will normally supply practices with strong plastic sacks for safe, leak-proof storage and transport of the cadavers. Individual cremation or burials are other options that may be offered by private companies.

Cleaning materials, disinfectants, and antiseptics

These are all likely to be well diluted before use and are discarded in relatively small quantities. Therefore they are disposed of in the sewerage system.

Controlled drugs

A Home Office Inspector or a member of a police drugs squad should witness destruction of any out-of-date or unusable controlled drugs. They should be contacted directly in these circumstances.

Domestic waste

This is general household refuse, which is collected by local authorities and disposed of in landfill sites. Note that many items of domestic waste may now be recycled, including empty pet food tins and unsoiled newspapers.

Offensive waste

This is a new category of waste. It covers waste that is non-infectious but may cause offence to those who come into contact with it. It includes faeces, urine, vomit and soiled bedding of animals *not* suffering from infectious disease. It also includes non-infectious disposable items (e.g. plaster casts, dressings). This waste is disposed of in landfill sites but is placed in a yellow/black striped bag to alert those in the disposal process as to its contents. Some of the waste produced in veterinary practice will now fall into this

new category. Many local authorities and private companies handling the waste further sub-categorize material. It is the responsibility of the producer (the practice) to check that their waste handler specifically agrees to collect offensive waste.

Isolation nursing

Isolation nursing is the name given to the methods used to prevent the spread of potential pathogens when nursing a patient suffering from a contagious or zoonotic disease. It is sometimes referred to as barrier nursing.

The aim of isolation nursing is to limit the likelihood of disease spread. This is particularly important in veterinary practice, as other animals at the surgery are likely to have reduced immune function due to stress, illness or surgery.

To achieve this aim there must be a protocol dictating where the patient is housed, how it is nursed, the cleaning procedures to be carried out and how waste generated is disposed of.

Terminology

There is often confusion concerning the terms infectious and contagious.

- **Microorganisms cause an infectious disease. This does not *necessarily* mean that the disease is transmissible to other animals, although many infectious diseases *are* also contagious.**
- **A contagious disease is one that may be transmitted from one animal to another.**
- **A zoonotic disease is a contagious disease that may also be transmitted from animals to humans.**

Examples:

- **Bacterial gingivitis is an infectious disease but it is not contagious**
- **Cat 'flu is infectious and contagious**
- ***Campylobacter* infection is infectious, contagious and zoonotic.**

The isolation unit

The provision of a dedicated isolation unit, preferably in a separate building to the main clinic, is obviously the best option for housing and treating patients suffering from contagious diseases (Figure 5.18).

In practice, there is not always the space available or a suitable separate building for a dedicated isolation unit. This makes nursing a patient with a contagious disease more complicated and may increase the likelihood of disease spreading to other areas or patients. In these circumstances careful thought should be given to where the patient will be housed to limit these risks as much as possible.

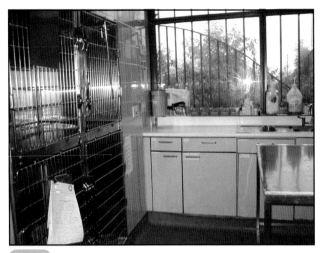

5.18 Isolation unit.

Many feline diseases are not contagious to dogs and *vice versa*. Bearing this in mind, the best option available for a small practice may be to house a dog with a contagious disease in a cat ward (or a cat in the dog ward). Barrier nursing methods would then be put in place for the entire ward.

The use of collapsible cages could also be considered when a dedicated isolation unit is not available. Collapsible cages are available in a variety of sizes and can be erected wherever it is deemed that spread of infection can most easily be controlled.

An ideal unit *must* be self-contained. It should contain facilities to:

- House the patient
- Carry out examination of the patient
- Give medical treatment
- Prepare food
- Wash and disinfect cages/bowls
- Dispose of waste.

Ventilation

Good ventilation is essential. Clean, fresh air will be beneficial to both the patient and the staff working in the unit. Airborne transmission is an important factor in cross-infection and so the unit should have a separate ventilation system to the other areas of the clinic.

Patient accommodation

There should be cages of suitable sizes to house a range of animal species and sizes. The cages should be easy to clean and disinfect. There must be no cracks or defects in them as these hinder effective cleaning and may harbour bacteria. For the same reason it must be possible to clean the cage front or bars thoroughly.

Examination area

The unit should have an area for examining patients and giving medication. An examination table with a non-slip top is recommended. Ease of effective cleaning of this area is essential.

Medications and treatments being received by the patient are stored in the treatment area. A pen or pencil should be kept in the unit for isolation staff to use and

should be discarded once the patient is discharged (this eliminates the need for staff to use their own implement, which could spread disease if they then used it elsewhere in the practice).

As the unit may be used only periodically, all medicines, disinfectants and food supplies must be checked to ensure that they are still in date.

Food preparation area

Food for the patients can be prepared before entry to the unit or in the unit itself. This is usually dependent on the type of food used. If tinned or dried food is fed, this can easily be prepared when required, in the unit. Home-cooked food will need to be brought into the unit each mealtime in a disposable container. The container is then discarded with the contaminated waste.

It is important to limit the quantities of food stocked in the unit (to reduce wastage, only enough for the patient's daily need should be stored) and to ensure that all food served is fresh.

Exercise area

Generally, to reduce the risk of contamination, there would not be access to exercise areas for these patients. However, many dogs are housetrained and will refuse to foul their cage. In these circumstances the patient should be taken to an area that other animals do not have access to and that is possible to clean thoroughly (not a grassed area). Faecal matter must be collected immediately and disposed of following the guidelines for the isolation unit.

After use, the area should be cleaned thoroughly with a suitable disinfectant.

Bedding

Disposable bedding is ideal for use in the unit, as it eliminates the need for washing contaminated material. However, this can prove to be expensive where a patient constantly soils the cage.

If non-disposable bedding is used, a set should be kept for exclusive use in the unit. The quantity of bedding required will depend on the condition of the patient. It is returned to the unit immediately after laundering. Non-disposable bedding should be rinsed clean of any gross soiling and soaked in disinfectant, in a bucket. After it has been soaked for the recommended contact time, it is placed in the washing machine on a hot cycle. Where possible, a separate washing machine should be provided for exclusive washing of this bedding.

Waste disposal

Most waste generated will be classed as infectious waste and disposed of as directed. It is important to ensure that no other person or animal will come into contact with this waste whilst it is awaiting collection. It is common practice to double wrap waste from isolation units to limit contamination by leakage.

Daily cleaning

Keeping a range of disinfectants in the unit enables staff to select the most effective chemical against the suspected pathogen.

In general, the daily cleaning regime discussed earlier in this chapter is suitable for the isolation unit, but it may be appropriate to use a more concentrated dilution of disinfectant (following the manufacturer's instructions on dilution rates).

Red paint nursing

This training aid can be used to assist in the understanding of how a staff member working in the isolation unit can themselves spread the offending pathogen to other areas of the clinic. The idea is as follows:

- **Imagine that the patient is completely covered in red paint (the paint indicates the contagious pathogen)**
- **The paint does not dry and will smear on to anything the patient touches**
- **Any secretions or excretions from the patient are also covered in red paint**
- **Any other animal that touches the red paint could themselves become infected with the disease or may act as a vector, spreading the red paint further**
- **If the staff member leaves the isolation unit without cleaning the red paint from their skin, their shoes or their uniform, they may also act as a vector, spreading the pathogen wherever they go next**
- **The red paint can be removed from both the environment and the staff member by *thorough* cleaning and disinfecting.**

Keeping this 'red paint' idea in mind while caring for a contagious patient gives a visual reminder of:

- **How areas of the unit and staff within it become contaminated**
- **Where contamination is at high levels (e.g. patient's bedding, particularly if soiled; staff members' hands after handling the patient)**
- **How the disease can be spread further**
- **How these areas and people can be decontaminated.**

Cleaning the unit on patient discharge

When a patient has been discharged, the unit must be cleaned thoroughly to ensure that all pathogenic organisms are destroyed. The cage walls, floor, bars and ceiling should be scrubbed clean and disinfected, ensuring that contact times are observed. All other working areas in the unit should be treated similarly. It may be advantageous to clean the unit daily for two or three days running. This is a useful technique because if an area is overlooked or inadequately cleaned on one day, the chances are that it will be picked up during the following day's cleaning.

Unused consumables that cannot be adequately disinfected must be disposed of.

Personal protective equipment

The use of PPE in the isolation unit will assist in preventing the spread of organisms by the person working within it, as well as protecting the staff member from contracting zoonotic diseases.

Clothing

A boiler suit and disposable apron should be worn to enter the unit. The boiler suit covers the clothes inside completely, offering good protection from contamination. When putting on and removing a boiler suit, great care must be taken to avoid the outside (potentially contaminated) fabric coming into contact with 'clean' clothing underneath.

Plastic disposable aprons can be used in conjunction with the boiler suit. These are designed for single use only. If an apron is used more than once, it is not usually clear which was the 'clean' inside after it has been removed. Putting the apron on 'inside out' would cause contamination of the clothes that it is supposed to be protecting.

All disposable PPE should be placed in the appropriate waste containers after use.

Non-disposable clothing, such as boiler suits or boots, should be cleaned of obvious soiling and left in the unit for the next visit. Boiler suits should be washed on a hot cycle of the washing machine at least once daily.

If clothing worn underneath the PPE becomes soiled, it should be changed on leaving the unit.

Gloves

Disposable gloves are used at all times within the unit. These should be discarded after single use and replaced if they become damaged or torn during use. Double gloving may be advisable when dealing with potential zoonoses.

Footwear

Disposable shoe covers can be used to protect the underside of the shoe. They are for single use only and should be discarded after each wearing.

Provision of boots that are for exclusive use within the unit is a more effective method of reducing cross-infection via footwear. They are put on as the unit is entered and removed upon exit, leaving 'normal' shoes outside, uncontaminated.

Foot dips

Foot dips are used in an attempt to remove pathogenic microorganisms from the sole of the shoe. A sponge soaked in disinfectant is stepped on with both feet as the staff member leaves the isolation area.

The underside of the shoe must be *clean* before the foot dip is used. Organic matter on the shoe will prevent the disinfectant from reaching all parts of the sole and will decrease the efficacy of the disinfectant. In addition, it is unlikely that contact times for disinfectants will be adhered to and so the usefulness of these dips is limited. Disinfectant must be freshly made up using correct dilutions and renewed at regular intervals (see manufacturer's directions).

Hats

Disposable hats are used to prevent contamination of the hair. This is particularly important if staff have long hair or are dealing with an animal that may jump up or rub against the staff member's face and hair (e.g. a playful puppy).

Face protection

A facemask may be required when dealing with zoonotic diseases, particularly those that may be spread by inhalation.

Goggles may be used to protect the eyes. This is important if dealing with any agent that may spray or splash into the eyes, particularly powerful disinfectants used at high dilutions.

Staff

One member of staff should be responsible for the running of the isolation unit. It may be necessary to have a second staff member available to assist with treatment, moving large patients or dealing with aggressive animals. This person can also provide care required during tea and lunch breaks.

Staff working in the isolation unit should not be involved with other high-risk patients, i.e. those that are very young or immunocompromised.

It may be appropriate for the patient's notes to be stored outside the unit so that members of staff can read or add comments to the record without actually going inside the unit. For the same reason, it is useful to have a porthole window in the door of the unit so that the patient can be viewed regularly.

It is on leaving the unit that the staff member is at the highest risk of acting as a vector and carrying the offending pathogen to other parts of the clinic. Therefore it is extremely important for them to carry out a thorough personal disinfection to minimize this risk. Hands should be washed for a *minimum* of 30 seconds, using a skin disinfectant that is effective at eliminating the suspected pathogen. All personal protective garments are removed as the unit is vacated.

References and further reading

Duquette RA and Nuttal TJ (2004) Methicillin-resistant *Staphylococcus aureus* in dogs and cats: an emerging problem? *Journal of Small Animal Practice*, **45**(12), 591–597

HSE (1994) Health and safety in small businesses. In: *An Introduction to Health and Safety*. Health & Safety Executive, Caerphilly

Lane D, Cooper B and Turner L (2007) *BSAVA Textbook of Veterinary Nursing, 4th edn*. BSAVA Publications, Gloucester

Masters J and Bowden C (2001) *Pre-Veterinary Nursing Textbook*. Butterworth-Heinemann, Oxford

6

Introduction to veterinary care

Joy Howell

This chapter is designed to give information on:

- How to perform a basic physical examination
- The regular health checks that are necessary and how to measure and record vital signs
- How to recognize the signs of good and poor health
- The correct terminology when describing normal and abnormal conditions
- Prediction of the common behavioural characteristics of the dog and cat, so that the most successful method of restraint will be used
- The principles of restraint, so that the animal is handled safely and without unnecessary stress for either the animal or the handler
- Types of restraint equipment
- The importance of regular grooming as a part of preventive healthcare management programmes
- Types of grooming equipment
- Basic grooming techniques
- The six basic nutrients and their role in supporting life

Introduction

Early recognition of signs of ill health during the initial stages of disease is vital to ensure diagnosis and treatment. In certain conditions, this early diagnosis is likely to lead to a more satisfactory long-term response.

Preventive veterinary healthcare includes the performance of a regular routine examination, in order to identify abnormal states. This entails methods of handling and restraint to allow examination of the animal; in addition, grooming is necessary to facilitate thorough examination of skin and to maintain coat condition. A further facet of healthcare and preventive medicine is nutrition, tailored to the animal's lifestyle and life stage.

Signs of health and disease

The early and successful recognition of signs of disease and ill health depends on the observation skills of the owner and, in the case of the hospitalized patient, those of the veterinary nurse in charge of inpatient care. These observational skills depend on a thorough understanding of any deviation from the normal state.

Regular health checks

Figure 6.1 shows the regular health checks and procedures to be used with companion animals and suggests how often they should be carried out.

Daily:
- Appetite
- Thirst
- Faecal production
- Urinary production
- Demeanour (bright, alert?)
- Abnormal signs evident.

Weekly:
- Condition of ear canals
- Condition of teeth and gums
- Colour of mucous membranes
- Coat and skin condition
- Abnormal discharges – prepuce, vagina
- Pain on palpation/movement of joints
- Presence and development of 'lumps'.

Monthly:
- Bodyweight
- Nails – dewclaws in particular
- Beaks – in birds and chelonians (tortoises, turtles).

Every 3–4 months:
- Carry out anthelmintic (worming) protocols as recommended.

Annually:
- Booster vaccinations
- Full physical examination by veterinary surgeon
- Annual blood tests may be recommended in some geriatric animals.

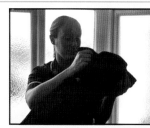
Checking ear canals.

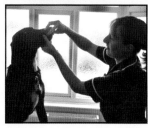
Checking teeth and gums.

6.1 Regular health checks and procedures and their suggested frequency.

In the case of elderly patients or those on long-term medication, full examination should be carried out more often, according to the animal's condition. With all health checks, including those that are not carried out on a daily basis, it is vital to be alert to any obvious signs of ill health at all times.

Physical examination

Figure 6.2 outlines the steps involved in performing a physical examination. The animal needs constant reassurance throughout the examination, especially prior to invasive techniques such as temperature taking.

- Assess the animal's temperament prior to handling.
- Talk in a reassuring tone.
- Allow the animal to feel comfortable with your presence before undertaking an examination.
- Start with the head:
  1. Examine both eyes for discharges or abnormal colour of conjunctiva.
  2. Examine both nostrils for abnormal discharges.
  3. Examine both ears for abnormal discharges, inflammation or smell.
  4. Examine the mouth – colour of the mucous membranes, capillary refill time, dental and gum condition, abnormal-smelling breath.
  5. Palpate submandibular lymph nodes.
- Gradually and systematically move down the body to examine:
  - all the limbs and tail for wounds or evidence of pain on palpation or movement
  - the feet for overgrown or unevenly worn nails, evidence of inflammation or wounds, or damage to the foot pads
  - the skin for signs of inflammation, ectoparasites, lesions or poor condition
  - all areas for any abnormal swellings or lumps (compare the animal symmetrically to identify abnormalities).
- Examine the genital tract of the male animal for:
  - asymmetrical size or shape of testicles (unneutered)
  - preputial discharge
  - inflammation or swelling of scrotal sac.
- Examine the genital tract of the female animal for:
  - evidence of being in season (unneutered) [a]
  - vaginal discharge
  - evidence of enlarged mammary glands
  - milk production.
- Examine anal region for swelling, inflammation and discomfort.
- Measure temperature, pulse and respiration rates (see Figure 6.3).

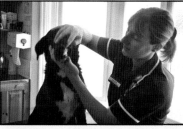
Examining the mouth.

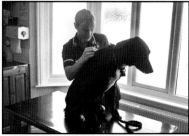
Examining the skin.

[a] Evidence of being 'in season':
- In the bitch:
  - swollen vulva
  - bloody or watery vaginal discharge
  - receptive to male advances
  - deviation of the tail and presentation of the vulva when the lumbar region is touched.
- In the queen:
  - persistent vocalization ('calling')
  - arched back with vulva presented ('lordosis').

6.2 How to perform a basic physical examination.

Some of these examinations can easily be demonstrated to the owner for carrying out at home. More detailed explanation is required for techniques such as the taking of temperature, pulse and respiration rates and these procedures are outlined in Figure 6.3. Normal values for these measurements are shown in Figure 6.4.

History taking

A programme of regular health monitoring establishes an accurate and detailed history, which will prove invaluable to the veterinary surgeon when an animal is presented with signs of ill health (Figure 6.5). The history supplies a record of the animal's normal characteristics and so allows any new sign that is truly abnormal to be highlighted (e.g. pale mucous membranes or red conjunctivae).

When taking the history of an animal's condition, it is important to consider the following points:

- Do not lead the questioning – ensure that the owner gives accurate information, rather than being led by a series of 'yes/no' questions that may encourage an answer although the owner is actually uncertain
- Rather than vague answers, gather information about actual quantities (of fluid intake, urine production, etc.)
- Confirm the accuracy of vital information, such as the reproductive status, vaccination status and age of the patient
- Confirm whether signs such as nasal discharge involve only one nostril (unilateral) or both nostrils (bilateral).

Taking temperature:
- Make sure the patient is suitably restrained
- Using either a mercury thermometer (which requires the mercury to be shaken down to the bulb of the thermometer prior to use) or by following carefully the instructions provided with a digital thermometer:
    1. Lubricate the end of the thermometer with petroleum jelly or water-soluble jelly.
    2. Gently insert the thermometer into the animal's rectum, with a twisting motion. The thermometer should be directed to the dorsal area of the rectum to avoid insertion into faecal material (which may alter the result).
    3. *Hold* the thermometer in the rectum for 1 minute.
    4. Remove from the rectum and clean, taking care *not* to hold the tip during this procedure.
    5. Now read the thermometer.

Taking the pulse:
- Make sure the patient is suitably restrained
- Locate the artery with the fingers. The femoral artery, which runs down the inside of the thigh, is commonly used for this procedure
- Apply firm pressure to the artery, using at least two fingers. Take care not to occlude the vessel
- Count the pulsations for exactly 1 minute.

Observing respiration rate:
- Make sure the patient is at rest but *not* sleeping or panting
- By observing movement of the chest, count *either* the breaths in *or* the breaths out (but not both) over 1 minute.

Measuring capillary refill time (CRT):
- Apply digital pressure to the mucous membranes of the gum until the area blanches
- Release the pressure to the mucous membranes and note the time taken for the capillaries to refill and the colour to return.

6.3   How to take temperature, check pulse and respiration rates and measure CRT.

Vital signs	Dog	Cat
Temperature	38.3–38.7°C	38.0–38.5°C
Pulse (beats per minute)	60–140 (lower part of range in large breeds, higher in small breeds)	110–180
Respiration (breaths per minute)	10–30	20–30
Capillary refill time	Almost instantaneous	Almost instantaneous
Water intake (per day)	40–60 ml/kg bodyweight	40–60 ml/kg bodyweight
Urine production (per hour)	1–2 ml/kg bodyweight	1–2 ml/kg bodyweight
Faecal production (per day): average amount when fed on canned foods (will be different for complete dry diets)	Miniature Dachshund: 70 g Beagle: 190 g Newfoundland: 500 g	
Faecal production (per day): frequency	Once or twice (but four times a day can be normal) Puppies: 2–6 times	

6.4   Normal ranges for vital signs.

Sign	Change evident	Possible normal cause	Possible abnormal cause
Temperature	Increase	Excitement After exercise Exposure to heat	Infection Heatstroke Convulsions Pain Some poisons
	Decrease	Exposure to cold Impending parturition	Shock Metabolic disorders (e.g. uraemia) Circulatory collapse Some poisons
Pulse	Increase	Exercise Excitement	Stress Pain Pyrexia (raised temperature) Early shock Hypovolaemia Hypoxia Sepsis
	Decrease	Sleep	Unconsciousness Debilitating disease Hypothermia (abnormally low body temperature)
Respiration rate	Increase	Excitement Exercise	Pain Pyrexia Poisons Hyperthermia (abnormally high body temperature)
	Decrease	Sleep	Poisons (sleep-inducing) Trauma to brain Hypothermia
Colour of mucous membranes	Pale	Normally pale individual (consider changes from normal)	Anaemia Shock
	Blue (cyanosis)		Hypoxaemia
	Brick red	Hyper-excitability	Sepsis Fever
	Yellow (jaundiced)		Accumulation of bilirubin, caused by hepatic disorder or bile duct obstruction
	Petechiation (red/brown spotting)		Clotting or bleeding disorders (e.g. platelet disorders, warfarin poisoning)
Capillary refill time (normally almost instantaneous)	Increase to > 2 seconds (indicates poor perfusion)		Hypovolaemia Shock Decreased cardiac output
	Increase to > 1–2 seconds (may indicate poor cardiac output and peripheral pooling of blood)	Anxiety	Fever Pain
Condition of coat	Poor	Moulting	Hormonal alopecia Neglect (lack of grooming by owner) Animal's inability to groom due to physical injury or disease Poor nutrition Endoparasite burden
Condition of skin	Poor	Ageing process	Parasitic skin disease Fungal infection Pyoderma Allergic skin disease Dietary deficiency

6.5 Signs of health and illness. (continues) ▶

Sign	Change evident	Possible normal cause	Possible abnormal cause
Condition of eyes	Discharges, irritation	Physical inability to groom Wearing Buster collar	Infections (bacterial, viral) Inflammatory condition Abnormal tear production Foreign body in or around eye
Condition of ears	Discharges, irritation	Physical inability to groom Wearing Buster collar	Infections (bacterial, fungal) Inflammatory condition Otodectes (ear mites) Foreign body in ear (e.g. grass seed)
Weight change	Increase	Normal growth rate in young animal Pregnancy Decreased activity level	Overfeeding Metabolic disease (e.g. hypothyroidism) Abnormal growth (e.g. tumour) Water retention due to metabolic or cardiac disease
	Decrease	Increased activity level	Underfeeding Metabolic disease (e.g. diabetes, hyperthyroidism) Endoparasites
Vomiting	True vomiting (movement of muscles of abdomen, chest or diaphragm in order to eject contents of stomach)		Eating unsuitable or decaying food Serious infectious disease, either contagious (e.g. parvovirus) or non-contagious (e.g. pyometra) Poisons Intestinal obstruction Travel sickness
	Regurgitation (more passive action, used to bring up sausage-shaped boluses of something eaten recently)	Demonstrated by some dogs when they bolt their food competitively if fed with others Demonstrated by some dogs if persuaded to feed when not hungry Nursing bitches and queens regurgitate partially digested food for offspring	Persistent regurgitation in older puppy or kitten or in adult may indicate obstruction or malformation of oesophagus
	Retching (involuntary spasm of vomiting, possibly accompanied by coughing; appears to be difficulty in swallowing food, which is quickly brought back covered in saliva)		Obstruction in mouth or throat Cough or acute sore throat
Dehydration		Lack of access to drinking water (neglect) Exposure to hot weather or environmental temperature increase	Inability to drink due to physical injury Diarrhoea/vomiting Metabolic disease Shock
Behaviour (normal: alert, bright, responsive, relaxed and comfortable)	Abnormal: dull, depressed, unresponsive, tense, restless	Introduction to strange environment or situation Lethargy after exercise Bitch in season Dog pining for bitch in season Grief after loss of animal or human companion	Pain Anxiety Underlying disease Lack of environmental stimuli (boredom) Subject of abuse or cruelty Inability to perform normal behaviour (e.g. no access to toilet facilities)

6.5 (continued) Signs of health and illness. (continues) ▶

Sign	Change evident	Possible normal cause	Possible abnormal cause
Appetite	Increased	Competitive feeding with other dogs Increased level of activity Change of diet, which has led to hunger Climatic change and therefore increased calorie requirement Pregnancy and lactation	Metabolic disease Endoparasite burden
	Decreased	Newly introduced foods Exhaustion after exercise Male dog may lose appetite when distracted by bitch in season Bitch will refuse food at certain stages in pregnancy (usually 24–36 hours before whelping)	Environmental stress (e.g. when strangers or new animals are introduced to environment; or during stay in strange environment such as boarding kennels) Pain Pyrexia Dental discomfort Physical discomfort in chewing and swallowing (dental, pharyngeal) Metabolic disease Loss of sense of smell; nasal congestion
Water intake	Increased	Change of diet to dry food containing less water	Diabetes insipidus Diabetes mellitus Renal failure Pyometra
	Decreased	Change of diet to food with greater moisture content	Physical discomfort preventing drinking or swallowing
Urine production	Increased		Metabolic disease Renal failure Diabetes insipidus Diabetes mellitus
	Decreased	Mild dehydration due to exposure to hot environment	Dehydration Nerve damage Trauma or obstruction to lower urinary tract Environment stress, such as kennel confinement
Faecal production	Increased	Change of diet	
	Decreased	Change of diet Decreased food intake Environmental effects (e.g. kennel confinement, soiled litter trays)	Rectal or colonic obstruction Prostate obstruction in male
	Constipation		Dehydration Impaction due to diet (e.g. bones eaten) Rectal or colonic obstruction
	Diarrhoea		Unsuitable diet or changes in diet Bacterial or viral infection Disease caused by protozoans Parasite burden

6.5 (continued) Signs of health and illness.

In addition to the details already noted during regular health monitoring, the veterinary surgeon will need further information to assist with diagnosis. This might include:

- Temperature, pulse and respiration rates
- Sex of the animal
- Whether the animal has been neutered
- Vaccination status
- Whether the animal has eaten recently
- In the case of a female, when she was last in season.

When reporting clinical signs, the abbreviations shown in Figure 6.6 are often used.

Abbreviation	Meaning	Examples and notes
T	Temperature	T 38.5°C (Celsius)
BPM	Respiratory rate: breaths per minute	30 BPM resp.
	Pulse: beats per minute	110 BPM pulse
	Heart rate: beats per minute	110 BPM HR
CRT	Capillary refill time	< 1 (less than 1 second) > 2 (more than 2 seconds)
mm	Mucous membrane	Used when noting colour of mucous membranes of mouth and conjunctiva in particular
DV	Diarrhoea and vomiting	Often followed by ++ to indicate amounts

6.6   Abbreviations.

Abnormal demeanour

Demeanour describes outward behaviour. In order to report on an animal's demeanour, it is essential to understand the normal behaviour patterns of the particular species. Owners who know their pet's character well are in a position to determine subtle changes in demeanour far earlier than an outside observer. Examples of abnormal demeanour include:

■ Reluctance to undertake normal activities (walking, playing, etc.)
■ Uncharacteristic aggression
■ Changes in normal patterns of:
   – Eating
   – Drinking
   – Urination
   – Defecation
   – Sleeping.

■ Unusual posture
■ Withdrawal and lack of response to familiar environments, people and other animals.

Recording clinical signs

During an initial consultation it is important to record abnormal signs and therefore it is essential to listen carefully to the information given by the owner, to ensure that any changes from 'normal' are particularly noted. For example, statements such as 'He normally only visits the litter tray a couple of times a day' or 'She has started to drink from the dripping tap and always seems to be looking for water' can be very informative and will direct the veterinary surgeon to a list of relevant diagnostic procedures.

If monitoring clinical signs over a period of time, changes in trends are particularly relevant. A well constructed record chart (Figure 6.7), especially one with graphs, can be very useful.

NANTWICH VETERINARY HOSPITAL DAILY HOSPITALISATION RECORD SHEET

ANIMAL:	CLIENT:	COMP NO :	DATE:
SPECIES:	BREED:	VET:	DAY NO:

COLOUR: | CLINICAL SUMMARY:
SEX: AGE:
WEIGHT: on admit | today

AM | PM

TIME
TEMP
PULSE
RESP
FEED (describe)
EATEN (Tick)
DRANK H2O (tick)
OUT/TIME
URINE
FAECES
VOMIT

IV CATHETER DAY 1 / 2 / 3	VET TO SPEAK TO OWNER Y / N	HOME TODAY Y / N	SEE OUT APPOINTMENT Y / N
MEDICATION			
PROCEDURES			
COMMENTS			

6.7   Example of daily hospitalization record sheet. (Courtesy of Nantwich Veterinary Hospital, Cheshire.)

Anatomical positions

It is essential to provide accurate descriptions, including precise references to anatomical positions, e.g. site of pain or position of wound (see Chapter 10).

Pain

Pain is a feeling of distress or suffering caused by stimulation of specialized nerve endings. Its purpose is chiefly protective: it acts as a warning that tissues are being damaged. Recognition of the signs of pain is an essential skill of the handler.

WARNING
It must not be overlooked that certain individuals will successfully disguise the signs of pain in order not to display vulnerability.

Signs of pain include:

- Vocalization
- Abnormal posture (huddled)
- Dilated pupils
- Lameness

- Panting
- Tachycardia (rapid heart rate)
- Pyrexia (raised body temperature)
- Inappetence
- Shivering
- Hiding.

Patient pain scoring

In order to improve awareness, and hence treatment, of acute pain it is constructive for veterinary practices to introduce a pain score to allow systematic assessment and recording of pain in all hospitalized patients (Figure 6.8). This scoring system can be explained to pet owners to allow accurate assessment to continue in the home environment. This will allow pain management to be tailored to the specific patient.

Information from owners

Accuracy in gaining information from owners and in reporting to the veterinary surgeon will ensure an enlightened assessment of the urgency of the case. An example of questions to ask an owner and assessment of the requirement for immediate action is given in Figure 6.9.

Score	Description	Level of pain
0	No pain at rest or on movement	None
1–3	No pain at rest; slight pain on movement	Mild
4–7	Intermittent pain at rest; moderate on movement	Moderate
8–10	Continuous pain at rest; severe on movement	Severe

6.8 Pain scoring.

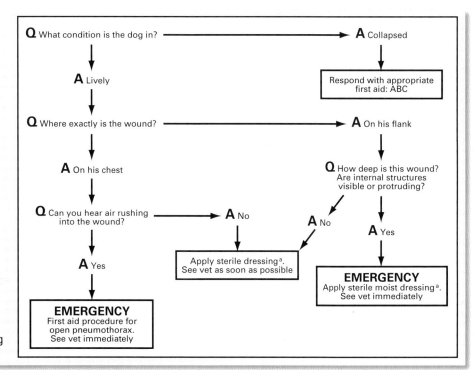

Owner's description: 'My dog has jumped through the patio window. There's not a *lot* of blood but he has got a large deep wound on his side.'

Questions (Q) to the owner, the sequence according to the owner's answers (A) and action to be taken (boxed) might be as follows.

Q What condition is the dog in? → **A** Collapsed
↓
A Lively
↓
Q Where exactly is the wound? → **A** On his flank
↓
A On his chest
↓
Q Can you hear air rushing into the wound? → **A** No

Respond with appropriate first aid: ABC

Q How deep is this wound? Are internal structures visible or protruding?
A No
A Yes

A Yes

Apply sterile dressing[a]. See vet as soon as possible

EMERGENCY
First aid procedure for open pneumothorax. See vet immediately

EMERGENCY
Apply sterile moist dressing[a]. See vet immediately

[a] With all dressings, advise regarding the possibility of embedded glass.

6.9 Assessing information from owners: an example.

Describing clinical signs

Figures 6.10 to 6.18 give definitions and guidelines for describing clinical signs relating to appetite, thirst, defecation, urination, abnormal discharges, coughing, vomiting, lameness and itching.

- A **sign** is an observable physical phenomenon that is associated with a given condition frequently enough to be considered indicative of the condition's presence.
- A **symptom** is any indication of disease perceived by the patient.

By these definitions, changes in animals are described as signs; only humans can have symptoms.

Definitions:

- *Polyphagia*: excessive ingestion of food
- *Anorexia* (anophagia, inappetence): lack or loss of appetite for food
- *Coprophagia*: ingestion of faeces
- *Pica*: craving for unnatural articles of food.

Questions to ask:

- What are the normal eating patterns?
- For how long has the appetite been abnormal?

6.10 How to describe appetite.

Definitions:

- *Polydipsia*: increased thirst
- *Adipsia*: absence of drinking.

The histories that accompany patients are often inaccurate on this point and the following details should be recorded:

- Measured water intake over 24 hours.

Questions to ask:

- Has a change in feeding occurred (e.g. from tinned food to dry)?
- Have glucocorticoids or diuretics been administered?

6.11 How to describe thirst.

Definitions:

- *Constipation*: failure to evacuate faeces
- *Diarrhoea*: frequent evacuation of watery faeces
- *Tenesmus*: ineffectual and painful straining (at defecation or urination).

Details to be recorded:

- Colour of faeces
- Smell of faeces
- Texture of faeces
- Volume and frequency of defecation
- Presence of blood, mucus or worms in faeces
- Recent changes in diet.

6.12 How to describe defecation.

Definitions:

- *Polyuria* [a]: excretion of a large volume of urine
- *Oliguria*: reduced output of urine
- *Anuria*: absence of urination
- *Dysuria*: painful or difficult urination
- *Haematuria*: presence of blood in the urine.

Other details to be recorded:

- Presence of urgency
- Frequency
- Tenesmus.

[a] Since polyuria and polydipsia often occur together, the abbreviation PU/PD is often used to describe this syndrome.

6.13 How to describe urination (micturition).

Be specific:

- Type:
  - purulent (containing pus)
  - mucoid (clear, tenacious)
  - serous (watery)
  - haemorrhagic.
- Colour
- Viscosity
- Origin:
  - nasal
  - ocular
  - vaginal
  - rectal
  - preputial
  - aural
  - wounds.
- Unilateral (affecting only one side)
- Bilateral (affecting both sides).

6.14 How to describe abnormal discharges.

Clarify:

- Sounds:
  - chesty/moist
  - throaty/dry ('hacking').
- Whether productive:
  - from bronchi (mucus)
  - blood.
- Is vomiting or regurgitation induced?
- Whether the coughing occurs:
  - first thing in the morning
  - after exercise
  - at night.
- Whether any foreign materials or abrasive items have been consumed.

Confirm vaccination status, particularly for:

- Distemper
- Canine contagious respiratory disease (kennel cough):
  - canine parainfluenza virus
  - *Bordetella bronchiseptica*.
- Feline upper respiratory tract disease (cat 'flu).

6.15 How to describe coughing.

Confirm whether the vomiting is:

- Projectile (vomited with great force)
- Regurgitation (casting up of undigested food with minimal effort)
- Retching (unproductive effort to vomit
- Dry (vomiting with ejection of gas only)
- With presence of blood (haematemesis)
- With presence of bile (yellow staining).

Confirm *when* vomiting occurs:

- Immediately after eating
- If not, actual length of time after eating
- Cyclical (recurring attacks).

Describe the *product* of vomiting:

- Food
- Bile (bilious vomit)
- Blood
- Faeces (stercoraceous vomit)
- Hair
- Bones
- Other foreign material.

Confirm further details:

- Vaccination status
- Any known consumption of foreign matter (bones, toxic substances, etc.)
- Patient's overall condition, including state of hydration
- Any other presenting signs:
  - polydipsia
  - polyuria
  - diarrhoea
  - pregnancy
  - last known oestrus.

6.16 How to describe vomiting (emesis).

Definitions:

- *Lame*: incapable of normal locomotion; showing deviation from the normal gait
- *Lameness*: the state of being lame
- *Gait*: the manner or style of locomotion
- Examples of abnormal gait:
  - *ataxic*: unsteady uncoordinated walk
  - *spastic*: a walk in which legs move in a stiff manner, the toes seeming to drag and catch
  - *antalgic*: a limp adopted so as to avoid pain on weightbearing structures.

Clarify:

- Was a known trauma involved?
  - road traffic accident (RTA)
  - fall.
- Which limb is involved?
- Chronic or acute? (This will aid in determining whether this is a fracture/dislocation that requires immediate veterinary intervention)
- Severity: partial or non-weightbearing
- Visible/palpable:
  - deformity of limb
  - swelling
  - bruising
  - heat in the region.
- When is the lameness worse?
  - after exercise
  - after rest.

6.17 How to describe lameness.

Confirm whether:

- Parasite control has been undertaken and note the product and schedule used
- There are particular zones:
  - ears, head and neck
  - anal region.
- The skin appears inflamed or abnormal
- The animal has been exposed to products not used before:
  - topical antiparasitics
  - shampoos
  - medications
  - home cleaning agents.
- The signs appear worse when the animal:
  - has walked among grasses
  - becomes hot.
- There has been any change to the diet.

6.18 How to describe pruritus (itching).

Handling and restraint

In order to handle animals safely and skilfully it is important to appreciate the behavioural differences between various species. Handlers (including veterinary nurses) must learn to avoid rushing in without first observing the animal's body language and assessing whether any obvious injuries are evident. This will prevent causing the animal unnecessary pain and will avoid unnecessary risk to the handler.

Dogs

Dogs are social pack animals and they look to a pack leader, in particular, to provide support and decision making. The veterinary nurse's aim is to take on the role of pack leader.

Body language is complex in the dog. Although they can signify much more than simply dominance or submission (Figure 6.19), these characteristics are the most important for a handler or veterinary nurse to recognize before approaching an unknown dog (see also Chapter 2).

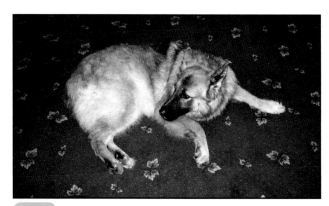

6.19 A submissive dog.

Training by owners

Whilst educating owners in the importance of responsible dog ownership and preventive healthcare, the veterinary nurse should emphasize how important it is that owners should:

■ Be able to examine their animal without causing distress or aggression

■ Realize the relevance of being able to examine *all* areas of the animal, including the feet, mouth and ears.

During a dog's life, it will have to be handled for many different reasons, such as:

■ Grooming and bathing
■ Examination of an injury
■ Administration of first aid
■ Administration of drugs prescribed by the veterinary surgeon (including those that the owner will need to give)
■ Weekly checks.

Responsible owners can prepare their animals for such handling from an early age. They can start by teaching the puppy to tolerate and even enjoy being examined. With particularly difficult areas, such as the paws and mouth, an animal that has been taught to tolerate examination will be a much easier patient for veterinary staff and owners alike.

Handling for examination

In order to be examined, the dog must be submissive. This means that the veterinary nurse needs to establish dominance over the dog. The first step is to interpret the animal's demeanour correctly. Then the dog can be approached, bearing the following guidelines in mind:

■ Approach the dog quietly but confidently
■ Use the dog's name
■ Talk in a reassuring manner
■ Lower yourself to the animal's level (in order to appear less threatening) but ensure that you can escape if necessary
■ Allow the dog to examine the back of your hand
■ Do not appear to trap the animal in a corner or at the back of the kennel.

WARNING
Do not make assumptions of aggression based on breed type alone. *All* types of dog can be equally aggressive.

If the dog shows signs of aggression, the handler's safety is paramount. Figure 6.20 explains how to deal with an aggressive animal.

Avoiding excessive restraint

In order to assess the need for active measures of restraint, it is important that the following considerations are made on admitting a dog to the hospital.

■ Discuss the animal's temperament (e.g. kennel guarding, only likes women, etc.) with the owner.
■ In the case of kennel guarding and uncertain temperament, do not remove the collar and lead. Instead, extend its length with another lead or rope and leave the extension outside the cage.

■ Personal safety is paramount – do not take unnecessary risks.
■ With a dog known to be aggressive, ask the owner to apply a muzzle before examination.
■ 'Kennel guarding' behaviour – secure all windows and doors and allow the dog out of the kennel before attempting to handle (this should only be attempted if it is certain that the aggression is kennel guarding!).
■ If the owner is present, ask them to leave, which may improve the animal's behaviour.
■ If the owner is absent, ask them to attend the surgery to calm the animal during administration of sedation to avoid unnecessary distress for the dog.
■ Carefully interpret body language – only use dominant behaviour (such as direct eye contact and standing over the dog) if the animal is adequately restrained.
■ Remember that often the aggression shown whilst the dog is injured or unwell may be uncharacteristic ('fear aggression') or an indication of pain, and the animal may therefore require less dominant handling techniques or analgesia.

 How to deal with an aggressive dog.

This will allow the handler to retrieve the lead safely and thus lead the animal out of the kennel without being bitten or distressing the animal.
■ Ensure that the kennel, case records and computer records are clearly marked with the details of the dog's temperament, so that all staff know the patient's character.
■ Discuss the animal's temperament with the veterinary surgeon *prior* to administration of routine premedicant drugs, as the anaesthetic regime may need to be adapted to allow for the difficulties in restraint.
■ Having discussed sedative or anaesthetic protocols with the veterinary surgeon, consider allowing the owner to stay whilst the animal is sedated, prior to admission to the hospital environment.

Restraint equipment

Collars and check chains

Before taking over control from an owner or admitting a patient to the hospital, certain procedures should be carried out to prevent patient escape or injury.

■ Always ensure that a check chain is fitted correctly, so that gravity ensures that the in-tension chain slackens.
■ Always check that a collar is fitted properly (often they are loose fitting and the patient is able to slip its head out and escape).
■ Always check that clips and fastenings are in good working order. If they appear broken or likely to snap, exchange them for a hospital collar and lead.
■ Never leave a trailing lead (for a kennel guarder) attached to a check chain, as this could result in asphyxiation (strangulation). Either clip or tie the chain into a locked position or exchange it for a collar.

> **WARNING**
> A struggling patient can inflict injury on a handler, even if the animal is muzzled and prevented from biting. Scratch wounds from dogs can be extremely painful. Dogs may also pull against the lead with which the handler is restraining them; therefore the handler should avoid wrapping the lead around the wrist, or fingers, as this could lead to personal injury.

Muzzling

As well as protecting staff from being bitten, a muzzle tends to distract the animal's attention. Types of muzzle (Figure 6.21) include:

- Tape muzzle
- Commercially available nylon muzzle
- Box muzzle
- Wire muzzle.

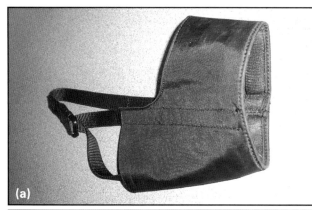

6.21 Types of commercial muzzle. **(a)** Nylon. **(b)** Box.

> **WARNING**
> Owners can fit muzzles to animals, but it is vital that muzzled animals are not left unsupervised. The handler or veterinary nurse must be aware of the dangers involved should an animal vomit whilst wearing a muzzle, or the possibility of injury to the front claws (dewclaws in particular) if the animal should attempt to remove the device.

Methods of handling a dog while a muzzle is being fitted are described in Figure 6.22.

If specifically designed muzzles are not available, a useful skill is that of applying a simple tape muzzle (Figure 6.23).

- Stand to one side of the animal, facing the same direction. Alternatively, stand astride larger dogs.
- Hold the scruff of the neck securely behind each ear.
- If the dog attempts to bring up its front feet to remove the muzzle, a second handler may be required to restrain its forelimbs.
- If the dog attempts to walk backwards out of the muzzle, both the handler and the person applying the muzzle should move with the dog or back into a corner or up to a wall to prevent further movement.

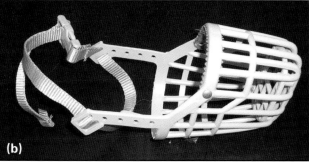

6.22 How to restrain a dog for application of a muzzle.

1. Select an adequate length of non-conforming bandage (conforming will stretch!).
2. Form a loop with a square knot.
3. Direct someone to restrain the dog correctly.
4. Approach from the side of the animal.
5. Slip the loop over the dog's nose with the knot being quickly tightened uppermost.
6. Cross the free ends under the jaw.
7. Bring the ends under the lower jaw and under the ears.
8. Tie in a quick-release bow around the back of the head.

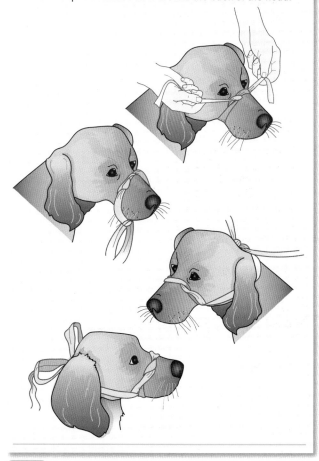

6.23 How to apply a tape muzzle.

Muzzling is unsuitable for most brachycephalic (short-nosed) breeds. For small breeds, such as Pug and Pekingese, a towel placed around the neck behind the ears is a suitable method of restraint that does not lead to prolapse of the eyeballs (an unfortunate risk when scruffing these patients).

In larger brachycephalic breeds, such as the Boxer, a specially adapted commercial muzzle is required or a modified version of the tape muzzle can be used.

Dog graspers (dog catchers)

The dog grasper (Figure 6.24) can be used as a last resort. However, the use of this equipment can be traumatic for both operator and animal, and alternative methods are usually considered first.

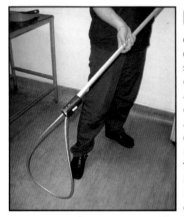

6.24 Dog graspers (or dog catchers) vary in complexity. The simplest form consists of a long handle with a lasso loop of rope or another material at one end. The other end of the rope runs up the handle so that the size of the loop can be controlled once the loop has been placed over the dog's head.

Alternative restraint techniques

The following techniques require more than one operator:

■ The lead is passed through a ring on the wall, pulling the dog's head up to the wall. An assistant holds the animal's body against the wall
■ The lead is passed through a doorway. Once the dog's head is through, the door is carefully held against the dog's shoulders
■ The lead is wrapped around the leg of a table to restrain the dog's head
■ The lead is pulled through kennel bars to restrain the dog's head.

These alternative techniques could facilitate:

■ Application of a muzzle
■ Injection of a sedative drug (if necessary, by means of a syringe pole – a tubular structure 1.6–1.9 m long with a fitment for a normal hypodermic syringe and needle at one end and an extended plunger at the other, thus allowing long-distance techniques).

Lifting

Once the dog has been secured (and muzzled, if required) it can be lifted. It is important to be careful when lifting, in order to prevent injury to the handler. For a larger dog, it is advisable to seek the assistance of another person (Figure 6.25).

Holding

When handling, the hands are not the only method of restraint. Holding an animal close to the handler's body will make the patient feel more securely held and will allow better control. Animals may require restraint in particular positions and for various procedures (Figure 6.26).

Unaided:
1. Prior to handling, determine the position of any injuries and take measures to avoid hurting the patient.
2. Grasp the animal around the front and rear legs.
3. Press the animal's body against the chest to prevent struggling.
4. With the knees bent and back straight, now carefully lift the patient up on to the examination table.

Small dogs can be supported by tucking the animal under the arm and supporting the barrel of the chest, without having to support the hindlimbs.

With an assistant:
■ One person can support the front quarters by placing one arm around the front of the animal's neck to restrain the head, whilst placing the other arm underneath the barrel of the chest
■ The second person can support the hindquarters by placing one arm under the abdomen and placing the other arm around the rump
■ Both handlers lift carefully and simultaneously.

6.25 How to lift a dog.

For examination:
1. Lift on to a table.
2. Stand to one side of the animal.
3. Wrap the arm nearest to the animal's head around its neck, in order to restrain its head.
4. The other arm can then be:
   - either pressed against the dorsal part of the neck to assist in restraint of the head
   - or placed underneath the chest or abdomen, to hold the animal against the handler's body to secure the patient.

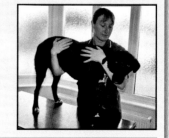

6.26 How to restrain a dog. (continues) ▶

On one side

On the floor:
1. Kneel to one side of the patient (with the patient standing).
2. Hold the front and hindlegs by placing the arms across the back and grasping the legs nearest the handler at the level of the tibia and radius.
3. Pull the legs away from the handler, whilst rolling the dog's body gently down the handler's lap and on to the floor.
4. Restrain by holding the limbs nearest to the floor and using the forearms and elbows to hold down the head and neck and the rump.

On a table:
1. Follow the same procedure as on the floor, but stand rather than kneel to one side of the patient.
2. Slide the patient gently down the chest rather than across the lap.

With large dogs two handlers may be required. As with lifting, one handler takes control of the forelimbs whilst the other controls the hindquarters. Once the animal is on its side (lateral recumbency) it may be possible for one handler to hold it down in position.

For an injection

Intramuscular and subcutaneous:
1. Use the technique for handling for examination.
2. On the floor 'scruff' the dog, with handler's legs straddled across the animal's shoulders to secure.
3. With an aggressive animal, dog graspers can be used.

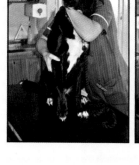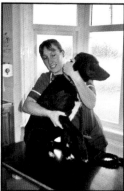

Intravenous injection or blood sampling:
Cephalic vein (forelimb)
1. Stand to one side of the patient, opposite to the site of the injection.
2. Patient is sitting or in sternal recumbency, handler places one arm around the neck and the other arm across the shoulders to restrain the limb used for venepuncture.
3. Hold the limb extended by grasping behind the elbow, which will prevent the elbow from bending.
4. Use thumb placed across top of limb to apply pressure and thus prevent venous return and achieve 'raising' of vein.

Saphenous vein (lateral aspect of tarsus)
- Dog restrained in lateral recumbency with leg to be used uppermost.

 (continued) How to restrain a dog.

Cats

Cats are agile, quick and independent by nature. This means that they may only tolerate handling for short periods. They have sharp teeth as well as four sets of claws and can inflict painful injuries to the handler.

The degree of restraint required depends on the individual cat. Most respond to a loose and gentle approach (rather than forceful restraint) gained by an unhurried but firm technique:

- Approach calmly but confidently
- Speak quietly
- If the cat is not hissing or growling, attempt to stroke its head and run a hand confidently along its back.

> **WARNING**
> **Take heed of aggressive behaviour such as hissing, lowered ears and swiping out with a paw.**

The body language of cats is illustrated in Figure 6.27.

To remove an unwilling cat from its container:

- Attempt to cover the cat's head with a towel
- Wrap the cat in the towel and gently lift it out of the container.

Avoiding excessive restraint

In general, cats respond best to light restraint (Figure 6.28). However, if the handler is acting alone, firmer restraint such as scruffing may prove necessary.

It is best to use only as much restraint as necessary, provided that firmer control can be applied rapidly if required. In some cases, once a cat has been scruffed briefly, a further attempt at a more gentle approach proves effective and can be tried if the handler is confident. It may be necessary to wrap the cat's body in a towel after scruffing, to protect the handler from the cat's claws.

To prevent the need for forceful restraint:

- Assess the patient's temperament
- If it is decided that sedative drugs will need to be administered before examination, place the cat directly into a crush cage

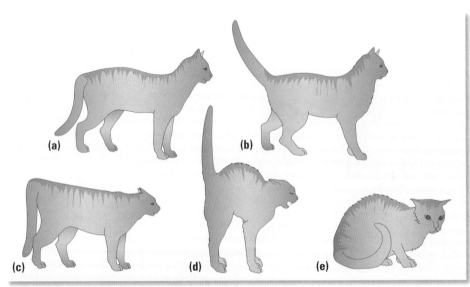

6.27 Cat body language. **(a)** Normal relaxed posture. **(b)** Friendly cat. **(c)** Aggressive cat. **(d)** Frightened cat. **(e)** Conflict. Redrawn after Thorne (1992).

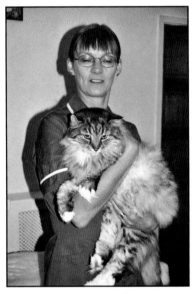

6.28 Minimal restraint of a cat. With one hand over the chest wall and the other supporting the rump, the cat is held firmly towards the handler's body.

■ To allow adaptation of sedative or anaesthetic protocols, discuss the animal's temperament with the veterinary surgeon prior to the administration of premedicant drugs.

Lifting and holding

Lifting techniques depend on the cat's bodyweight and temperament, and from where the cat is being lifted (Figure 6.29). Figure 6.30 describes techniques for holding a cat for examination.

Restraint equipment

In order to avoid injury to the handler, it might be necessary to wear handling gloves. A more aggressive cat might require restraining aids such as a crush cage, muzzle, cat bag or cat grasper.

■ Crush cages have a movable internal wall that can be eased across gently to hold the patient against the wire side of the cage, allowing injection through the wires.
■ Cat muzzles are fitted in the same manner as a dog muzzle but they also cover the eyes like a blindfold, thus subduing the animal.

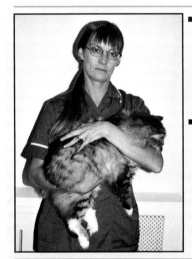

■ Pass one hand over the chest wall and support the sternum, whilst the other hand supports the abdomen from the other side.
■ To retrieve from a basket, gently grasp both forelegs from the elbow and pull free.

6.29 How to lift a cat.

For examination of the head
■ Hold the cat under the arm or against the handler's chest, whilst holding the forelegs to prevent the person examining the cat from being scratched.
■ The free hand can be used to hold the cat's chin in order to support the head.

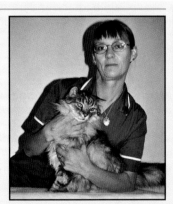

For examination of the body

Depending on the cat's temperament:

■ Either gently hold the cat's shoulders and forelegs
■ Or hold the head under the jaw and use the other hand to hold the cat against the handler's body and restrain the forelegs.

6.30 How to hold a cat for examination.

- Cat restraining bags are specially designed zip-up bags with holes to expose the head or limbs as required.
- Cat graspers are like a pair of tongs, used to grasp the animal by the neck; a towel is used to wrap up the limbs (Figure 6.31).

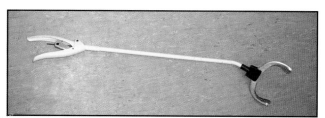

6.31 Cat grasper. Unlike dog catchers, cat graspers do not incorporate a loop to lasso the animal but are designed like a set of tongs to grasp the cat by the neck. They should only be used in extreme cases. *Never* lift the unsupported body by the neck (use a towel to wrap up the limbs).

> ⚠️ **WARNING**
> **Cat graspers should only be used in extreme cases. It is essential that the cat's unsupported body should *never* be lifted by the neck.**

Techniques for removing an aggressive cat from its kennel are described in Figure 6.32.

- Attempt to cover the cat's head with a towel, wrapping the animal in the towel and gently lifting it out of the kennel.
- In extreme cases the cat's head can be restrained by use of a cat grasper around the neck, to enable wrapping the animal in a towel to remove it from the kennel.
- Slide a cat basket into the kennel, trapping the cat between the cage back and the basket. Once the cat has entered the basket, slide a towel between the cage back and the basket to prevent escape. Now slide the cat basket out of the kennel, close the lid of the basket and withdraw the towel before fastening.

6.32 How to retrieve an aggressive cat from a kennel.

Administration of injections

Cats can be restrained for injections in a similar manner to that used in dogs, but with extra precautions to prevent handler injury from claws (Figure 6.33).

A technique that can be implemented when giving an *aggressive* cat an intramuscular injection is:

- Scruff the neck with one hand
- Extend the hindlimbs with the other hand
- This stretches the cat's body and thus prevents movement.

6.33 How to hold a cat for injection.

Grooming and coat care

Reasons for grooming

Regular grooming accustoms an animal to being handled and also enables the early identification of a range of health problems. Motives for grooming include:

- To clean the coat and remove dead shedding hair
- To prevent the coat from matting or soiling with faeces, urine or discharges
- To allow regular inspection for signs of:
    - External parasites (lice, fleas) (Figure 6.34)
    - Hair loss in particular regions
    - Poor skin condition
    - Wounds/injuries
    - Abnormal swellings or lumps
    - Pain or discomfort when moving or touching any part of the body
    - Overgrown nails (particularly dewclaws).
- To enforce dog pack hierarchy and form a bond with the animal (dogs lower in the pack order submit to grooming by a more dominant member).

Fleas are notoriously difficult to see and even harder to catch. Therefore it is more appropriate to examine for the evidence of fleas in the form of flea dirt (faeces).

- Place a white sheet of paper on the floor or table top.
- Mist over with water.
- Stand the animal on the paper and groom with fingertips or comb.
- Examine particles that have landed on the moist paper.
- Flea dirt is formed from excreted blood and will stain the paper red or brown.

6.34 How to examine for fleas.

A carefully managed grooming protocol ensures a successful grooming session. Procedures for commencing and carrying out grooming are outlined in Figures 6.35 and 6.36.

- Ideally, introduce the pet to grooming from an early age, as a continuation of the grooming administered by the animal's mother.
- Start with brief grooming sessions and gradually increase.
- Allow the animal to enjoy being examined, before using grooming equipment. Incorporate handling in your stroking of the animal, several times every day when it is calm and relaxed.
- Initially pretend to brush, but use your hand instead of a brush.
- Do not aim to cover all of the body: do a little at a time, reward the animal for being good and then stop.
- Keep a titbit or toy to hand to retain the pet's interest and reward the animal with it at the end of the session. Try smearing a foodstuff (such as pâté, cheese spread, etc.) on a wall or cupboard door at nose height in front of the animal, which will lick at this while you introduce handling of feet, tail, etc.

6.35 How to introduce grooming to a new animal. (continues) ▶

- If a dog tries to 'mouth' you, say 'Ow!' in a very hurt way and reward them for stopping.
- Gradually increase the time spent grooming and handling each day and introduce other examinations, such as:
  - examining the mouth (including opening it and looking down the throat)
  - examining the eyes
  - wiping the inside of the ears with cotton wool (do not insert cotton buds down the ear canal)
  - examining the tail and anal area
  - examining the vulva/prepuce
  - checking the pads and between the paws.
- Do not try to teach tolerance of all of these procedures at once – concentrate on a different one at each session.
- Always reward good behaviour – with a titbit, play session or just a cuddle and verbal praise.
- Remember the independent nature of cats – it is often extremely difficult to teach them to tolerate a lot of handling or grooming, and it often depends on whether they have been introduced to handling at an early age.

6.35 (continued) How to introduce grooming to a new animal.

- Assess the animal's temperament – is muzzling, sedation or anaesthesia indicated?
- Have all the necessary equipment to hand, including titbit rewards for the animal.
- Carry out a physical inspection of the animal to ascertain that there are no wounds or injuries that need to be avoided or treated prior to grooming.
- Put on an overall or apron.
- Loosen dead hair, using fingertips.
- Use a comb to remove tangles and further loosen dead hair in longhaired animals.
- Brush the coat with the appropriate brush or hound glove required for the hair type (not all hounds require a 'hound' glove: for instance, the Saluki has long fine hair).
- After combing and brushing, a smooth or silky medium coat can be finished off by using a damp cloth, a smooth hound glove or a piece of velvet or chamois cloth.
- It may also prove necessary to pluck excess hair carefully from the ear canal in breeds prone to overgrowth.

6.36 How to carry out grooming.

Hair growth

Unlike humans, whose hair grows continuously and therefore has to be cut, dogs and cats periodically shed their coats (moult). The hair grows in cycles:

- Growth phase (brief)
- Resting phase
- Shedding phase.

The average rate of hair growth is 0.5 mm per day. A number of factors can affect hair growth and moulting:

- Central heating:
  - Animals kept in centrally heated houses will often moult continuously.

- Seasons:
  - In the spring: summer coat produced, winter coat moulted
  - In the summer: increased sebaceous gland activity to allow air circulation through the coat
  - In the autumn: winter coat produced, summer coat moulted
  - In the winter: reduced sebaceous gland activity, increased density of insulating coat.
- Hormones:
  - Oestrogen slows hair growth (bitch on heat)
  - Thyroid deficiency: slow-growing dull rough coat with bilateral flank alopecia (hair loss)
  - Hormonal alopecia is also occasionally seen during pregnancy and lactation, and after neutering.
- Poor diet:
  - Insufficiency of nutrients or an imbalance of nutrients, such as amino acids and essential fatty acids, or vitamin and mineral deficiencies, such as zinc and iodine.
- External parasites such as fleas, mites and lice
- Ill health: various chronic diseases may affect hair growth.

Coat types

A variety of coat types are seen in dogs and cats (Figure 6.37). The choice of grooming equipment needs to be correct for each type.

Animal	Type of coat	Breed examples
Dog	Smooth: ■ Short fine ■ Intermediate or coarse dense	Boxer, Dachshund German Shepherd Dog
	Wire	Wire-haired terriers
	Double	Rough Collie Longhaired German Shepherd Dog
	Single: ■ Medium ■ Long fine	Spaniels Afghan Hound
	Woolly	Poodle Irish Water Spaniel
	Corded	Hungarian Puli Komondor
Cat	Longhair	Chinchilla Persian
	Semi-longhair	Birman Maine Coon
	Shorthair	Manx Siamese

6.37 Examples of coat type.

Grooming equipment

Choice of equipment (Figure 6.38) depends on the coat type to be groomed.

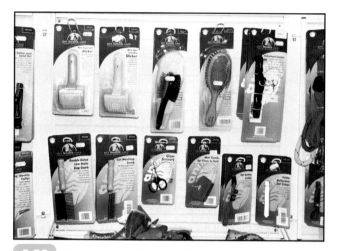

6.38   A selection of grooming equipment.

Brushes

Brushing takes time and effort, especially when dealing with longhaired, dense or matted coats.

Pin brushes

Pin brushes have a series of pins mounted on a rubber-backed cushion, with a wooden or plastic frame. Sometimes the ends of the pins are coated in plastic to minimize scratching of the skin during grooming. A pin brush cannot break or pull out hair, so the coat must be free from knots and tangles. The main function of a pin brush is to keep the coat sleek and glossy by distributing natural coat oils from the skin.

Bristle brushes

Bristle brushes are very similar in design and function to the pin brush except that the grooming surface consists of either manmade or natural bristles instead of metal pins.

Slicker brushes

Slicker brushes consist of hooked wire pins mounted on a rectangular pad with a handle. Care should be taken when brushing in areas where hair cover is thin, such as the axillae (armpits). Slicker brushes are excellent for use on matted and tangled coats, as their design and shape enable them to pull out dead hair and break down mats.

Hound gloves/mittens

These brushes resemble gloves or mittens. They remove dead hair from the undercoat and give the outer coat a polish. The grooming surface of the glove consists of rubber bumps, wires or bristles. Because the glove fits the hand like a mitten, the grooming process is as easy as stroking. Gloves and mittens are especially useful and effective on smooth shorthaired breeds and on short wire-haired terrier coats.

Rubber grooming devices

Available for both dogs and cats, these one-piece handheld grooming aids have large bumps along the grooming surface. They are useful for short-coated breeds such as the Labrador Retriever.

Combs

The several different types of comb can be divided into two basic groups: traditional and special function combs.

Traditional combs

These are available either with or without a handle. They have rigid metal teeth that are rounded at the tip and are available in various tooth widths. The most commonly used traditional comb has coarse tooth widths at one end and fine tooth widths at the other. Traditional combs are only to be used along the lie of the hair, at an angle of 45 degrees, to remove dead hair, to groom long silky hair behind the ears and to untangle and break up mats.

Dematting combs

Designed to cut through mats without destroying too much of the coat, these combs usually consist of a series of metal teeth that are bladed on one side and blunt on the other. The comb is introduced between the mat and the skin. With the sharpened side of the blade facing towards the groomer, a firm but gentle sawing motion is adopted. As the blade works through the mat it breaks it down into smaller mats, which can then be combed out. This type of comb allows the maximum amount of coat to be preserved once the mat is removed.

Rake combs

Rake combs have rigid metal teeth with round ends perpendicular to the handle. Care should be taken not to inflict skin trauma. Rake combs are used in dense coats for the removal of dead undercoat and the breaking up of some small mats.

Flea combs (nit combs)

Available either with or without a metal, wooden or plastic handle, these have very finely separated metal teeth. They are used to eradicate fleas, lice and their eggs (nits are lice eggs).

Untanglers

These devices have a plastic grip with metal pin teeth that can roll, thus preventing pull on the tangles.

Scissors

The routine clipping or trimming of some areas in longhaired dogs will assist in maintaining cleanliness. Clipping, hand stripping and trimming of specific breeds should be carried out by a trained groomer. However, the veterinary nurse or owner can carry out maintenance of specific problem areas. For example:

■ Trimming between the toes, to prevent mat formation and the trapping of grass seeds during the summer and autumn
■ Trimming the ears, particularly the underside, to prevent mat formation and the trapping of grass seeds and to prevent soiling with food in breeds with pendulous ears

- Trimming the anal region and feathering of the tail and hindlegs to prevent mats and faecal soiling
- Trimming pregnant bitches around the vulval region and hindlegs to prevent excessive soiling during whelping.

Trimming scissors

Trimming scissors have long and very sharp blades that taper to a point. They are used to trim around the edges of ears.

Toe scissors

Toe scissors have short blades with blunt ends and are used to trim delicate areas between the toes.

Thinning scissors

Thinning scissors have either a single serrated and a single plain blade, or two serrated blades. The specialized blades cut small amounts of hair and leave an equal uncut amount at intervals. This action thins the coat without leaving steps (for example, to enhance features such as the shoulder).

Clippers

Cosmetic clipping for specific breeds should be carried out by a trained groomer, but veterinary advice is often sought in the case of elderly or difficult-to-handle patients. Sedation prior to professional grooming may be required or anaesthesia may be the only course open to facilitate the dematting of a patient. In these circumstances the use of clippers (Figure 6.39) is recommended over the use of scissors, which in inexperienced grooming hands can lead to accidental skin wounds.

- Choose an appropriate blade size for the required clip, following manufacturer's guidelines.
- Hair must be completely dry, as wet hair blunts the blades.
- Do not force clippers through a thick coat or matting – use a slicker comb first to break up mats.
- Allow clippers to cool down whenever they become hot during use.
- Thoroughly clean and oil after each use, using only manufacturer-recommended lubricants and cleaners.

6.39 How to use electric clippers.

Dematting

Important points that should be borne in mind before dematting a coat include the following:

- In order to prevent misunderstandings, always discuss thoroughly with the owners (prior to the procedure) the amount of hair that will be removed
- Avoid scissors if at all possible, as skin wounds are easily inflicted when cutting away large mats
- Depending on the weather conditions, make appropriate arrangements for the animal whilst the coat is regrowing:

   – Avoid exposing shaved skin to excessive sunlight (use sunblocks)
   – Protect from the cold (use coats).

Bathing

Bathing is not normally carried out routinely on animals (particularly cats) without specific indications. However, it should not be overlooked as an important process in encouraging owners to check regularly every area of their pet – particularly in longhaired animals, where skin wounds and the development of swellings and lumps can easily be undetected.

Indications for bathing include:

- Preparation of show animals prior to exhibition
- Ectoparasite control
- Medication of specific skin problems
- Cleaning of soiled coats
- Removal of unpleasant or unwanted odours.

The appropriate steps in bathing a dog are given in Figure 6.40.

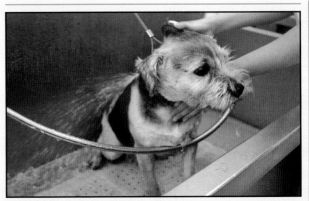

1. Apply a collar and lead, which can be used to restrain the animal whilst it is in the bath.
2. Prepare all the required equipment.
3. Groom the dog before bathing.
4. Wear the required protective clothing (often includes impervious gloves).
5. Place the animal carefully in the bath.
6. Having prepared the correct flow and temperature of the water from the shower fitment, carefully apply the water to soak the dog's coat.
7. Apply shampoo and massage in.
8. Follow manufacturer's guidelines regarding contact time and dosage.
9. Rinse thoroughly.
10. Squeeze out excess water.
11. Lift dog from the bath (do *not* encourage the dog to jump out as this may cause injury).
12. Towel dry.
13. Use hair dryer.
14. Now carry out final grooming and finishing.

6.40 How to bath a dog.

Types of bath include:

- Domestic bath (not ideal, as it might be easily damaged by claws)

- Baby bath (useful for smaller animals but can be easily tipped over)
- Metal bath or specifically designed grooming bath.

For all types of bath, certain requirements should be considered:

- Ease of getting animal into and out of the bath
- Non-slip surface (a bath mat to give additional protection)
- Shower fitment available for rinsing
- Access to adjustable water and heat controls
- Easy to clean and maintain.

Shampoos

There are several different types of shampoo:

- Cleansing, for general-purpose cleaning and conditioning
- Insecticidal, used for control of ectoparasites
- Medicated, for treatment of specific skin ailments.

When using shampoos, the following precautions are important:

- Follow the manufacturer's directions precisely
- When using new products, carry out a patch test: apply to one small area, following directions, and then observe for any adverse reactions before using on the entire coat
- Particularly with medicated products, wear protective apron, gloves and mask and use in a well ventilated area, if directed to do so
- Wear non-slip footwear to avoid accidents
- Transfer shampoo from glass bottles to unbreakable receptacles in order to apply without risk of breakages
- Protect delicate areas of the animal from shampoo:
  - Put cotton wool into ear canals (remember to remove later)
  - Apply barrier cream to delicate anal, vulval, preputial and scrotal areas
  - Take measures to prevent shampoo from running into eyes (apply non-medicated eye ointment).

Dryers

Dryers range from the very cheap to the very specialized and expensive. Types of dryer include:

- Handheld dryers
- Floor or stand dryers
- Forced-air dryers or blasters
- Cage or kennel dryers
- Cabinet dryers.

Handheld dryers

For normal domestic or veterinary purposes, handheld dryers are the most commonly used. They are light, simple and cheap, but are slow when used to dry a large heavy-coated dog and, being handheld, they limit the groomer to only one free hand.

Floor or stand dryers

Dryers mounted on stands are generally more powerful and larger than handheld ones. They therefore dry the coat more quickly as well as leaving the groomer with both hands free.

Forced-air dryers or blasters

These do not have a heating element, as they rely on the velocity of air coming out of the nozzle to force the water and dead hair out of the coat. They are very noisy and therefore unsuitable for cats or smaller nervous dogs.

Cage or kennel dryers

These dryers are attached to the front of standard kennels, thus allowing the dog to be dried whilst the groomer is doing something else. However, the dog needs to be moved at intervals to ensure that all of the coat dries, especially the underside.

Cabinets

Heated drying cabinets, into which the animal is placed, are often used in large professional grooming parlours. They must be carefully monitored to prevent the animal becoming hyperthermic (overheated). The cabinets have built-in drying elements and viewing doors. The dog stands on a false floor with integrated vents through which warm air flows.

Claw maintenance

The claws of a healthy animal do not normally require regular clipping. Trimming may be necessary for animals that appear not to wear down their claws naturally or for practical reasons:

- Dogs that do not have access to hard ground that would naturally wear down their nails
- Animals that are inactive (e.g. elderly)
- Paraplegic animals
- Those with disease conditions of the foot or nail that have led to abnormal growth
- Those with abnormal nail position or uneven wearing down of nails due to lameness or uneven gait
- Cats that damage furniture (scratch posts are a solution in the long term)
- Puppies, to prevent trauma to bitch's mammary region.

Also, regular observations must be made of the length of dewclaws. These are usually slow growing (see Chapter 2) but, because they are not routinely worn down by daily exercise, the owner needs to ensure that they do not become overgrown.

Nail clipping equipment includes:

- Suitable nail clipper for the size of the animal
- Cotton wool and a silver nitrate pencil (in case of inadvertent cutting of the quick and subsequent bleeding).

The technique for nail trimming is described in Figure 6.41.

- Gather equipment together.
- Suitably restrain the animal.
- Hold the foot firmly and examine the claws to be trimmed.
- In cats, gentle pressure to the foot will expose the normally retracted claws.
- If the quick is visible, cut below the quick.
- If the quick is not visible (black claws), estimate where the quick should be by examining how much claw exceeds the bottom of the pad. Cut with care, avoiding cutting too high up and causing bleeding.
- If bleeding occurs, apply silver nitrate via styptic pencil and cover with cotton wool.
- Continue until all claws (including dewclaws) have been trimmed.

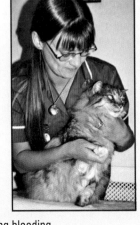

6.41 How to cut claws.

Dental hygiene

When carrying out grooming and coat care, the opportunity arises to maintain good dental hygiene. The teeth of dogs and cats were designed for killing prey and for tearing and chewing raw flesh. With changes in feeding protocols and the consistency of many pet foods, it has become evident that regular oral hygiene is required in many pets. For optimum results, oral hygiene routines should become a daily event.

As with grooming and handling, it is best to commence these techniques in young animals. However, if introduced gradually and with patience, many animals will accept dental cleaning later in life (Figure 6.42).

- Firstly assess the animal's temperament.
- Begin by handling the animal's mouth daily for several days and praising good behaviour.
- Gradually start to mimic tooth brushing with the finger alone, for several days.
- Begin to apply specific canine or feline toothpaste (human preparations are unsuitable) with the finger for several days.
- Now very gradually replace the finger with a toothbrush.
- Once the animal has learnt to tolerate dental cleaning, it may prove possible to clean the inner surfaces of the teeth as well as the outermost (finger brushes are helpful with this).

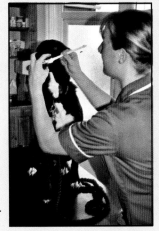

6.42 How to introduce dental hygiene.

Other aids to oral hygiene include:

- Specifically designed dental chews
- Oral hygiene gels and pastes
- Specifically designed dental biscuits.

Introduction to nutrition

In order to maintain optimal body health, it is essential that the body receives adequate nutrition. This requirement comes second only to the requirement for water and air.

It is important to have a good understanding of normal nutritional requirements before considering those specific to various life stages.

Basic nutritional requirements

During various disease states and stages of life, the nutritional and energy requirements of animals will vary. However, the basic nutritional requirements of all animals are:

- To meet energy requirements without excess
- To meet all nutrient requirements without incurring detrimental excesses.

Animals can be classified as:

- Carnivores: eating primarily flesh
- Herbivores: eating plants and plant products
- Omnivores: eating both plant and animal foods.

Although they belong to the order Carnivora, dogs are actually omnivorous. They can feed not only on animal tissue such as meat, but also on vegetable matter. Cats, however, are true carnivores and must have animal tissue in their diets. Cats cannot be vegetarians.

Why cats cannot be vegetarian but dogs can follow a vegetarian diet

- **Cats have a higher protein requirement than dogs. This appears to be due to a high rate of protein breakdown, which the cat cannot 'adapt' (re-forming amino acids into new proteins) if fed a low-protein diet.**
- **One of the amino acids in particular is essential in the cat's diet. Cats cannot metabolize it, as dogs can. This essential amino acid is taurine and it is only found in meat sources. If the diet is deficient in taurine, it can lead to retinal degeneration, which can lead to blindness.**
- **There are three essential fatty acids (EFAs) found in dietary fat, which are required for many metabolic functions in the body. Dogs can convert any one of the EFAs into another within the body tissue, which means that if a dog were to be fed only one EFA in a sufficient amount, the other two could be** ▶

manufactured. Cats, however, require *all three* EFAs, as they are unable to metabolize in this way and a dietary deficiency could occur, resulting in problems such as scurfy skin and poor growth.

- **Most mammals can convert carotenoid (a substance that can be converted into active vitamin A). Cats cannot carry out this reaction and therefore require a source of pre-formed vitamin A in the diet, which is found only in animal materials and *not* in vegetable matter.**

Meeting energy requirements

Animals eat to obtain energy and it is therefore important that all nutritional requirements are balanced to the calorific level of food, as the animal will only eat to meet calorific requirements.

The smaller an animal is, the greater is its body surface area (relative to the environment) and the higher is its energy requirement. For example:

- A Chihuahua needs more calories per kilogram of bodyweight per day than does a Great Dane
- A Labrador puppy is a small version of the mature Labrador and therefore needs more calories per kilogram of bodyweight per day (approximately twice as much).

Hunger

Hunger is a craving for food. It is stimulated by:

- Decrease in blood glucose
- Decrease in circulating amino acids
- Increase in gastric motility.

Nutrients

A nutrient is a substance assimilated from the gastrointestinal tract and utilized by cells of the body to support life. It may be:

- Non-essential – manufactured within the body and therefore not an essential daily dietary requirement
- Essential – must be provided in food, because the nutrient is either not synthesized by the body at all, or the rate of synthesis is too slow to meet demands.

The function of nutrients is to supply:

- Energy
- Materials for growth, repair and reproduction
- Substances that regulate the processes involved in energy production or the utilization of materials for growth, repair and reproduction.

Classes of nutrients are:

- Water
- Protein
- Fat
- Carbohydrate
- Minerals
- Vitamins.

Water

Every body cell requires a continuous water supply in order to function. In total, water makes up 70% of the animal's bodyweight.

- Intracellular water (inside the cells) makes up 50% of the animal's bodyweight.
- Extracellular water (inside the body but not inside the cells) makes up 20% of the animal's bodyweight.

Functions of water

- Digestion: protein, fats and carbohydrates are digested by hydrolysis in water.
- Transport: water-soluble materials are transported in the gut and bloodstream.
- Body temperature regulation: water is an ideal medium to transfer heat.

Water intake

The body cannot store water for long periods and an intake is therefore required to meet demands. Water intake and output *must* be in balance.

Water sources

- Water drunk (as fluid).
- Water in food.
- Metabolic water.

Alternatives to water

Some cats enjoy drinking cow's milk but there are individuals that react adversely to it; they have difficulty digesting it and may develop diarrhoea. For all cats, the milk provided should be limited, as cats find digesting single-unit sugars easy but digesting disaccharides, notably lactose, more difficult. Commercially available 'cat milk' has been developed with a reduced level of lactose (only 5% of that found in normal cow's milk), and can be administered to cats that enjoy milk, without the unpleasant dietary side effects.

Metabolic water

When carbohydrates, proteins and fats are broken down in the body, they release a certain quantity of water. Each nutrient will yield a different amount of water from every gram that is oxidized. Fat creates more water in the body than the weight of fat actually eaten. Therefore if an animal eats a high-fat diet it needs to drink less.

Water output

Water is normally lost in:

- Urine
- Faeces
- Evaporation from the skin
- Expiration from the lungs
- Milk (when a female is lactating).

Water can also be lost abnormally, in:

- Vomit
- Discharges, such as from pyometra
- Diarrhoea.

Oral electrolyte solutions

When the body has lost fluids abnormally, various ions are also lost. A method of both fluid and ion replacement is to give oral electrolyte solutions, which come as powders that are reconstituted with water prior to administration.

Protein

Proteins are very large molecules that consist of hundreds of simple single units called amino acids, joined together to form chains. Each amino acid can be thought of as a building block used to make up a particular protein. Digestion is involved in the breakdown of this protein into its component blocks (amino acids). The body can then assimilate (rebuild) these amino acids into new proteins to form body tissue.

Functions of protein

- Production of energy.
- Tissue building and maintenance.
- Regulation of metabolism (enzymes and some hormones).
- Formation of antibodies.

Protein sources

- Animal sources: meat, fish, eggs, milk.
- Plant sources: soya, cereals.

Protein output

- Energy production.
- Utilized in the body.
- Faeces.
- Urine.
- Hair.
- Skin.
- Sweat.

Protein metabolism

Digestible protein is that part that is absorbed through the gut wall into the body and not lost in faeces. This can range from as low as 50% in some cereals to over 95% for milk or egg protein.

Much protein metabolism takes place in the liver. Unlike fat and carbohydrate, protein contains nitrogen molecules and urea is one of the few safe forms in which nitrogen can be eliminated from the body. Nitrogen is converted to ammonia and eventually urea. This urea can be safely transported in the blood and excreted via the kidneys.

Amino acids

There are 23 amino acids, of which 10 are classified as essential in the dog. These amino acids must be supplied in the diet as the animal is unable to synthesize them from other materials in sufficient quantity to meet its needs.

Non-essential amino acids can be made in the body from other raw materials.

Taurine

In cats, as well as the essential amino acids there is a nutritional requirement for taurine (an aminosulphonic acid). Taurine is only available as a dietary source from animal-derived proteins.

Protein quality

Protein quality is governed by certain characteristics. A high-quality protein should:

- Be well digested and absorbed
- Have a balanced amino acid profile.

Examples of high-quality protein include:

- Eggs
- White fish
- Meat.

Protein deficiency

Lack of one or more amino acids, or an inadequate quantity of protein, can result in deficiency diseases. Signs of protein deficiencies include:

- Lack of appetite
- Poor growth, loss of bodyweight
- Impaired immune function
- Loss of coat condition
- Retinal degeneration (taurine deficiency in cats).

Fat

Fats are made up of a mixture of triglycerides and cholesterol. Each triglyceride is composed of a glycerol backbone with fatty acids attached. The difference between one fat and another is mostly a result of the different combinations of fatty acids attached to this backbone. Some fatty acids are essential (must be ingested) but most can be synthesized in the body.

Fats contain 2.25 times more energy per unit of weight than proteins and carbohydrates. Fats are therefore an extremely good source of concentrated calories.

Functions of fat

- Provides energy.
- Provides essential fatty acids.
- Carrier of fat-soluble vitamins (A, D, E, K).
- Increases dietary palatability.

Fat sources

- Animal sources: dairy produce, meats (variable), fish.
- Plant sources: seed oils, nuts.

Fat output

- Energy production.
- Faeces (a few hydrogenated fats are poorly digested).
- Hair coat condition.
- Deposition in the body.

Essential fatty acids (EFAs)

- Linoleic acid: required by *all* animals.
- Linolenic acid: synthesized from linoleic acid by both cats and dogs.
- Arachidonic acid: essential in the cat; other species can synthesize from linoleic acid. Arachidonic acid is a constituent of animal fat and is not present in plant products of any type.

Signs of EFA deficiency include:

- Poor coat condition
- Skin lesions
- Reproductive failure.

Carbohydrate

Carbohydrates are classified as:

- Polysaccharides: starches and cellulose
- Disaccharides: paired monosaccharides (e.g. sucrose)
- Monosaccharides: simple sugars (e.g. glucose).

The long polysaccharide and short disaccharide chains have to be broken down into simple sugars in order to be digested. The polysaccharide starches are broken down into their component sugars, but cellulose (because of the way the sugars are linked) is not easily digested by single-stomached animals.

Functions of carbohydrate

Carbohydrates are not generally considered to be an essential nutrient in dogs and cats but they are a cheap source of energy.

Carbohydrate sources

- Animal sources: milk sugar (lactose), meat (very small amount, quickly lost after death).
- Plant sources: fruit sugars, cereal starches, root vegetables.

Carbohydrate deficiency

Carbohydrate deficiency is not seen in dogs and cats.

Dietary fibre

Dietary fibre describes the portion of foodstuffs that cannot be broken down by intestinal enzymes and juices of monogastric (single-stomached) animals, and therefore passes through the small intestine and colon undigested. It is mainly composed of cellulose (the skeleton of plants), lignin, pectin and other carbohydrates. It is essential to maintain the health of the gastrointestinal tract.

Minerals (ash)

Minerals are inorganic elements that can be divided into two groups:

- Major minerals: needed in quite large quantities (Figure 6.43)
- Trace minerals: (also know as trace elements) needed in very small amounts (Figure 6.44).

Mineral	Source	Function	Deficiency	Excess
Calcium	Bones, milk, cheese	Bone formation, nerve and muscle formation	Poor growth, rickets, convulsions	Bone deformities
Phosphorus	Bones, milk	Bone formation, energy utilization	Rickets (rare)	Similar signs to calcium deficiency
Potassium	Milk, meat	Water balance, nerve function	Poor growth, paralysis, kidney and heart lesions	Muscular weakness, heart failure
Sodium	Salt, cereals	Water balance, muscle and nerve activity	Poor growth, exhaustion	Thirst, increased blood pressure
Magnesium	Cereals, bones, green vegetables	Bone formation, protein synthesis	Anorexia, vomiting, muscle weakness	Diarrhoea

6.43 Major minerals.

Mineral	Source	Function	Deficiency	Excess
Iron	Eggs, meat (liver), green vegetables	Part of haemoglobin	Anaemia	Weight loss, anorexia
Iodine	Fish, dairy produce	Part of thyroid hormone	Hair loss, apathy, drowsiness	Unknown
Copper	Meat, bones	Part of haemoglobin	Anaemia	Hepatopathy in Bedlington Terriers
Zinc	Meat, cereals	Digestion, tissue maintenance	Hair loss, skin thickening, poor growth	Diarrhoea

6.44 Trace minerals.

Functions of minerals

- Major structural components (e.g. calcium and phosphorus in the skeleton).
- Maintenance of fluid balance (e.g. sodium and potassium).
- Regulation of metabolism through enzyme function.

Mineral balance

It is vital to remember that the balance of minerals in the diet is as important as the quantity.

Calcium and phosphorus

- The calcium to phosphorus (Ca:P) ratio should be 1–1.5:1.
- Pure meat diets have adverse Ca:P ratio of 1:20.

Supplementation

If a good quality prepared pet food is used, there is no need for supplementation in the normal healthy animal. Foods rich in calcium include milk and cheese.

> ⚠️ **WARNING**
>
> **Indiscriminate supplementation with one or even several minerals is likely to be more harmful than beneficial, and is the main cause of mineral imbalances in dogs and cats.**
>
> **For example, over-supplementation with calcium may lead to the development of skeletal abnormalities. It will also interfere with zinc absorption, so that the animal will become zinc deficient.**

Vitamins

Vitamins (Figure 6.45) are complex organic molecules involved in most essential body functions. They are usually needed in only very small quantities.

Fat-soluble vitamins

Fat-soluble vitamins (Figure 6.46) require fat for their absorption, utilization and storage. Once in the body, unused fat-soluble vitamins are not excreted and are therefore potentially quite dangerous if over-supplemented. The storage ability of the fat-soluble vitamins prevents the need for a daily supply.

Water-soluble vitamins

Water-soluble vitamins (B group and vitamin C) (Figure 6.47) are not stored and are therefore required on a daily basis. Unlike humans (and guinea pigs), dogs and cats can produce vitamin C from glucose in the liver to meet their needs.

Feeding a balanced diet

With an awareness of nutritional requirements, one can understand the impact that good and poor nutrition can have on the animals in our care. It is important to feed a balanced diet, which is one that provides all the necessary nutrients at optimal levels. Types of diet are summarized in Figure 6.48. The optimal levels of nutrients will differ between species, and will also change throughout life and are affected by activity level. Feeding an animal a balanced diet throughout life is known as life-stage feeding.

- A **complete diet** is one that contains all the nutrients necessary for a balanced diet. Most commercial foods are complete, including both moist and dry foods.

Vitamin	Name
A	Retinol
B1	Thiamin
B2	Riboflavin
B6	Pyridoxine
B12	(Cyano)cobalamin
C	Ascorbic acid

Vitamin	Name
D2	Ergocalciferol
D3	Cholecalciferol
E	Tocopherol
K1	Phylloquinone
K2	Menaquinone
K3	Menadione

6.45 Common names for vitamins.

Vitamin	Source	Function	Deficiency	Excess
A	Fish oil, liver, vegetables	Vision in poor light, skin maintenance	Night blindness, skin lesions	Anorexia, bone pain (malformation)
D	Cod liver oil, eggs, animal products	Calcium balance, bone growth	Rickets, osteomalacia	Anorexia, calcification of soft tissue
E	Green vegetables, vegetable oils, dairy produce	Reproduction	Infertility, anaemia, muscle weakness	Not known
K	Spinach, green vegetables, liver	Blood clotting	Haemorrhage	Not known

6.46 Fat-soluble vitamins.

Vitamin	Source	Function	Deficiency	Excess
B1	Dairy products, cereals, liver and kidney	Release of energy from carbohydrate	Anorexia, vomiting, paralysis	Not known
B2	Milk, animal tissue	Utilization of energy	Weight loss, weakness, collapse, coma	Not known
B6	Meat, fish, eggs, cereal	Metabolism of amino acids	Anorexia, anaemia, weight loss, convulsions	Not known
BI2	Liver, meat, dairy produce	Division of cells in bone marrow	Anaemia	Not known
Folic acid	Offal, leafy vegetables	Division of cells in bone marrow	Anaemia, poor growth	Not known
C	Fruit, green vegetables	Synthesis of collagen, osteoblast function	Scurvy, gingival haemorrhage, anaemia, epiphyseal fractures	Not known

6.47   Water-soluble vitamins.

Diet	Advantages	Disadvantages
Homemade	Can be made cheaply More control over ingredients used Ingredients such as additives, preservatives and GM foods can be avoided Variety	Time-consuming Detailed understanding of nutrition required to ensure balanced diet is fed
Commercial canned	Balanced diet Easy to measure quantity required Usually palatable	Expensive Difficult to store as bulky Heavy to carry from retail outlet Owners perceive that mixer biscuit must be given (despite most canned food being complete diet), which can lead to overfeeding Once opened, needs to be used quickly If not eaten immediately, can go stale, attract insects, etc.
Commercial dry	Balanced diet More economical, as less wastage Easy to store in airtight containers Can be left in food bowl for access during day without risk of going stale or attracting insects, etc.	Some animals find less palatable More difficult to measure required amounts Owner's perception that animal would prefer moist foods
Commercial semi-moist (sealed packets containing soft processed food)	Individual portion ensures accurate feeding amounts Food remains fresh, as no unopened cans to store High palatability	Expensive

6.48   Types of diet.

- A **complementary diet** is one that is *not* balanced if fed alone. This type of diet needs to be fed in addition to another food. An example is a complementary tinned food fed in conjunction with a complementary biscuit.

Supplementation

Supplements, such as vitamins, minerals and bone meal, are *not* required for routine feeding if a good quality commercial 'balanced' or complete diet is fed. In fact, supplementing a good quality complete diet may lead to nutrient excesses or imbalances. In particular the use of supplements such cod liver oil and bone meal can cause skeletal abnormalities.

Nutritional supplements may be required for managing a specific condition and should be pre-scribed by a veterinary surgeon. This also applies to a wide range of prescription diets, which are used to support conditions such as renal failure, and have adjusted levels of nutrients.

Quantity and frequency of feeding

The quantity of food given must provide all the nutrients in balance, along with the required amount of calories. Therefore, the amount of food needed will depend upon the calorie density. The more calories that are found in a gram of food, the less is the amount of that food required to meet the animal's daily energy requirement.

Commercially available diets provide feeding guides but it is very important that animals are weighed regularly. If there is any undesirable change in bodyweight, the amount fed must be adjusted accordingly.

The suggested feeding pattern for dogs and cats is at least twice per day. It is thought that once daily feeding can cause gastric overload and this can lead to regurgitation.

Fresh water must be available to dogs and cats at all times.

Feeding and water bowls and utensils

Commonly used materials include ceramic, stainless steel and plastic. The advantages and disadvantages of each are summarized in Figure 6.49. Various designs are used and are outlined in Figure 6.50.

All equipment for food preparation should be used only for animals. It should be kept separate during washing and storage, for hygiene reasons.

Type of bowl	Advantages	Disadvantages
Ceramic	Durable Heavy, so difficult to tip over (which prevents spillage)	Breakable Expensive Difficult to clean Heavy, so unsuitable for young animals (could injure themselves)
Steel	Durable Easy to clean Can be sterilized in autoclave	Can be chewed by animal Noisy Lightweight, therefore spillage common
Plastic	Cheap Easy to clean	Can be chewed by animal Lightweight, therefore spillage common

6.49 Advantages and disadvantages of types of food and water bowls.

Type	Description
Standard	Straight-sided bowl for everyday usage
Inward-sloping	Inward-sloping sides, useful for long-eared breeds
Outward-sloping	Outward-sloping sides, suitable for brachycephalic breeds
Raised	Bowl fits into raised platform so that dog does not have to bend over to eat or drink Useful for breeds susceptible to gastric dilatation/torsion as it decreases amount of air swallowed Also useful for animals with neck pain or injuries, or recovering from head, neck or throat surgery
Timer	Bowl with timer-operated lid, allowing controlled feeding over a period of time
Inflatable	Very useful for providing water when travelling away from home in car or on foot
Disposable	Cardboard disposable bowls, very useful when feeding animal with contagious condition
Travel	Bowl with removable rim, which prevents spillage during movement
Litter-feeding system	Litter-feeding system for puppies. Unique segregating stalls that allow each puppy to eat its fair share of food in communal situation, promoting even growth, preventing spillage and allowing medication to be given individually	Litter-feeding system. (Courtesy of Weanafeeda.)

6.50 Types of bowl design.

Water fountains

In kennels, specially adapted water fountains can be installed, where dogs activate the flow of water by licking at the dispenser. This is an excellent system to ensure that water is always fresh and at a suitable temperature.

Water fountain bowls, where a pump ensures that fresh cold water is always flowing, are a particular favourite with cats.

Animal behaviour during feeding

Cats are opportunistic feeders that evolved in circumstances where they had little control over the timing and size of their meals. They have a relatively simple digestive system capable of dealing with large quantities of food in a short period, but given free choice they will nibble several small meals throughout the day and night. Even so, they are excellent at adjusting their energy intake so that it is roughly equal to their energy expenditure. This is why obesity is less common in cats than in dogs.

Dogs are pack animals and it is important that dog owners are aware that they make up the members of their pet's pack. They must therefore consider the importance of 'pecking order' in the feeding regime. The pack leader *always* eats first; therefore, human pack members *must* eat first to ensure that they maintain their dominance within the pack hierarchy.

Many animals become protective over their food, leading to aggression towards their handler. This behaviour is not acceptable, as the handler should be established as pack leader.

Dogs (and sometimes cats) can behave differently at meal times due to excitement. Feeding more than one dog in the same area can lead to fighting and bullying over meals. Each dog should be fed in a separate area to avoid aggression and prevent competitive eating, as the latter encourages dogs to bolt down their food. Bolting leads to regurgitation or aerophagia (swallowing excessive amounts of air), which can result in severe complications in breeds prone to bloating, such as deep-chested breeds (e.g. Great Danes).

Nutrition in life stages

Gestation and lactation

The bitch

Malnourishment of the bitch before and during gestation is thought to contribute to 20–30% of neonatal deaths. However, provided that the bitch is receiving a nutritionally well balanced diet, there is no need to alter the regimen until 5–6 weeks into the pregnancy, when the fetuses start to grow.

Most fetal weight gain occurs in the last 3 weeks of pregnancy. Up to this point in pregnancy, little extra feeding is required. A palatable balanced maintenance diet is suitable, fed at normal rates. From the 5th–6th week onwards, the ration should be increased by 10–15% per week. In late pregnancy, feeding smaller meals of higher-density diets may be required due to the reduced space available in the abdomen for the stomach to expand.

Lactation is the biggest nutritional test of a bitch (and of a queen). Energy requirement depends on litter size, with the maximum demand occurring 4 weeks after the litter is born. Small meals of highly palatable, highly digestible food are required for bitches. In general it is necessary to feed a diet that is specifically formulated for lactation (increased energy-density).

Figure 6.51 gives guidance on feeding pregnant or lactating bitches.

Do:

- Feed a diet formulated for growth or lactation
- Increase calorie intake by 10% weekly until whelping (from 5–6 weeks of pregnancy)
- Feed at frequent intervals during the last 10 days of gestation (as the stomach capacity may be limited by the enlarged uterus)
- Feed 1.5 times maintenance requirement for the first week of lactation
- Feed 2–3 times maintenance requirement during the 2nd and 3rd week or allow free-choice feeding at this stage
- Always allow free access to fresh drinking water, especially during peak lactation
- Commence weaning the puppies from 3 to 4 weeks of age by giving them supplementary feeding and thus decreasing the demand on the bitch.

Do not:

- Give supplements when feeding a good quality prepared growth/lactation diet (calcium or vitamin D supplements can cause soft tissue calcification and physical anomalies in puppies)
- Give unsupplemented meat diets, which are low in calcium
- Increase calorie intake until the 5th–6th week of pregnancy onwards.

6.51 How to feed a pregnant or lactating bitch (with average litter size).

The queen

A pregnant or lactating queen should be fed in a similar manner to the bitch, except that calorie intake should increase from the 5th week of pregnancy. With a growth or lactation diet, it is recommended that the queen should be allowed free-choice feeding at all times.

Growing animals

Pre-weaning

Ideally a puppy or kitten feeds on the bitch's or queen's milk; if this is not possible, the next best approach is fostering. If kittens or puppies are to be hand reared, a proprietary milk substitute is required in the long term as both cow's and goat's milk give inadequate levels of nutrients.

Puppies

Weaning (separation from the mother) normally occurs at 6 weeks of age and preparation for this can start as early as 3–4 weeks of age. Specialized weaning diets are available, or milk replacements and liquidized growth diets can be used, gradually increasing the viscosity of the diet until the puppies are on solid food.

The aim is to reach a growth rate of 2–4 g/day per kilogram of anticipated adult bodyweight. Most puppies attain 50% of their adult weight by 5–6 months of age, but maximal growth does not mean optimal growth. The energy demands of a growing puppy are high and need to be met by frequent meals to enable the necessary volume to be consumed (e.g. a 20 kg 12-week-old puppy needs about 2.5 kg of wet food per day). Puppy food needs to be energy dense and highly digestible, with a suitable amount and balance of vitamins and minerals, particularly calcium and phosphorus.

Mature bodyweight is reached at about 7–8 months of age in small breeds, but not until about 18–24 months of age in giant breeds. Therefore a Chihuahua can move straight from puppy food to adult food. Labradors and larger breeds need an interim food between puppy and adult and these are often described as junior diets.

Figure 6.52 summarizes how to feed a growing puppy.

Do:
- Commence weaning at 3–4 weeks of age
- Aim to reach a growth rate of 2–4 g/day/kg adult weight for the first 5 months of life
- Allow 20–30 minutes to eat each meal
- Offer four meals a day from 4 weeks of age
- Gradually reduce the number of meals to one or two meals per day as the animal approaches adult bodyweight
- Feed toy breeds 3–4 times per day until 6 months of age (they are susceptible to hypoglycaemia)
- Gradually (over 3–4 days) change from one diet to another when required.

Do not:
- Overfeed to increase growth rates – maximum growth rate is not in the best interest of the dog. Adult body size is not determined by growth rate as a puppy
- Supplement with minerals and vitamins when a suitable good quality pet food is used
- Allow the puppy to become overweight – a fat puppy becomes a fat adult
- Allow free-choice feeding until the dog has reached 80–90% of anticipated adult weight
- Allow food not eaten within 30 minutes to remain available
- Change from one diet to another rapidly, as this can lead to dietary disturbances and subsequent diarrhoea.

6.52   How to feed a growing puppy.

Kittens

Kittens may be fed on a free-choice basis on a growth diet from 3 weeks of age. As with puppies, supplementation should be avoided. Energy requirement/kg bodyweight peaks at about 10 weeks of age but tends to be lower than that of puppies, as the percentage increase over birth weight is smaller, although they achieve a higher percentage of adult weight (75%) by 6 months of age.

Maintenance

Average maintenance requirements can be estimated and are indicated on all good quality pet foods. Some of the terms used in these estimations are as follows:

- Basal metabolic rate (BMR); also called basal energy requirement (BER): the minimal energy expended for the maintenance of respiration, circulation, peristalsis, muscle tone, body temperature, glandular activity and other body functions
- Resting energy requirement (RER): energy required at rest
- Maintenance energy requirement (MER): energy required in an active animal.

Factors that affect maintenance energy requirement include:

- The animal's life stage
- Pregnancy and lactation
- Illness or disease
- Environmental conditions (e.g. temperature)
- Level of activity
- Reproductive state (MER often decreases after neutering).

Obesity

It is important to realize that regular assessment of an individual's weight is required in order to prevent under- or (more commonly) overfeeding. Many commercial pet foods are now available to cater for animals prone to obesity; the foods provide reduced calories but still satisfy hunger.

- Dogs are pack hunters and therefore tend to eat voraciously whenever food is available; they are therefore prone to obesity.
- Cats are solitary hunters; they eat every few hours and are therefore unlikely to overeat when offered free-choice food.

Working dogs

Working dogs have an increased energy requirement, as a result of their lifestyle. Depending on the level of activity, dogs may have, in general, requirements as much as 2–3 times their adult maintenance. These increased energy requirements are often met by feeding a calorie-dense high-fat diet. Few dogs, despite many owners' beliefs, are truly active. A 5 km run will increase a dog's requirements by around 10%. Maximum demands occur in dogs travelling long distances in cold conditions, where they have an energy requirement of 4–5 times maintenance.

Diets should meet the needs for muscular work and stress. For short-burst athletic dogs, such as greyhounds, increased carbohydrates are required; for sustained effort, particularly at low temperatures, energy needs are best met through high-fat, low-carbohydrate diets. There is no evidence that an increase in dietary protein is required. It has been suggested that working dogs may have an increased requirement for iron, vitamin E and selenium.

Generally, working dogs need a highly palatable, energy-dense, highly digestible and nutritionally balanced diet.

Older animals

In general, older animals are less active. This can lead to energy requirements being 20% less than their previous maintenance level. For this reason, it is clear that a reduction in calorific intake is required in order to prevent obesity.

Older animals are also prone to conditions such as constipation, and for this reason other nutritional considerations are made when preparing food for the ageing animal (Figure 6.53). There is now a wide range of diets available for all stages of life, including those designed for the older animal.

- Reduce energy intake if weight gain is evident.
- Reduce fat intake, again in order to prevent obesity.
- Divide total daily food allowance over two to three meals to aid digestion.
- Increase fibre intake if constipation is evident.
- Feed highly palatable and easily digested foods.
- Consider that alterations in the gastrointestinal tract and general metabolism may result in increased requirements for vitamins A, B1, B6, B12 and E.
- Seek veterinary surgeon's advice on the need to reduce sodium, phosphorus and protein levels if clinical examination indicates organ failure (for example kidney, liver or heart).

6.53   How to feed ageing pets.

The requirements for vitamins, particularly water-soluble vitamins (B and C), may be increased, due to increased water turnover. A decrease in energy requirements and nutrient density needs to be balanced against the tendency to a poorer appetite. A compromise of a highly palatable diet with mildly reduced nutrient density and increased vitamin levels is currently recommended. Increasing the number of feeds per day is also desirable.

Clinical diets

A clinical diet is one that has been formulated to control or treat a specific condition (Figure 6.54). There are many different ranges of clinical diets, which are available only from veterinary surgeons: an appropriate diet can be prescribed for a given condition.

Condition	Specific nutritional requirements
Renal failure	Moderated levels of high-quality protein Low phosphorus Potassium levels increased for cats Moderate sodium restriction Increased B-complex vitamins
Liver disease	Moderated levels of high-quality protein Increased zinc, B-complex vitamins and vitamin E Restricted copper Moderate fat restriction and increased fibre
Congestive heart failure	Moderately restricted high-quality protein Salt restriction generally felt to be beneficial Magnesium supplementation Potassium supplementation or restriction, depending on serum levels
Cardiomyopathy	Feline taurine-deficient dilated cardiomyopathy: taurine supplementation Canine dilated myopathy: L-carnitine may be of value

6.54   Examples of clinical conditions and their specific nutritional requirements. (This is not an exhaustive list as the range of conditions for which the importance of dietary support has been acknowledged has developed considerably over recent years and is constantly expanding.)

References and further reading

Anderson RS and Edney ATB (1991) *Practical Animal Handling*. Butterworth-Heinemann, Oxford

Blood DC and Studdert VP (1990) *Baillière's Comprehensive Veterinary Dictionary*. Baillière Tindall, London

Earle KE (1990) Feeding for health. *Journal of Small Animal Practice* **31**, 477–481

Evans JM and White K (1992) *The Doglopaedia*. Henston, Guildford

Lane D, Cooper B and Turner L (2007) *BSAVA Textbook of Veterinary Nursing, 4th edn*. BSAVA Publications, Gloucester

Masters J and Bowden C (2001) *Pre-Veterinary Nursing Textbook*. Butterworth-Heinemann, Oxford

O'Farrell V (1992) *Manual of Canine Behaviour*. BSAVA Publications, Cheltenham

Thorne (1992) *The Waltham Book of Dog and Cat Behaviour*. Pergamon Press, Oxford

7

Use of medicines

Sally Anne Argyle and Heather Roberts

This chapter is designed to give information on:

- The definition of the term 'veterinary medicines'
- The main categories of veterinary medicines
- The main routes used for the administration of drugs
- The advantages and disadvantages of each route of administration
- The equipment used in the administration of medicines
- Practical information regarding the administration of drugs
- The legislation and practicalities regarding the safe handling, storage and dispensing of veterinary medicines

---

Veterinary medicines

According to the Veterinary Medicines Directorate (www.vmd.gov.uk) and based on European Community law, a veterinary medicine is defined as: (a) any substance or combination of substances presented as having properties for treating or preventing disease in animals; or (b) any substance or combination of substances which may be used in or administered to animals with a view either to restoring, correcting or modifying physiological functions by exerting a pharmacological, immunological or metabolic action or to making a medical diagnosis.

The main categories of veterinary medicines are listed in Figure 7.1.

Category	Definition	Examples
Anaesthetics	Used to produce unconsciousness, immobility and a loss of sensation such as pain	Injectable agents such as propofol and thiopental Inhalation agents such as halothane and isoflurane
Analgesics	Designed to relieve pain	Opioids such as pethidine and morphine NSAIDs such as meloxicam and carprofen Local anaesthetics such as lidocaine
Antiarrhythmics	Used to abolish or control abnormal heart rhythms	Lidocaine, procainamide

7.1 Examples of some of the main categories of veterinary medicines. (continues) ▶

Category	Definition	Examples
Antibacterials	Kill (bactericidal) or inhibit the growth of (bacteriostatic) bacteria	Bacteriostatic: sulphonamides and tetracyclines Bactericidal: ampicillin, amoxicillin and streptomycin
Antidiarrhoeals	Used in the treatment of diarrhoea	Loperamide, kaolin
Anti-emetics	Prevent vomiting	Metoclopramide, maropitant
Anti-epileptics	Used to prevent or abolish seizures	Phenobarbital, primidone
Antifungals	Kill (fungicidal) or inhibit the growth of (fungistatic) fungi	Orally administered preparations such as griseofulvin Topically administered preparations such as miconazole
Anti-inflammatory drugs	Used to reduce inflammation	Non-steroidal anti-inflammatory drugs (NSAIDs) such as meloxicam and carprofen Corticosteroids such as prednisolone
Antineoplastics	Treat neoplasia	Cyclophosphamide, vincristine
Antitussives	Suppress coughing	Butorphanol
Anti-ulcer drugs	Used for treatment and prevention of gastric ulcers	Cimetidine, sucralfate, omeprazole, misoprostil
Bronchodilators	Dilate the bronchial smooth muscle	Etamiphylline, clenbuterol
Cardiac drugs	Exert their effect on the cardiovascular system	Digoxin, enalapril
Diuretics	Enhance water loss through the kidneys	Furosemide, spironolactone, hydrochlorothiazide
Ectoparasiticides	Used in the treatment and prevention of external parasite infestation (e.g. flea control)	Imidacloprid, fipronil, selamectin
Emetics	Induce vomiting	Xylazine, apomorphine
Endoparasiticides	Used in treatment and prevention of internal parasitic infections (e.g. tapeworm, roundworm)	Fenbendazole, praziquantal, pyrantel
Hormones	Substances produced endogenously (within the body) by endocrine glands. Naturally occurring or synthetic substances may be administered exogenously	Estradiol benzoate, proligesterone, methyltestosterone
Laxatives	Aid the passage of faecal material	Liquid paraffin, lactulose, bran
Sedatives	Used to calm animal, often prior to anaesthetic induction or for minor procedures such as radiography	Acepromazine, xylazine
Vaccines	Stimulate the animal's active immunity to an organism, such as bacterium, virus or parasite	Canine parvovirus vaccine, leptospirosis vaccine, parainfluenza virus vaccine

7.1 (continued) Examples of some of the main categories of veterinary medicines.

Routes of administration

The most frequently used routes of administration of drugs are summarized in Figure 7.2.

Oral administration

This is a frequently used route of administration.

Drugs to be administered orally are most often in a solid form such as a tablet or a capsule. They may also be in a liquid form, such as a suspension or a solution.

- In a **suspension** the drug is dispersed in the fluid in the form of fine liquid or solid particles; the drug particles have a tendency to settle at the bottom of the container when the vessel in which the drug is contained is left standing.
- In a **solution** the drug is dissolved in the liquid, giving a homogenous mixture.

Common sense should be exercised when handling any drugs. Special care should be taken by individuals with known sensitivities to particular drugs. For

Route	Detail	Advantages	Disadvantages
Oral	Tablets, capsules or liquid	Often well tolerated by the animal Owner may administer drug at home	Some drugs cannot be given orally (e.g. penicillin G, which may be broken down by gastric acid) Animal may not be compliant, making dosing difficult especially if drug cannot be administered with food Gastrointestinal disease may interfere with drug absorption
By injection (parenteral)	Solutions or suspensions Examples of routes: ■ Intradermal (i.d.) ■ Subcutaneous (s.c.) ■ Intramuscular (i.m.) ■ Intravenous (i.v.) ■ Intraperitoneal (i.p.)	Rapid systemic drug levels achieved, especially with i.v. route No reliance on gastrointestinal function	Animal may experience pain on injection Local reaction to injection may occur Risk of self-injection Generally not suitable for owner administration Risk of damage to internal organs (e.g. i.p. injection) Risk of perivascular injection with the i.v. route
Intraosseous	Useful for administration of fluids and drugs to neonates or where not possible to access peripheral vessel	Rapid access Useful in neonates	Strict aseptic technique is essential
Intranasal	Limited to certain vaccines		Resented by many animals
Rectal	Infrequently used. Mainly confined to laxatives and some anti-epileptics	Good vascular supply ensures rapid absorption	
Transdermal	Mainly used for drugs metabolized by liver so rapidly that oral administration is prevented	Ease of application	Risk of absorption by administrator
Topical	Examples include drugs formulated as lotions, ointments, gels and shampoos	Ease of administration Direct delivery to required site Owner can administer	Absorption of drug through skin of administrator Animal can lick drug Limited to sites that can be accessed (e.g. skin, ears, eyes)
Inhalation	Limited to inhalation anaesthetics such as halothane, and some drugs administered by nebulization (e.g. gentamicin)	Direct delivery of drug to site of action in the case of nebulized drugs for respiratory disease	Limited application Specialized equipment required

7.2   A summary of the main routes used for drug administration.

example, penicillin sensitivity is widespread in the general human population and owners asked to administer drugs to their animals need to be informed. Ideally, gloves should be worn at all times, preferably latex free.

It should be determined whether or not the drug should be given with food. For example, the absorption of the antifungal drug griseofulvin is enhanced by the presence of fatty food, whereas the antibacterial drug ampicillin is best given on an empty stomach.

Tablets and capsules

Figure 7.3 illustrates how an animal may be restrained for the administration of a tablet or capsule:

1. The mouth is held open and the medicine is dropped or placed at the back of the tongue.

2. The mouth should then be allowed to close but the head held slightly tipped back.

3. Once the mouth is closed, the animal will swallow as a reflex action to the tablet or capsule on the back of the tongue.

Capsules should not be split. Some tablets (for example, many of the cytotoxic drugs used to treat neoplasia) should not be divided.

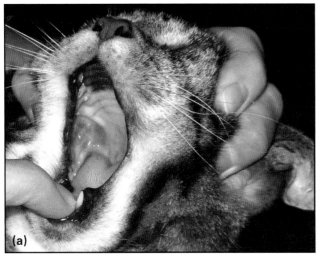

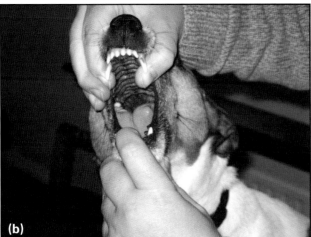

7.3 Methods of restraint for oral administration of tablets and capsules. **(a)** Cat. **(b)** Dog.

Liquids

- Liquid suspensions should be well shaken to re-suspend drug particles that will have settled to the bottom of the container.
- Administration of liquid medication is best performed with a syringe; with some preparations a plastic dropper is provided.
- Liquids are best administered into the side of the mouth, at a slow rate, allowing the animal to swallow frequently.

Other methods of oral administration

A crop tube may be used for the oral administration of drugs to birds (see Chapter 4). A similar approach may be used in chelonians.

Some drugs may be administered in the drinking water. This can be useful for the medication of large numbers of animals but is unreliable due to the inevitable variability in water intake.

Parenteral administration

This is a commonly used route of drug administration. The term parenteral refers to a route of administration of drugs into the body that bypasses the enteral (i.e. gastrointestinal) tract. Most commonly, this involves drug administration by injection.

Equipment

Hypodermic needles and syringes are the items of equipment used to administer drugs parenterally. Figure 7.4 illustrates examples of hypodermic needles and syringes.

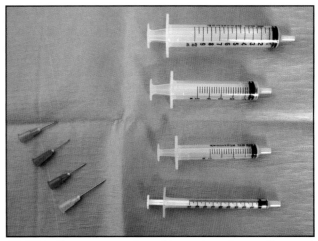

7.4 Some examples of hypodermic needles and syringes used for parenteral administration of veterinary medicines.

- Needles are sized according to their gauge (G).
- The gauge determines the bore of the needle. Commonly used sizes are 25 G, 23 G, 21 G, 20 G, 18 G, 16 G and 14 G. The bore of the needle decreases with increasing gauge size. The needles have a bevelled end, which facilitates entry through the skin.
- Each gauge can also come in a variety of lengths, commonly used ones being 5/8 inch (15.9 mm), 1 inch (25 mm) and 1.5 inches (40 mm).

For intravenous administration of drugs, intravenous cannulae may be used (Figure 7.5).

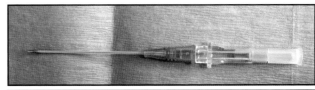

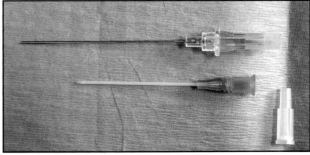

7.5 An example of an over-the-needle catheter. **Top**: A fully assembled catheter. **Bottom**: The various components comprising: the rigid stylet used to insert the catheter; the Teflon catheter which remains in the vein; the bung which is used to seal the catheter when not in use.

Practical points on parenteral administration

- Drugs for injection may come as solutions, emulsions or suspensions. Suspensions should be well shaken to re-suspend the drug before use, and should never be given by the intravenous route.
- All equipment used for parenteral administration should be sterile and should not be reused.
- As far as possible drugs should not be mixed in the same syringe, to avoid cross-contamination.
- Bottles containing drugs for parenteral administration are usually equipped with a rubber bung (Figure 7.6). To withdraw the drug from the bottle or vial:
  1. The bottle should be inverted.
  2. The needle on the end of the syringe should be inserted into the bottle.
  3. It is usually good practice to inject a volume of air equal to the volume of drug to be withdrawn to prevent a vacuum developing in the air-tight sealed bottles. It is important, however, not to inject *too much* air as this may cause the drug to spray out through the seal.
  4. The plunger of the syringe should then be drawn out of the barrel of the syringe, drawing the drug into the syringe.
  5. Excess air should be removed from the syringe by inverting the syringe (needle uppermost) and gently tapping the barrel to bring the air to the top. The air can then be gently expelled without spraying the drug. The use of a sterile gauze pad to absorb any drug leakage from the needle is useful.
- Drugs for parenteral administration may also come in individual glass vials.
- Care should be taken to avoid accidental self-injection and skin contact with the drugs being used (gloves should be worn).
- After use, all needles should be disposed of in a sharps bin (Figure 7.7).

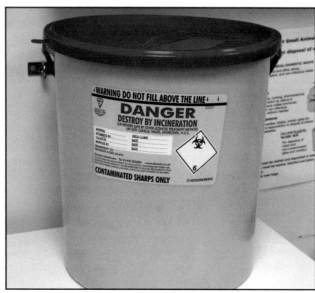

7.7 Example of a yellow container used for the disposal of 'sharps' (such as used hypodermic needles). Once full, the container is sealed and incinerated.

Sites for injection

> **WARNING**
> Follow the manufacturer's directions with regard to the route of administration. For example, some drugs are highly irritant and can only be given intravenously, or drugs recommended for intramuscular administration may be too poorly absorbed to achieve adequate levels in the blood if they are given subcutaneously.

Intradermal injection

This route is used primarily for allergy testing and is therefore a less common parenteral route in small animal practice. Figure 7.8 demonstrates the site of the dermis in relation to the other skin layers. Only very small volumes can be injected into the dermis.

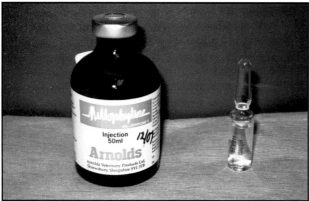

7.6 Injectable containers. **Left:** A typical multi-dose bottle containing a drug in liquid form for parenteral administration. A rubber bung seals the bottle and the needle is inserted through this to draw up the drug at each use. It is good practice to note the date of first use on multi-use bottles as once opened they have a limited shelf-life. **Right:** A glass vial designed for single use. The top is snapped off and all parts disposed of in a sharps bin once the drug has been used.

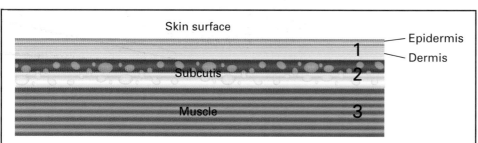

7.8 The layers of the skin and underlying tissues, illustrating the sites of: (1) intradermal injection; (2) subcutaneous injection; and (3) intramuscular injection.

Subcutaneous injection

This is often performed at the scruff of the neck but may be performed at any site where there is sufficient loose skin. Figure 7.8 shows the location of the subcutis in relation to the other skin layers. Figure 7.9 illustrates the technique for subcutaneous injection.

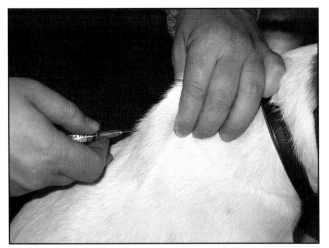

7.9 Example of a subcutaneous injection site. The dog's head is to the right, tail to the left. The injection is made under the loose skin overlying the shoulders, into the skin 'tent'.

1. The skin is raised with one hand to form a 'tent'.
2. The needle is inserted under the skin.
3. Negative pressure should be applied by withdrawing the plunger slightly to ensure that the needle has not been placed in a blood vessel.
4. The plunger should then be depressed slowly to discharge the drug from the syringe. If resistance is met, this may suggest that the needle is not in the subcutaneous layer.

Subcutaneous injections tend to elicit less pain than other parenteral routes, but absorption of the drug is relatively slow from this site and is sometimes unreliable. Certain conditions such as shock or dehydration, in which the peripheral circulation is constricted, may further prolong or reduce absorption from this site, and this should be a consideration when medicating very sick animals.

Intramuscular injection

This is injection of the drug into a muscle mass. The best sites are those with a large muscle bulk.

■ A commonly used site in the dog and cat is the quadriceps muscle mass at the front of the thigh (Figure 7.10); another is the epaxial muscles which run along the length of the spine.
■ In birds, the pectoral muscles (those overlying the breast) are preferred.

Because of the greater blood supply, absorption from this route is generally much faster and more reliable than from the subcutaneous route. However, intramuscular injection is quite painful and only small volumes can be injected at a given time. For example,

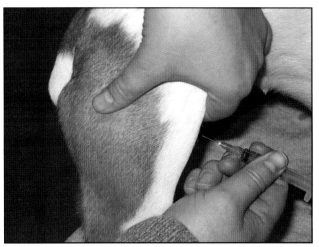

7.10 Site for intramuscular injection in the hindlimb of the dog.

approximately 1.5 ml would be the maximum *desirable* volume for intramuscular injection into the hindlimb of a medium-sized dog.

Care should be taken to avoid blood vessels (negative pressure should be applied on the syringe prior to injection). The inadvertent insertion of the needle into a blood vessel is much more likely using this route than the subcutaneous route.

Intravenous injection

This involves injection directly into a vein.

■ The most commonly used vessels in dogs and cats are the cephalic vein, the jugular vein and the lateral saphenous vein (Figures 7.11, 7.12 and 7.13).
■ The marginal ear vein is commonly used in rabbits (Figure 7.14).

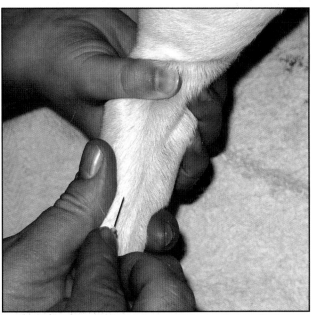

7.11 The cephalic vein runs down the anterior aspect of the forelimb. Note how the person restraining the animal raises the vein with their thumb. The person administering the injection uses their thumb alongside the vein to stabilize it while the tip of the needle is inserted.

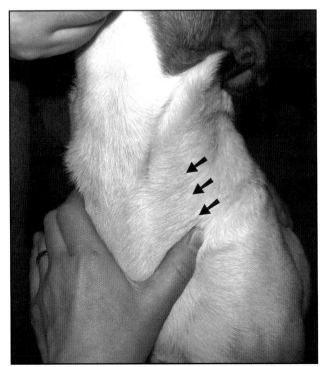

7.12 Method for restraining an animal to allow injection into a jugular vein. The animal could also be restrained in lateral recumbency. The thumb of the person administering the injection is used to apply pressure to raise the vein (arrows demonstrate approximate location of the jugular vein).

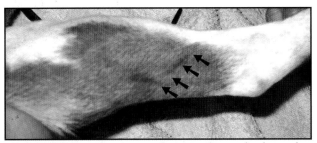

7.13 The saphenous vein runs down the lateral aspect of the hindlimb. Usually the animal is held in lateral recumbency and the vein is raised by applying pressure behind the stifle joint (arrows show location of the saphenous vein).

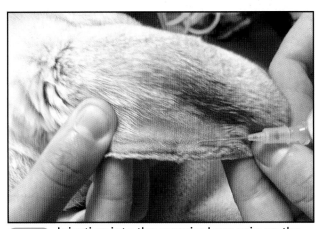

7.14 Injection into the marginal ear vein on the outer aspect of a rabbit's ear. The vessel is raised by application of pressure at the ear base. (Reproduced from *BSAVA Manual of Rabbit Medicine and Surgery, 2nd edn.*)

This route of administration bypasses the need for drug absorption into the bloodstream and so rapid systemic drug levels are achieved, often taking effect within seconds. The route is suitable for the administration of large volumes of a suitable drug.

1. To allow the vessel to be seen accurately and to improve aseptic technique, hair overlying the vessel should be carefully clipped away.
2. The vein is raised by an assistant.
3. The skin is swabbed with a skin preparation fluid (e.g. Hibiscrub or surgical spirit) and the tip of the needle is placed into the vein.
4. At this point it should be confirmed that the needle tip is correctly positioned in the vein by applying negative pressure on the syringe plunger to draw blood back into the hub of the needle (the 'flashback').
5. The assistant then removes pressure from the vein so that the drug may be injected.
6. Injection of the drug should be performed slowly unless it is specified otherwise by the manufacturer.

Intravenous cannulae should be used at all times for the administration of drugs into the jugular vein, as due to the mobility of the vein the risk of perivascular leakage is too great when using a needle.

> ⚠ **WARNING**
> **Some drugs are extremely irritant. This includes many of the cytotoxic drugs,** such as vincristine and doxorubicin. These should be administered using intravenous catheters, to avoid the risk of perivascular leakage of the drug. It is best to flush these catheters with non-heparinized 0.9% sterile saline as some of the drugs (e.g. doxorubicin) precipitate in the presence of heparin.

Intraperitoneal injection

This is administration of the drug into the peritoneal cavity of the abdomen. It provides a large surface area for drug absorption and is mainly used for the administration of fluids in small patients and neonates, and the administration of injectable anaesthetics in small mammals. There is a risk of penetration of abdominal viscera.

The best position is with the animal's forelimbs raised off the ground. The needle is inserted just caudal to the umbilicus, angling the needle cranially.

Intraosseous injection

This is used to deliver the drug directly into the bone marrow cavity. It is a useful route when it is not possible to access a peripheral vein such as the cephalic or the saphenous (a common situation in neonates).

Sites used include the trochanteric fossa of the femur, the proximal tibia and the greater tubercle of the humerus.

Intranasal administration

This route is used for the administration of certain vaccines, such as the *Bordetella bronchiseptica* vaccine. A special delivery nozzle is supplied with the vaccine for delivery into the nasal cavity. The nozzle is attached to the syringe containing the vaccine.

- With the animal's head tipped upwards, the tip of the nozzle is inserted gently into one of its nostrils.
- The vaccine is then delivered into the nasal cavity. It is wise to keep the head tilted upwards for a few moments following administration.

Rectal administration

This route of drug administration is less frequently used in animals than in humans. The lining of the large intestine provides a large surface area for the absorption of drugs delivered by this route. An example would be diazepam for a dog suffering an epileptic seizure.

- Enema solutions are delivered per rectum.
- Gloves should be worn.
- Urinary catheters or rubber tubing, in conjunction with syringes, may be used for the administration of solutions that are not already supplied in long-nozzled delivery tubes designed for the purpose.

Transdermal administration

This route, in which the drug is applied to the skin to be absorbed through the skin and act systemically, is not commonly used in veterinary medicine. Examples of drugs administered in this way are fentanyl (a drug used for pain relief) and glyceryl trinitrate (a drug used in heart failure to dilate the veins).

- Care should be exercised to protect the administrator from absorbing the drug. Gloves must be worn.
- The drug is usually applied to a site that is largely inaccessible to the animal and that has minimal hair cover (such as the inner aspect of the ear pinna). Clipping may be required.

Topical administration

This commonly used route encompasses the administration of drugs to the ear, the eye and the skin. It is commonly used in the treatment and prevention of skin conditions.

- Care should be taken to avoid contact with the skin of the person administering the treatment – gloves should be worn.
- Excess hair may need to be clipped from the site to allow access to the skin.

There is a wide variety of formulations for topical administration, including the following:

- Creams: water-miscible; non-greasy; are easily removed by washing and licking
- Ointments: greasy; insoluble in water and generally anhydrous; more difficult to remove than creams

- Dusting powders: finely divided powders
- Lotions: aqueous solutions or suspension, evaporate to leave a thin film of drug at the site
- Gels: semi-solid aqueous solutions; easy to apply and remove
- Sprays
- Shampoos.

Ophthalmic administration (application to the eye)

Figure 7.15 demonstrates the administration of an eye preparation. The eyelids are held apart with the thumb and the index finger.

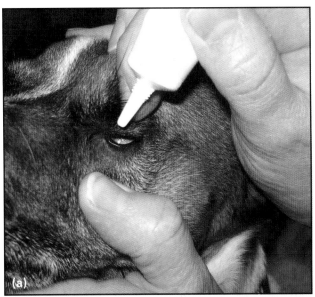

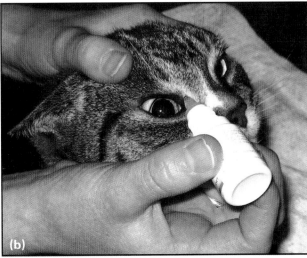

7.15 Administration of **(a)** eye ointment in a dog and **(b)** eye drops in a cat.

- **Liquid solutions** (eye drops) are dropped on to the surface of the eye, following the manufacturer's recommendations on how many drops to apply and at what frequency.
- **Eye ointment** is semi-solid and greasier in consistency. A length of ointment can be squeezed on to the lower palpebral surface (lower eyelid border); when the animal blinks, the ointment is distributed over the eye surface.

> **WARNING**
> Care should be taken to avoid contact between the dispenser/container and the surface of the eye, as this would contaminate the container and may also traumatize the eye.

Aural administration (application to the ear)

Ear disease is extremely common in small animals and this is a frequently used route of administration.

1. Any loose dirt or debris should be removed from the ear using tissue, gauze or cotton wool.
2. The pinna of the ear is grasped gently and pulled upwards while the animal is well restrained.
3. The tip of the dispenser is then placed into the vertical canal of the ear and the drug is administered to the ear (Figure 7.16).
4. The base of the ear is gently massaged to distribute the medication within the ear canal.

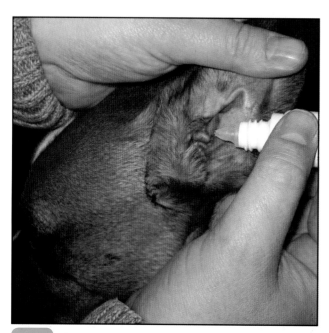

7.16 Administration of ear ointment.

> **WARNING**
> Do not poke anything like a cotton bud into the ear canal. As a general rule, avoid inserting anything smaller than the little finger into the canal, to avoid damage to the ear drum.

Inhalation

Administration of drugs by inhalation is mainly confined to gaseous and volatile anaesthetics, such as halothane, isoflurane and nitrous oxide. The equipment required for the administration of these is covered in the *BSAVA Manual of Practical Veterinary Nursing*.

Nebulization

Nebulization is useful in the treatment of respiratory disease as an adjunct to systemic treatment. A nebulizer (Figure 7.17) produces small droplets forming a mist in which the drug is contained. The mist can then be inhaled by the animal.

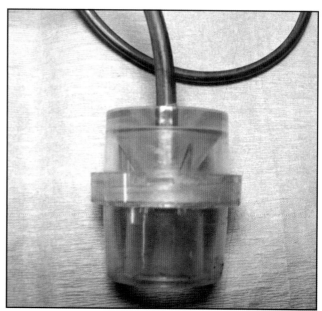

7.17 A nebulizer. It unscrews so that the drug solution can be placed in the central chamber. One end is then connected to an oxygen supply and the other to a facemask. The oxygen flowing through creates a mist containing the drug, which is inhaled by the animal.

This route is useful for the administration of drugs that are very toxic when administered systemically. A good example of this would be gentamicin, an antibacterial drug that can be associated with nephrotoxicity (toxicity to the kidneys) when administered systemically. Care must be taken to prevent exposure of personnel.

Legislation

The legislation regarding the handling, usage, storage, dispensing, disposal and prescribing of veterinary medicines is covered in some detail in the *BSAVA Manual of Practical Veterinary Nursing*. Due to the importance of this topic, pertinent points are also outlined here.

The legislation is constantly changing, most recently on 30th October 2005 when The Veterinary Medicines Regulations 2005 superseded the Medicines Act 1968.

Relevant legislation includes:

- Veterinary Medicines Regulations 2005
- Health and Safety at Work etc. Act 1974
- Control of Substances Hazardous to Health Regulations 2002 (enacted under the Health and Safety at Work etc. Act 1974)
- Misuse of Drugs Act 1971 (Modification) Order 2001.

Figure 7.18 lists the legal categories of veterinary medicines.

Category	Definition
AVM–GSL	*Authorised Veterinary Medicine – General Sales List* Sale of these is unrestricted. May be sold by a veterinary surgeon to anyone, whether they are a client or not. May also be sold by other retailers, e.g. supermarkets. Will roughly be equivalent to the original GSL category
POM–VPS	*Prescription Only Medicine – Veterinarian, Pharmacist & Suitably Qualified Persons* May be prescribed by an RQP (registered qualified person, which includes a registered veterinary surgeon, a registered pharmacist or a suitably qualified person (SQP)[a]). A clinical assessment of the animal is not a prerequisite prior to prescribing
NFA–VPS	*Non-Food Producing Animals – Veterinarian, Pharmacist & Suitably Qualified Persons* Applies to products intended for non-food producing animals. A clinical assessment is not a prerequisite and these medicines may be supplied by an RQP (registered veterinary surgeon, registered pharmacist or SQP[a])
POM–V	*Prescription Only Medicine – Veterinarian* Prescribed by a veterinary surgeon to animals under their care following clinical assessment. May also be supplied by a registered pharmacist or other registered veterinary surgeon in accordance with a written prescription from the animal's own vet
Controlled drug (CD)	Drugs capable of being abused. Under the control of the Misuse of Drugs Act; divided into five Schedules: **Schedule 1** Veterinary surgeons have no authority to possess these. Examples: cannabis, LSD **Schedule 2** A requisition in writing is required to obtain these and they need to be recorded in a register and kept in a locked receptacle. Examples: morphine, pethidine **Schedule 3** As for Schedule 2 but transactions do not need to be recorded in a register. Examples: phenobarbital, buprenorphine **Schedule 4** Exempt from most restrictions of controlled drugs. Example: benzodiazepines **Schedule 5** Exempt from all controlled drug requirements except the need to keep invoices for two years. Example: preparations containing codeine and morphine at less than a specified amount

7.18 Legal categories of veterinary medicines. [a] = Veterinary nurses may only be classed as a Suitably Qualified Person (SQP) if they have studied and passed the appropriate training module. This module is available as a separate 'top-up' course for qualified veterinary nurses.

Handling of veterinary medicines

Control of Substances Hazardous to Health Regulations 2002

COSHH regulations relate to work involving substances that are deemed to be hazardous to health. These include certain veterinary medicines and animal products. It is the employer's responsibility to perform a risk assessment for each of these substances used. Manufacturers of veterinary products provide a product safety data sheet to aid this risk assessment. *The employer must aim to prevent or control exposure of employees to these substances by information, instruction and training.* A responsibility also extends to the client and the client should therefore be clearly informed with regard to the safe handling and disposal of the medicine.

> ⚠ **WARNING**
> **Anyone involved in the handling or dispensing of veterinary medicines should be sufficiently trained.**

Practical points for handling and dispensing of medicines

- Direct contact between the skin of the person dispensing the drug and the drug itself should be avoided. This can be achieved through wearing protective clothing, such as disposable gloves, or by using pill counters.
- The veterinary surgeon should be notified of skin abrasions and the dispensing of drugs should be avoided under these circumstances.
- Particular care should be taken with drugs marked **teratogenic** (capable of causing a malformation in the developing embryo) or **carcinogenic** (capable of causing cancer).
- The data sheet should always be consulted, especially if the individual dispensing the drug is not familiar with the particular drug in question.
- Drugs should be appropriately labelled and dispensed in an appropriate container (see 'Labelling' and 'Containers', below).
- The client should be given clear instructions with regard to the safe handling, storage and disposal of the medicine (for example, some products

should be kept refrigerated). It may be necessary to give the client disposable gloves for the application of certain externally used products.

Cytotoxic drugs

Cytotoxic drugs, such as cyclophosphamide, require extreme care in handling and administration as many are highly toxic and irritant.

- Appropriate protective clothing should be worn.
- The drugs should be prepared in a designated area.
- Tablets must never be divided or crushed.
- These drugs should not be handled by pregnant women.

Figure 7.19 illustrates a self-contained fume hood which may be used to dispense cytotoxic drugs. All procedures are carried out within the hood, which is provided with a filter, thereby protecting the individual from inhalation of the drug. It also clearly allows the designation of an area in which cytotoxic drugs are to be handled. These units are not commonplace in veterinary practice.

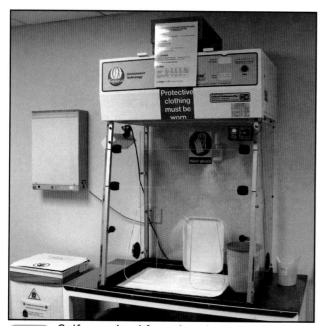

7.19 Self-contained fume hood used solely for the dispensing of cytotoxic drugs. The hood contains a sharps bin and a filter is attached to the top of the hood. A removable tray allows for easy cleaning.

Labelling

Details covering prescription writing and labelling are given in the *BSAVA Manual of Practical Veterinary Nursing*. Figure 7.20 gives an example of a dispensing label for a veterinary drug. Abbreviations commonly used in prescription writing are shown in Figure 7.21 (see also Chapter 10).

Essential information that *legally must be provided* on the label includes:

For Animal Treatment Only
Mr Ebb's dog Flo
21 Seaside Lane
Beach Town
1/1/2000

20 Ampicillin tablets 250 mg
1 tablet twice daily without food

Keep all medicines out of the reach of children

S.A. Argyle, MRCVS
Veterinary Surgeon
1 Seaside Lane
Beach Town

7.20 Example of correct labelling of a veterinary medicine.

Abbreviation	Latin phrase	Meaning
o.d.	*omni die*	Once daily
sid	*semel in die*	Once daily
b.d.s.	*bis die*	Twice daily
bid	*bis in die*	Twice daily
tid	*ter in die*	Three times daily
qid	*quater in die*	Four times daily

7.21 Abbreviations commonly used in veterinary practice.

- The statement 'for animal treatment only'
- The name and address of the owner and the identity of the animal (i.e. the animal's name)
- The date
- The statement 'Keep out of the reach of children'
- The name and address of the veterinary practice.

Information that it is *recommended* should appear on the label includes:

- Details of the drug (name, strength and amount)
- Instructions for administration
- Instructions for storage.

Containers

Many veterinary medicines may be dispensed from bulk containers and should therefore be packaged in suitable containers when dispensed to the public.

- Resealable child-resistant containers made of light-resistant glass, rigid plastic or aluminium should be used. Elderly or infirm clients may require more easily opened containers and discretion may be used in these circumstances.

- Blister-packed medicines may be dispensed in paperboard cartons or wallets.
- Paper envelopes and plastic bags are not acceptable as sole containers of products.
- Creams, dusting powders, ointments, powders and pessaries should be supplied in wide-mouthed jars made of glass or plastic.
- Light-sensitive medicines should be dispensed in opaque or amber-coloured containers.
- Liquids dispensed for oral medication should be in plain, smooth-sided bottles, whereas those for external use only should be in ribbed bottles, to allow the blind owner to differentiate.

Calculation of drug dosages

The ultimate responsibility for the calculation of the correct drug dosage for an animal currently rests with the veterinary surgeon. Nurses performing this task should always check with the veterinary surgeon responsible for the case.

The calculation of a dose for a particular animal is usually worked out in terms of the weight of the drug per kilogram bodyweight of the animal.

Calculation of drug dosages is covered in more detail in the *BSAVA Manual of Practical Veterinary Nursing*.

Example 1

A puppy weighing 5 kg requires worming with piperazine citrate. The dose rate is 125 mg/kg. The tablets give 500 mg each. How many tablets are required to worm this puppy?

The dose will be the dose rate multiplied by the weight of the puppy:

Dose = 125 x 5 = 625 mg.

The number of tablets will be the dose divided by the tablet weight:

Number of tablets = 625 ÷ 500 = $1\frac{1}{4}$ tablets.

Example 2

A dog weighing 26 kg requires clindamycin following dental treatment. The dose rate is 5.5 mg/kg, twice a day. The tablets come in 25 mg, 75 mg and 150 mg. The dog requires a seven-day course. What would you dispense?

The dose will be the dose rate multiplied by the weight of the dog:

Dose = 5.5 x 26 = 143 mg. Therefore 150 mg capsules would be appropriate.

One capsule twice a day: 2 x 7 days = 14 capsules would be dispensed.

Example 3

A cat weighing 4 kg requires an injection of carprofen following surgery. The dose rate is 4 mg/kg and the drug is available in a 50 mg/ml solution. How much would you prepare for injection?

The dose will be the dose rate multiplied by the weight of the cat:

Dose = 4 x 4 = 16 mg.

To calculate how much to draw up from the bottle, divide the amount of drug by the concentration:

16 mg ÷ 50 mg/ml = 0.32 ml.

Storage of veterinary medicines

Drugs should be stored in accordance with manufacturers' instructions. They should be stored correctly for several important reasons:

- To ensure the optimum shelf-life of the drug and to protect it from damage due to inappropriate storage
- To protect the public from access to potentially dangerous drugs and to protect the employer and employees on the premises
- To allow effective monitoring of drug stocks, which is essential for stock control and the monitoring of expiry dates.

Storage area

- The designated storage area must be inaccessible to the public.
- Storage areas should be kept clean and should be well ventilated.
- Eating or drinking should be forbidden in this area.
- Refrigeration must be available and maintained between 2°C and 8°C. Refrigerators should be fitted with a maximum/minimum thermometer to allow monitoring of the temperature. Insulin and vaccines are examples of products that must be kept refrigerated.
- Flammable products should be stored in appropriate cabinets.

Stock control

- An effective stock control system should be implemented that allows routine checking and detection of products requiring reordering or approaching their expiry date. The legislation that came into effect in October 2005 requires more data to be stored relating to stock purchase and usage; in particular, records of batch numbers and expiry dates are required.

- For multi-use products, date of first use should be marked on the product.
- Products returned by clients should not be reused as they may have been inappropriately stored.

Controlled and POM drugs

- Controlled drugs (see Figure 7.18) in Schedule 2 and some in Schedule 3 must be stored in a locked cabinet that is fixed in position, e.g. attached to a wall. Keys for this cabinet should only be available to the veterinary surgeon or an authorized person designated by the veterinary surgeon. It is recommended that other drugs such as ketamine, which are liable to abuse although not as yet classed as controlled drugs, should also be stored in a locked cabinet.
- Drugs in consulting rooms and in vehicles should be kept to a minimum and should not include controlled drugs.
- POM drugs may only be advertised to restricted categories of people. In the case of POM-V drugs this includes veterinary surgeons, pharmacists and professional keepers of animals. In addition, POM-VPS categories of drugs may also be advertised to Suitably Qualified Persons (see Figure 7.18), other veterinary healthcare professionals and owners or keepers of horses.

- This means that POM drugs and posters advertising them may not be displayed in waiting rooms. Price lists are excluded, however, from the advertising restrictions provided that no single product is seen to be promoted above any other.

References and further reading

Bishop Y (2004) *The Veterinary Formulary, 6th edn.* Pharmaceutical Press, London

Lane D, Cooper B and Turner L (2007) *BSAVA Textbook of Veterinary Nursing, 4th edn.* BSAVA Publications, Gloucester

Meredith A and Redrobe S (2002) *BSAVA Manual of Exotic Pets, 4th edn.* BSAVA Publications, Gloucester

Moore M (2001) *Calculations for Veterinary Nurses.* Blackwell Science, Oxford

Orpet H and Welsh P (2002) *Handbook of Veterinary Nursing.* Blackwell Science, Oxford

Roberts H and Argyle SA (in press) Practical pharmacy for veterinary nurses. In: *BSAVA Manual of Practical Veterinary Nursing*, ed. E Mullineaux and M Jones. BSAVA Publications, Gloucester

Tennant B (2005) *BSAVA Small Animal Formulary, 5th edn.* BSAVA Publications, Gloucester

8

Animal first aid

Sue Dallas

This chapter is designed to give information on:

- Definition of the term first aid and its limitations
- Reasons for patient evaluation
- The need for obtaining a good case history, and what should be included
- Emergency procedures that may be performed to maintain life until the veterinary surgeon arrives
- Basic resuscitation techniques
- Emergency procedures for common first aid situations

Introduction

First aid is defined as the immediate treatment of injured animals or those suffering from sudden illness, with a view to preventing worsening of disease or death.

Although veterinary nurses do not have greater legal powers than lay people, in situations requiring first aid they will have far greater knowledge of anatomy and physiology, and of the specific emergency first aid techniques required. In practice, nurses may be faced with emergency situations requiring evaluation and stabilization until the arrival of the veterinary surgeon. Due to the nature of these emergencies it is important that:

- A part of the practice is set up with the required equipment and drugs
- A triage of treatment is formulated (the process of examination and rapid classification of emergency cases by the urgency with which treatment is required) (Figure 8.1)
- A plan for initial evaluation of a severely injured animal is established and followed.

Life-threatening

- Cardiopulmonary arrest (heart and breathing have stopped)
- Airway obstruction
- Respiratory arrest
- Haemorrhage from a major artery or vein
- Anaphylaxis (acute allergic reaction).

Immediate action

- Multiple deep lacerations, haemorrhage, with hypovolaemia (low blood volume circulating in the blood vessels)
- Profound shock
- Penetrating wounds of the thorax or abdomen
- Head injuries
- Respiratory distress
- Spinal injury.

8.1 Evaluation and urgency. (continues) ▶

Urgent

- Extensive muscular or skeletal injuries
- Acute to overwhelming infection
- Compound fractures
- Dystocia (difficulty during parturition)
- Spinal cord injury with paralysis
- Shock (early stages)
- Collapse due to accident or illness.

Less urgent

- Fractures and dislocations
- Severe diarrhoea and vomiting
- Deep puncture wounds
- Foreign body in ear or eye.

8.1 (continued) Evaluation and urgency.

Purpose and limitations of first aid

The aims of first aid are:

- To preserve life
- To prevent further suffering
- To promote recovery.

In order to manage the situation the first aider should:

- Be calm and confident
- Be in command of the situation
- Use initiative
- Show sympathy.

Background information that is useful includes:

- An understanding of the anatomy and physiology of the body
- Knowledge of one's own limitations in situations requiring first aid
- Knowledge of how much a nurse can legally do
- Safe handling procedures to ensure that no one is injured by the patient or by the situation.

Unusual problems arise in first aid situations. For example, the person reporting or arriving with the animal may not be the owner, or the owner may be upset and require sensitive handling and support.

The basis of triage

Triage is performed immediately on arrival and presentation of an injured animal. It should take less than 5 minutes to perform. The procedures in triage include:

- Evaluation of the main body systems (e.g. respiratory, cardiovascular, renal and central nervous)
- Obtaining a brief history of the incident
- Assessment of extent of obvious injury/wounds.

The purpose of triage is to decide whether the animal is stable or unstable and plan the support of vital organ systems.

Handling and transport of injured animals

Initially it is important that an injured animal is not moved until it has been examined. An exception to this rule is if the animal's or first aider's life would be in danger if it was not moved.

Injured animals are usually in pain, shocked and frightened. This means that they may attack anyone who tries to approach or handle them.

- Slow deliberate movements are essential.
- When approaching, use a calm soothing voice.
- Ensure that there is no danger from electrocution.
- The animal should be handled as little as possible. If the animal is not already at the clinic, the owner should be instructed to transport it with consideration to obvious injuries at all times (Figure 8.2) and to maintain its body temperature (Figure 8.3).
- If the owner can check the airway, breathing and heart rate before transport, initial help can be given at an early stage. This assists nursing staff in preparing for the patient's arrival.

- Do not obstruct breathing or airway by bending the animal's neck.
- Support the animal's back and body.
- Retain its body temperature.
- Keep the weight off any obviously fractured limb.
- Muzzle a dog if necessary (unless contraindicated) to prevent injury from biting.

WARNING
Muzzling is contraindicated in cases of dyspnoea (difficulty in breathing) or epistaxis (bleeding from the nostrils) and for brachycephalic (short-nosed) breeds.

8.2 Basic rules of transportation.

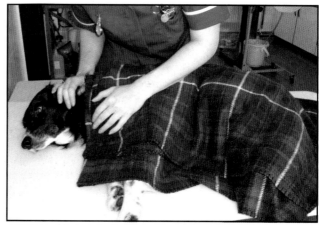

8.3 Maintain body temperature to prevent shock from becoming established.

Protective equipment

In order for the animal to be examined and transported, it must be restrained and in some cases muzzled to ensure the safety of the handlers. Types of muzzle include:

▪ Tape or bandage muzzle
▪ Commercial nylon muzzle
▪ Wire and box muzzle.

Other useful protective equipment includes:

▪ Thick leather gloves
▪ Disposable gloves (in case of suspected zoonosis)
▪ Plastic disposable apron
▪ Face visor
▪ Dog/cat graspers
▪ Crush boxes/cages.

Methods of transport

Small animals

Small dogs, cats and smaller pets are safely transported in a basket or pet carrier. If a container is not available, the animal should be picked up in a manner that provides support around its chest and hindquarters. It should be supported by the handler's body.

Medium-sized dogs

Medium-sized dogs with a minor injury may be able to walk. If this is not possible, they should be lifted into the handler's own body with an arm around the front of the forelegs and an arm around the hindlegs (provided this is not contraindicated by the injuries) (Figures 8.4 and 8.5). Dogs weighing under 15 kg can be lifted by one person; dogs weighing over this amount must be lifted by two people for health and safety reasons.

Large dogs

Large and giant breed dogs that are unable to walk should be lifted by at least three people (Figure 8.6) or by using a stretcher or blanket and four people:

1. The blanket should be spread beside the animal.
2. The animal should be slid on to the blanket (taking care not to lift the body up), still in the position in which it was lying.
3. The corners of the blanket can now be lifted by two to four people, depending on the size of the animal.

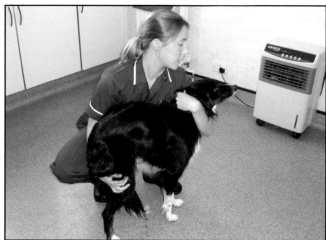
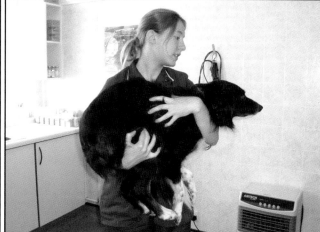

8.4 Lifting a medium-sized dog: the safe-lift technique, protecting the handler's spine.

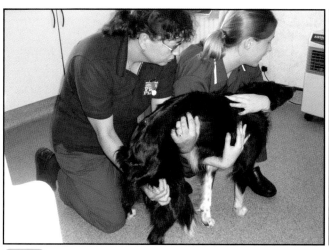
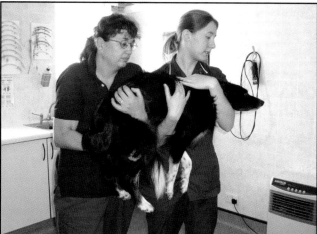

8.5 Two people lifting a dog. Each handler should keep their back straight for safety during lifting.

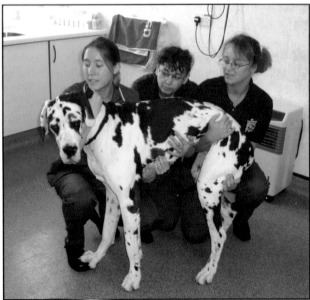

 Lifting a giant breed of dog requires at least three people.

> **WARNING**
> Always lift in a correct manner, so that the handler's own back is not at risk (see Figure 8.4).

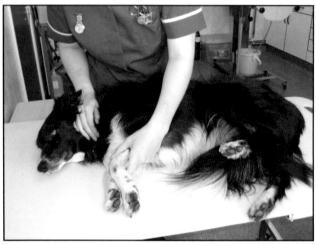

8.7 Placing an animal in the recovery position. The tongue should now be drawn forward and the collar removed.

> **WARNING**
> It is not advisable to put an animal in the recovery position if a head or spinal injury is suspected, as moving the patient may cause further damage. In this instance the animal is best left in its own position until a veterinary surgeon is able to assess the patient fully.

Procedure on arrival of a first aid case

A key element of triage is that, when evaluating the patient, it must be borne in mind that some situations will allow plenty of time to attend to the injuries or problems, whereas other situations are so severe that the animal will die if urgent and emergency care is not initiated immediately (see Figure 8.1).

If possible, always have a detailed case history ready for the veterinary surgeon's arrival. This should include:

- Name and address of owner
- Telephone numbers (home, work, mobile phone)
- Species, breed, age and sex of injured animal
- Initial evaluation of the extent of injury
- Time of admission
- Change in patient's status since admission
- Nature of first aid treatment given.

General procedure on arrival at the clinic

Recovery position

Unless it is contraindicated, always start by placing the animal into the recovery position (Figure 8.7):

1. Lie the animal on its right side.
2. Ensure that its head and neck are straightened.
3. Draw the tongue forward so that it hangs out of the side of the animal's mouth.
4. Remove any collar or harness.

Evaluation and examination

The initial positioning should be followed by evaluation of all areas of the animal using the CRASH PLAN protocol (Figure 8.8). All findings should be recorded, including:

- External haemorrhage (bleeding)
- Colour of mucous membranes (Figures 8.9 and 8.10)
- Capillary refill time (when the gum over the top canine tooth is pressed, the time it takes to go pink again, i.e. for the blood vessels to refill)
- Rate and quality of pulse
- Breathing – note whether it is normal speed, slow or fast, and whether there is evidence of dyspnoea
- Body temperature – take the rectal temperature
- Level of consciousness
- Unusual odours (on the body or coming from the mouth)
- Evidence of vomiting or diarrhoea.

Basic initial nursing

- Maintain respiratory and cardiovascular function.
- Body temperature must be kept within normal limits.
- Clean wounds.
- Arrest haemorrhage.
- Tender loving care (TLC).
- Observation (monitor and record temperature, pulse and respiration, mucous membrane colour and capillary refill time).

A	**A**irway	Check airway is patent
C	**C**ardiovascular	Check the apex beat of the heart
R	**R**espiratory	Presence/absence of breathing
A	**A**bdomen	Look but do not palpate
S	**S**pine	Look for any deformity but do not palpate
H	**H**ead	Look for deformity and level of consciousness
P	**P**elvic and anal areas	Look for sign of injury
L	**L**imbs	Check for deformity
A	**A**rteries and veins	Check for signs of dehydration and shock
N	**N**erves, peripheral	Check for ability to move limbs and tail

8.8 A CRASH PLAN.

Description	Colour	Cause
Pale		Shock, haemorrhage or anaemia
Cyanotic	Blue tinge	Lack of oxygen at tissue level
Jaundiced	Yellow tinge	Excess bile pigment in the circulation
Injected/red	Bright red	Over-exercise
Congested	Dark red	Cardiovascular insufficiency

8.9 Colour of mucous membranes.

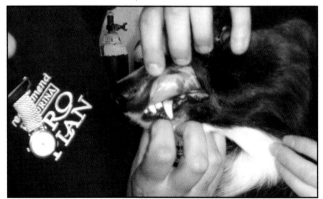

8.10 Checking the colour of mucous membranes and capillary refill time.

Contents of an animal first aid box

- **Cotton wool for padding.**
- **Antiseptic solution and 0.9% sodium chloride solution.**
- **Sterile swabs.**
- **Sterile dressings and bandages.**
- **Adhesive tape.**
- **Scissors.**
- **Thermometer.**

Cardiopulmonary resuscitation (CPR)

Cardiopulmonary resuscitation (Figures 8.11 to 8.14) should be initiated following all cardiac arrests, unless otherwise directed by a veterinary surgeon or owner. Cardiopulmonary arrest is when the heart and breathing have stopped. The object is to restore circulation and respiration and to prevent irreversible brain damage. Following cardiac arrest, this damage would usually occur within 3–4 minutes; therefore being adequately prepared is the most important step in managing a cardiac emergency.

A	**A**irway	Clear it of any obstructions, such as saliva, vomit, the patient's own tongue or any other material that could block the trachea or throat
B	**B**reathing	Start artificial respiration (see Figures 8.12 and 8.13) and assist with oxygen if available
C	**C**irculation	If the heart has stopped, start cardiac compression (see Figure 8.14)

8.11 ABC – the basic cardiopulmonary technique.

1. Place in recovery position – on its right-hand side, with head and neck extended and tongue drawn forward (see Figure 8.7).
2. Clear airway.
3. Place hand over ribs, behind shoulder bone, and compress chest with sharp downward movement (see Figure 8.13).
4. Allow chest to expand and then repeat the downward movement at intervals of 3–5 seconds, until breathing restarts.

8.12 Artificial respiration.

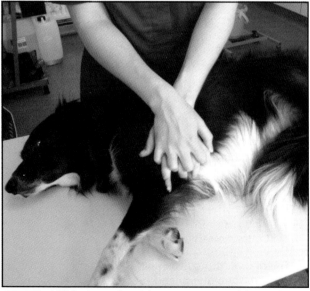

8.13 With the animal in recovery position, place hands over ribs, behind shoulder bone, and compress the chest.

Small dogs and cats

1. Place in recovery position (see Figure 8.7).
2. Take hold of chest (thorax) between thumb and fingers of one hand, just behind elbows. Support the animal's body with the other hand on spine to prevent it moving away.
3. Squeeze thumb and fingers of first hand together over heart, to compress chest and heart.
4. Repeat this action at rate of approximately 120 times per minute.

Medium-sized dogs

1. Place animal in recovery position (see Figure 8.7).
2. Put heel of one hand on its chest, just behind elbow, and place other hand on top of first hand.
3. Press down on chest with firm sharp movements.
4. Repeat this action at rate of about 80–100 times per minute.

Large or fat dogs

1. Put dog on its back, with head lowered.
2. Place heel of one hand on abdomen end of chest and put other hand on top of that hand.
3. Press firmly on chest, pushing hands forwards (towards animal's head). This method requires some strength.
4. Repeat chest pressure at rate of 80–100 times per minute.

Whatever size of animal

- Apply compressions for about 15 seconds at a time
- Then stop and check for a pulse
- Continue until pulse returns
- Seek veterinary attention as soon as possible.

8.14 Cardiac compression techniques.

Recognition and first aid procedures for specific emergencies

Asphyxia (suffocation)

Interference with respiration or breathing can occur in the upper respiratory tract (nose, mouth and throat) or lower respiratory tract (trachea, bronchi and lungs). It can involve a simple physical blockage of air conduction to the lungs or interference with the transference of air through the alveoli (air sacs), preventing gaseous exchange.

Signs and causes

Signs of asphyxia (which is suffocation, resulting from failure to oxygenate the blood) include:

- Cyanosis (blue mucous membranes)
- Dyspnoea (difficulty in breathing)
- Tachypnoea (increased rate of inspiration, which is also shallow)
- Absence of breathing
- Cardiac arrest.

The respiratory and cardiovascular systems are closely linked and so a change in one is usually reflected in the other. Change in breathing ability can be mirrored in the pulse rate (speed) and character (strong, weak or thready), and in the colour of the mucous membranes, as the blood gas levels become abnormal.

Causes of asphyxia include:

- Obstruction of the airways
- Pressure on the chest or neck region, possibly due to a road traffic accident (RTA), causing collapse of the airway
- Conditions that cause fluid build-up in the thorax (e.g. heart failure)
- Paralysis of the respiratory muscles caused by electrocution, spinal injury or poisons
- Direct thoracic injury
- Drowning
- Inhalation of poisonous gases, such as carbon monoxide, which will interfere with the uptake of oxygen
- Diseases of the central nervous system (CNS).

Dyspnoea

Damage or disease to any part of the respiratory system makes breathing difficult and painful. In addition, diseases not associated with the respiratory tract, such as heart disease, anaemia (lack of red cells or haemoglobin in the blood) or gastric dilatation and torsion (when the stomach fills with gas and twists), can have an effect on the breathing.

Whatever the cause of dyspnoea, it should be taken very seriously and viewed as an emergency. If breathing has stopped, it must urgently be restarted.

Resuscitation methods include the use of drugs that stimulate the heart and the breathing, but these must be administered only by a veterinary surgeon. For first aid, therefore, manual techniques such as Airway/Breathing/Circulation (ABC) apply (see Figure 8.11). It is important to reassure the patient and allow it to settle as any stress will worsen the dyspnoeic animal.

Drowning

Drowning happens when the lungs of an animal become flooded with fluid, preventing air inhalation. Affected animals will often also swallow amounts of water and other debris as they begin to weaken following immersion. First aid measures for drowning include:

- Recover the animal, drain water from its mouth and pull tongue forward (see Figure 8.7)
- Small dog: hold dog upside down to assist in draining water
- Large dog: lay dog on its side with head lowered and raised hindlegs
- Check for heart beat
- Allow 30–40 seconds for drainage, then commence artificial or mouth-to-nose resuscitation (see Figure 8.12) until the animal starts to gasp
- Dry and treat for shock.

Haemorrhage

Haemorrhage is bleeding from a damaged blood vessel in any part of the body due to injury or a disease condition. Even slight bleeding over a long period could result in eventual death, and certainly sudden severe blood loss will cause death.

It should be remembered that many owners will overestimate the extent of blood loss and this must always be borne in mind.

Signs

General signs of life-threatening haemorrhage include:

- Pale mucous membranes
- Rapid weak pulse and altered breathing pattern
- Subnormal temperature
- Slow capillary refill time
- Inability to rise.

Evaluation

Information on the following should be recorded:

- Type of blood vessel damaged (whether an artery, vein or capillary)
- When the bleeding started (for example: immediately; within the past 24–48 hours; several days before)
- In relation to the body, is the bleeding visible (external) or is internal haemorrhage suspected? Internal haemorrhage can be recognized by pale mucous membranes, poor capillary refill time and general lethargy of the patient over time.

Different types of haemorrhage are described in Figure 8.15.

Type	Description
Arterial	Bright red blood, in spurts synchronized with heart beat
Venous	Dark red blood, with definite bleeding point and steady flow
Capillary	Bright red blood, oozing slowly with no definite bleeding point
Primary	Haemorrhage as direct result of a blood vessel having been damaged
Secondary	Haemorrhage that restarts several days after injury, due to infection
Reactionary	Haemorrhage that restarts within 24 hours of the initial injury, due to rise in blood pressure that displaces clot formation
External	Haemorrhage seen on surface of body or coming from body opening (mouth, nose, urethra, anus)
Internal	Haemorrhage into a body cavity, therefore unseen during examination

8.15 Types of haemorrhage.

Action

Methods of haemorrhage control include applying digital pressure, the use of pressure bandages, using pressure points or (rarely) applying a tourniquet.

Digital pressure

Fingers are used to control the bleeding (Figure 8.16), but care is required to ensure that there is no foreign body embedded in the wound, as the pressure would push it deeper into the tissues.

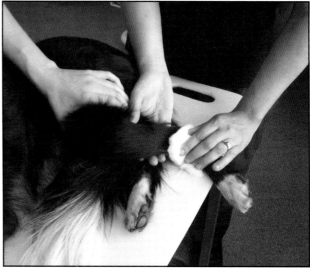

8.16 To inhibit bleeding, press a pad of swabs on the affected area.

Pressure bandages

These are applied to extremities, such as limbs, and are used to constrict the surface circulation temporarily, helping to limit the loss of blood. A pressure bandage is applied over plenty of padding material backing the wound dressing, tightly bandaged in place until a veterinary surgeon arrives. Pressure bandages should not be used over the head, neck or thorax, as further injury or dyspnoea may result.

Useful pressure points

Pressure is applied on an artery (where it passes over a bone) to the body extremities. The supply of blood to forelimbs, hindlimbs or tail can then be temporarily constricted to reduce blood loss. The pressure applied must be sufficient to prevent the flow of blood through the artery. Pressure points are:

- The brachial artery – distal third of humerus, medial to the shaft
- The femoral artery – proximal third of the femur, medial aspect of the thigh
- The coccygeal artery – underside of the tail, at the root or base.

Tourniquet

Historically, a tourniquet was used to cut off the circulation supply to the tissues below its application site. However, this technique should *not* be employed.

Unconsciousness

Unconsciousness may render the brain:

- *Inactive* – as seen in central nervous system injury (head injury or resulting from asphyxia as in drowning), with flaccidity of the patient
- *Active* – seen in convulsions or epileptic-type fits and in electrocution.

Causes of unconsciousness include:

- Epilepsy
- Respiratory or cardiac arrest
- Poisoning
- Electrocution.

Action for flaccid unconscious patient

- Place in recovery position (see Figure 8.7).
- ABC (see Figure 8.11).
- Examine for signs of injury.
- Keep warm.
- Do not leave unattended.

Action for fits or seizures

- Do not restrain (to avoid injury to the patient or handler).
- Subdue light and reduce noise.
- Clear a space by moving furniture back.
- Observe but do not handle.
- If the animal's breathing becomes obstructed, clear the airway.
- Handle only when the animal responds to its name or attempts to stand.

Seizures that last longer than 5 minutes or start again following recovery require urgent veterinary attention.

Wounds

A wound is a break in the continuity of a tissue anywhere in the body, internal or external. In a first aid situation this will usually mean a break in the skin or mucous membrane, but the term also applies to damage to other tissues or organs in the body. Wounds may be:

- *Open* – damage to the skin and underlying tissues
- *Closed* – they do not penetrate the whole thickness of the skin.

Action

- Arrest any haemorrhage.
- Check for foreign bodies.
- Flush the wound, preferably using 0.9% sodium chloride (normal saline).
- Cover with a sterile non-adherent dressing.
- Keep the animal warm.
- Comfort and monitor the patient.
- Apply a bandage in selected cases (see *BSAVA Manual of Practical Veterinary Nursing*).

Bandaging

Indications for bandaging:

- **Protecting a wound from further injury or contamination**
- **Prevention of self-mutilation and interference**
- **Supporting soft tissues (muscle or ligament) in sprains and strains**
- **Arresting bleeding (pressure bandage).**

The layers of a bandage:

1. **Primary layer: *dressings* – placed against the wound to provide a sterile contact material, which will not allow further contamination of the site.**
2. **Secondary layer: *padding* – provides the absorption and padding (i.e. cotton wool).**
3. **Tertiary layer: *bandage* – secures the above layers and protects them from the environment and the patient.**

Aims when bandaging:

- **Patient comfort – if applied too tightly the animal will try to remove the bandage, or the surface tissues will be damaged by the animal's constant chewing and licking**
- **Prevention of patient interference with the area under the bandage**
- **Restriction of movement – in the case of broken bones or tissue damage (and therefore limits pain).**

After application of the bandage the following should be monitored:

- **Discomfort**
- **Interference or self-mutilation to try to remove the bandage**
- **The bandage getting wet or dirty.**

Rules for bandaging:

- **Wash hands before starting (to prevent introducing infection)**
- **Get all the materials together before restraining the animal**
- **Never stick adhesive tape on to the animal's coat or hair as it is hard to remove**
- **Do not use safety pins or elastic bands to secure the ends of any bandage. Use narrow adhesive tape on the bandage surface**
- **In the case of a leg bandage include the foot, otherwise it will swell**
- **If unsure of temperament, always muzzle for safety**
- **Suspected fractures of the upper limbs should not be bandaged.**

Penetrating wounds to the thorax
Signs

- Breathing painful and often rapid and shallow.
- Affected animals often reluctant to move.
- May adopt a sitting position.

Action

- Cover the wound.
- Keep the animal quiet and calm.
- Allow it to choose its own resting position.
- Keep it warm.

Penetrating wounds to the abdomen
Signs and causes

An open wound to the abdomen is seen, allowing abdominal tissues and organs to protrude. Complications include:

- Drying of exposed tissues
- Swelling of exposed tissues
- Contamination or infection
- Self-inflicted damage (animals will attempt to eat exposed organs).

Causes of abdominal rupture include:

- Road traffic accident
- Bite wounds
- Stab or stake injuries
- Breakdown of surgical site (dehiscence).

Action

- Clean the wound.
- Cover exposed tissue with swabs soaked in saline warmed to body temperature, or in cooled boiled water.
- Do not leave unattended.
- Treat for shock.
- Seek veterinary help urgently.
- Prevent self-mutilation.

Burns

Burns cause destruction of tissue by extreme localized *dry* heat. The severity of a burn is measured by the depth of tissue and the proportion of surface area affected. The full extent of the injury is often not apparent until several days after the accident.

Signs

- Loss of coat or fur; skin change.
- Swelling.
- Redness and heat.
- Local infection.
- Pain and signs of shock.

Evaluation

The depth of the injury may be described as:

- *Superficial* – penetrating no deeper than the skin surface
- *Deep* – penetrating through the skin, subcutaneous tissues, fat, muscle and even to bone.

The physical extent of the injury is also important, as the extensive pain and fluid loss (in the form of plasma from the damaged blood vessels) can lead to serious dehydration and shock.

Action

While waiting for the arrival of a veterinary surgeon:

- Cool and flush the area with cool water for at least 10 minutes if immediately post-injury. This will reduce the swelling and plasma loss, and also provide some pain control
- Avoid wetting the patient as a whole (to avoid hypothermia)
- Cover burn with moist sterile dressing or clingfilm to prevent any contamination
- Prevent self-mutilation
- To prevent shock, keep the animal warm (but do not use direct heat)
- Restrict the animal's movement to lessen the pain
- Do not leave unattended
- Comfort the patient
- Prepare fluid therapy equipment if burns are extensive or shock is severe.

Scalds

Scalds are caused by *moist* heat, such as steam or hot liquids. The signs of scalds can be similar to those of burns, but with scalding the coat is not singed.

It is important with both types of injury that the area affected is covered with a dressing to prevent contamination.

Shock

Shock is a term used to describe a very complex and potentially fatal clinical syndrome that always involves insufficient blood flow to the tissues, resulting in hypoxia (lack of oxygen to the cells) which can be fatal if not corrected.

When blood is lost from the body in bleeding from a damaged blood vessel, the body tries to compensate by redistributing blood to vital structures such as the brain and heart at the expense of other organs such as kidneys, skin, intestines and muscles. The resulting tissue hypoxia can cause organs to be severely damaged.

The causes of shock vary. Examples include:

- **Blood loss from damaged vessels**
- **Pain**
- **Heart disease that interferes with the normal pumping action of the heart**
- **Overwhelming infection.**

▶

The signs of shock include:

- **Pale mucous membranes**
- **Cold extremities**
- **The animal becomes weak and may become unconscious**
- **Increase in the heart and respiratory rate**
- **Slow capillary refill time of longer than 2 seconds.**

Shock has three phases:

1. *Impending* – shock is anticipated because of the events or injuries suffered by the animal.
2. *Established* – shock is in place. The animal must have urgent medical treatment to prevent death.
3. *Irreversible* – treatment is unlikely to save the animal's life because body systems are irreversibly damaged.

Treatment is aimed at not allowing shock to move on beyond the impending phase. Useful steps to achieve this are:

- **Maintain body temperature by wrapping in blankets or towels. (Never use artificial heat as the animal's temperature may get too high and cause peripheral vasodilation, which may worsen the situation)**
- **Position the head slightly lower than the body to encourage blood flow to the brain**
- **Stop any further blood loss**
- **Assist the animal to breathe by placing in recovery position, and if required give artificial respiration if breathing stops**
- **Record the pulse**
- **Seek veterinary attention as soon as possible.**

Hyperthermia (heatstroke)

Heatstroke results from an excessive rise in body temperature caused by high environmental temperatures. Due to their dense coats and lack of sweat glands, dogs and cats do not lose body heat through the skin. They eliminate excess body heat through the respiratory system, inhaling cool air through the nose and exhaling hot air from the body through the mouth. The faster this exchange occurs, the faster their body will cool down, which is why dogs pant after exercise.

Heatstroke is rarely seen in cats, and in dogs it is usually because the animal has been confined, on a hot day with no access to shade, or in a vehicle with insufficient ventilation.

> ⚠️ **WARNING**
> **On a hot or sunny day, the temperature in a car soon becomes higher than the environmental temperature even if windows are left open.**

Heatstroke may affect any dog, but those most at risk if exposed to excess heat are:

- Those with thick dense coats
- Overweight animals
- Short-nosed breeds
- Animals with heart conditions
- Elderly animals
- Animals with medical conditions that affect breathing.

When the environmental temperature exceeds the animal's body temperature it becomes impossible ultimately to maintain body temperature within normal limits for that animal.

As the environmental temperature rises, panting becomes ineffective and the body temperature will rise rapidly. Death follows quickly if the body temperature is not immediately reduced.

Signs

- Excessive panting and salivation.
- Bright red mucous membranes (check the gums).
- Vomiting.
- Excitement/anxiety.
- Disorientation.
- Collapse/inability to stand.
- High body temperature (41–43°C).

Action

It is essential to reduce body temperature urgently.

1. Remove the animal from the hot environment.
2. Cool the animal by:
   - Holding a frozen pack of vegetables or ice pack on neck area
   - Wrapping in towel/blanket soaked with cold water
   - Using fans or air conditioning.
3. Monitor the animal's body temperature.
4. If collapsed, put into recovery position to assist breathing.
5. If conscious, encourage to drink restricted amounts of water continuously (if unrestricted the animal may swallow too much too fast and cause vomiting).
6. Treat for shock if temperature goes below normal temperature.
7. Prepare equipment for fluid therapy.
8. Avoid extreme measures such as hosing the patient or applying ice directly to the patient (place ice in a bag or wrap in a cloth to avoid burns).

Hypothermia

Hypothermia is most commonly seen in young or small animals due to an inability to control body temperature within normal limits. This may be caused by illness or exposure to cold or wet environmental conditions.

Signs

- Animal appears sleepy or lethargic.
- Movements become weaker.
- Unconsciousness.
- Eventually, respiratory or cardiac arrest.

Action

■ If the animal is wet, dry it by rubbing vigorously with a towel.
■ Wrap using a lightweight covering to preserve heat (e.g. reflective blanket or fleece).
■ Increase the environmental temperature but do not overheat. Warming the inspired air is particularly effective.
■ Monitor constantly by taking temperature and do not leave unattended.

Skeletal injuries (fractures and dislocations)
Signs

■ Pain/lameness.
■ Shortening or lengthening of limb.
■ Deformity of the limb.
■ Abnormal position of bone or joint.
■ Loss of use of the part.
■ Crepitus (crackling sensation on palpation).

Causes of fracture

A fracture is a break in a bone. Causes include:

■ *Direct violence* (such as in an RTA) – the bone breaks at the place to which violence is applied
■ *Indirect violence* – the fracture occurs some distance from the area where force was applied (for example, an animal landing on a hard surface with the break occurring to bones further up the limb)
■ *Muscular action* or *fatigue fracture* – seen after muscular contraction during a race, particularly in the Greyhound and Whippet
■ *Pathological* or *spontaneous fracture* – may be due to an existing bone disease or a condition that weakens the structure of the bone. These fractures often occur during a normal limb movement.

Causes of dislocation

Dislocation refers to the displacement of one or more bones forming a joint. Causes of dislocation include:

■ Direct violence (e.g. RTA)
■ Indirect violence (e.g. falling)
■ Pathological displacement (e.g. hip dysplasia, an inherited condition – the joint and bone that should be in contact are so deformed that they cannot stay in contact)
■ Congenital displacement (e.g. luxating patella – the patella, i.e. kneecap, is dislocated from the groove in the femur, often due to poor alignment in the stifle joint).

Action

Emergency treatment for fractures and dislocations is as follows:

■ Arrest any haemorrhage
■ Clean any wounds to the area and cover with sterile dressing to prevent contamination
■ Confine the animal to prevent movement

■ Monitor and observe until arrival of a veterinary surgeon
■ Apply a supportive bandage (e.g. Robert Jones).

Sprains and strains

Sprains always involve a joint, with damage to ligaments and other tissues that are stretched and torn during the injury. Recovery and repair of some of these tissues are slow, due to continued use of the area and because some of the tissues (e.g. ligaments) are naturally slow to heal. Sprains occur most commonly in the lower limbs to the carpus (wrist) area and the tarsus (hock) area.

Strains involve tearing and stretching damage to muscles, often close to joints. They can occur anywhere in the body.

Signs of both sprains and strains include localized pain, swelling or lameness.

Action

■ Initial care involves the application of a cold compress to the area, to reduce the swelling and pain.
■ Prevent use of the affected limb.
■ Confine to a kennel with plenty of bedding.
■ Comfort the patient.
■ Treat for shock if suspected.

Poisons

A *poison* or *toxin* is a substance that, on entry to the body in sufficient amounts, has a harmful effect on the individual. An *antidote* is a substance that counteracts a poison.

Animals can be poisoned by any of a multitude of potentially toxic substances. Sources include poisonous plants, and toxic chemicals used on or stored near the animal (e.g. in kitchen or utility room cupboards). These chemicals might be pesticides for the garden, paint, cleaning solutions or drugs (either medicinal or substances of abuse).

Signs

Very few poisons produce distinctive signs. Most cause non-specific signs, such as:

■ Excitement or depression
■ Weakness or ataxia (unsteady on the feet)
■ Salivation
■ Development of vomiting or diarrhoea
■ Abdominal pain
■ Convulsions.

Evaluation

The following should be ascertained from the owner:

■ Whether there have been any changes in routine at home or in the walk route
■ Whether any medication has been given
■ Full details about the animal concerned – age, sex, breed and species
■ Details of clinical signs and any actions taken by the owner

- A full case history (this is very important to the veterinary surgeon's diagnosis, unless the chemical is already known and named).

Any material passed by the animal (vomit, urine or faeces) should always be saved for forensic testing if required. The owner should be asked to bring the suspected toxin to the veterinary surgery, if possible.

Action

If the owner is able to tell staff what the poison was, treatment should be started sooner rather than later:

- Place the animal in the recovery position (see Figure 8.7)
- Keep it warm to reduce shock (see Figure 8.3)
- Provide comfort companionship and never leave the patient unattended (in case its condition suddenly worsens)
- Prepare equipment for fluid therapy and gastric lavage (stomach tube and warm water).

WARNING
The animal should not be made to vomit, except on instructions from a veterinary surgeon.

Insect stings

Most insect stings are painful but harmless. However, it is possible that an animal may have an allergic reaction to insect venom; therefore any stings near the face in particular must be considered serious. Appropriate action for anaphylaxis (life-threatening allergic reaction) should be initiated (ABC – see Figure 8.11).

WARNING
Never squeeze the venom sack if it is embedded in the animal's skin. Such action may inject more venom into the animal.

Action

- *Wasp stings* are alkaline, therefore treat with an acid solution (e.g. a vinegar compress).
- *Bee stings* are acid, therefore treat with an alkali (e.g. bicarbonate of soda compress).

If it is unclear what the biting insect was, a cold compress should be applied to reduce the pain and swelling of the affected area.

Snake bites

Snake bites are uncommon and will rarely be observed as they happen.

Signs

The signs that a bite has occurred include:

- Animal is upset, trembling, salivating and may be vomiting
- Pupils may be dilated
- Collapse

- Pain and swelling at the bite site
- Lameness.

Venomous snake bites may leave two visible puncture marks at the site (bites are often located on the legs or head).

Action

- Calm the animal.
- Apply an ice pack to the swollen area to constrict the surface blood vessels and slow the spread of the poison.
- Treat for shock.

Eye injuries
Signs and causes

Both eyes should be examined and compared, and any differences noted. Signs include:

- Obvious loss of vision
- Tissue swelling (oedema) (Figure 8.17)
- Bleeding around the eye
- Abnormal size and position of the eyeball within the orbit.

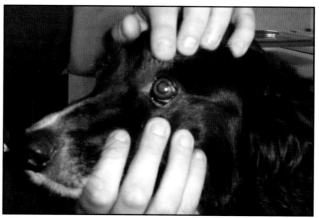
8.17 Examining the eye for signs of tissue swelling.

Causes of eye injury include:

- Direct violence
- Indirect violence
- Chemical exposure
- Foreign bodies.

Evaluation

A history should be taken from the owner, concerning:

- The type of trauma
- When it occurred
- Whether there has been any exposure to chemicals
- Whether there are any pre-existing eye problems.

The animal should be approached slowly – and should be warned of any approach. Most eye injuries are quite painful, and if the animal has considerable sight impairment it will also be frightened and could injure any handler.

Action

For emergency treatment:

- Keep the eye moist with sterile water or normal saline
- Prevent self-mutilation (by restraining the patient or applying an Elizabethan collar)
- Do not leave unattended
- Keep warm and quiet.

> **WARNING**
>
> In cases of prolapse: do *not* attempt to force the eye into the socket. Pull eyelids over gently, to cover the eye.

Death

Signs and recognition of death

- Absence of heart beat – check by palpation of thorax, pulses and use of stethoscope.
- Absence of breathing – observe for movement of the thorax or evidence of air flow at the nose or mouth.
- Loss of corneal reflex – test only using a wisp of moist cotton wool touched on to the cornea.
- Loss of blink reflex – check by touching the inner corner of the eyelids.
- Loss of light reflex – check by darkening the room and shining a penlight into each eye.
- Eyeball becomes glazed – check by observation.

- Cooling of the body – using hands, check by feeling extremities and body.
- Rigor mortis – stiffening of the body.

Action if death is suspected

Death can be difficult to confirm, particularly in cold blooded animals or in cases of hypothermia. A veterinary surgeon should examine the patient if any doubt exists.

If death is suspected the owner should be advised, but a veterinary surgeon should make the final decision.

References and further reading

Andrews B and Boag A (in press) Triage and emergency nursing. In: *BSAVA Manual of Practical Veterinary Nursing*, ed. E Mullineaux and M Jones. BSAVA Publications, Gloucester

Bell C (1993) *First Aid and Health Care for Dogs*. Lutterworth Press, Cambridge

Bryant C and Phillips D (in press) Wound management, dressings and bandages. In: *BSAVA Manual of Practical Veterinary Nursing,* ed E Mullineaux and M Jones. BSAVA Publications, Gloucester

Kirk B and Bistner S (1985) *Handbook of Veterinary Procedures and Emergency Treatment*. WB Saunders, Philadelphia

Lane D, Cooper B and Turner L (2007) *BSAVA Textbook of Veterinary Nursing, 4th edn*. BSAVA Publications, Gloucester

9

Organization and communication skills

Maggie Shilcock

This chapter is designed to give information on:

- The organization of a veterinary practice
- Communication skills
- Basic reception work
- Nurses working with clients

Introduction

Good communication with clients is an essential part of the service that a veterinary practice provides. The aim of the veterinary practice and its staff is to create a good working relationship with clients so that the client feels they are part of the practice and that the practice staff really care about them and their animals.

Clients are looking for convenience, confidence, help, advice, understanding and care when they come to the practice. Receptionists and nurses are usually the first point of contact for a client, either on the telephone or in the reception area, and their communication skills have a great effect on the client's first impressions of the practice. It goes without saying that these impressions must be good. Client expectations from any kind of business or service are constantly increasing and as the competition between veterinary practices is becoming more fierce the need for effective communication (which is the basis of good client care) becomes ever more important.

Organization of a veterinary practice

Veterinary practices vary in size from the small one-owner practice, with perhaps two nurses and a receptionist, to multi-site practices employing teams of veterinary surgeons, nurses, receptionists and administrative staff.

Although there are still quite a lot of mixed veterinary practices, specialization is increasing. Many practices are now for small animals only, some are purely equine and a smaller number specialize in exotic animals and birds or are referral practices carrying out veterinary work in specific veterinary areas, such as dermatology, cardiology or orthopaedics.

Roles and responsibilities of the veterinary team

Good teamwork is essential to the success of a veterinary practice. Whether a practice is large or small, to work effectively it has to operate as one team of people working together to provide the best veterinary service for the client.

The veterinary practice team is made up of all or a combination of the following members:

- Owners
- Practice managers
- Veterinary surgeons
- Nursing staff
- Reception staff
- Administrative staff.

Owners

The owners of the practice take responsibility for running the business and keeping it financially successful. Most are veterinary surgeons but non-veterinary surgeons can also own veterinary practices. They are responsible for the health and safety of the staff they employ and for complying with all other legislation relating to a small business; they also take the ultimate responsibility for any clinical errors or client complaints.

Practice managers

Many veterinary practices now employ a practice manager to relieve the owners of the basic management of their practice, enabling them to devote more time to their clinical role. In smaller practices the practice manager may take responsibility for human resources, health and safety, office management, marketing and financial management. In very large practices there may be a number of managers, each concentrating on a specific aspect of management.

Veterinary surgeons

The veterinary surgeons' role is to carry out the clinical and medical work of the practice. They are responsible for maintaining the health of clients' animals, by advising clients on how to keep their animals healthy and treating the animals when they are sick.

Nursing staff

There is a variety of nursing roles in veterinary practice. The qualified veterinary nurse (Figure 9.1) gives clinical and surgical support to the veterinary surgeon, provides expert nursing care to hospitalized animals and often helps to train fellow nurses. Many run their own nurse clinics, advising clients on various aspects of pet healthcare. Animal nursing assistants (ANAs) and veterinary care assistants (VCAs) give practical nursing support and animal care. Many nurses also carry out reception duties (Figure 9.2).

Reception staff

Receptionists (Figure 9.3) provide an interface between the client and the practice, and they have one of the most varied roles in the practice. They are responsible for answering telephone enquiries, booking appointments and operations and giving general veterinary advice as well as promoting the practice and its services to the client. Another key responsibility is ensuring that clients pay their bills at the end of their animal's treatment.

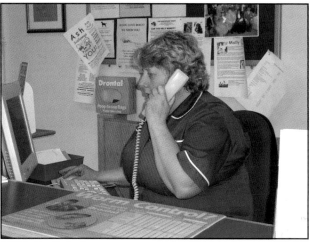

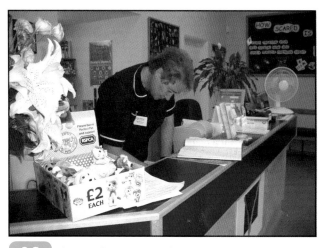

9.2 Veterinary nurses are often required to perform some reception duties.

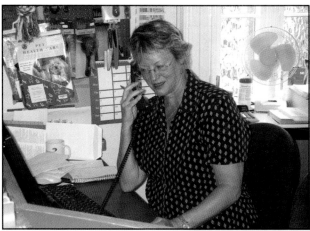

9.3 A veterinary receptionist.

Administrative staff

No medium-sized or large practice can operate without the help of administrative staff (Figure 9.4), whose role is to carry out the basic administration of the practice. They are usually responsible for sending out large animal accounts, chasing unpaid bills, paying practice bills, keeping practice accounts and general record keeping and secretarial support.

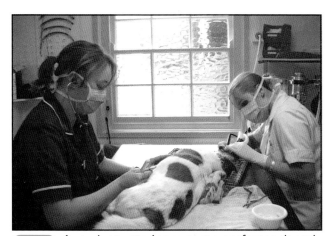

9.1 A student veterinary nurse performs dental hygiene treatment whilst being supervised by a qualified veterinary nurse, who is also monitoring the animal's anaesthetic.

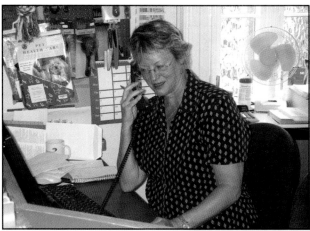

9.4 A member of the practice's administration team.

Communication skills

Veterinary care involves caring for animals, but each animal has an owner, whose needs and expectations must also be cared for. Many clients are worried or concerned about their pet; they need help, advice, information and reassurance, all of which need to be communicated to them in the most effective and efficient way. People skills and good communication are a very important part of the roles of receptionists and nurses.

Importance of customer care

Good client care is one of the best ways to attract clients to the practice and to ensure that they keep coming back. It is good client care that creates the relationship with clients. They cannot easily judge the veterinary care that their pet receives, but they can judge the client care that they are given. The better they are treated by practice staff, the better they will assume their animal will be treated. Customer expectations are constantly increasing and veterinary practice staff must meet these expectations and higher standards. The practice and its staff depend on the client for their livelihood and if clients are not happy with the service or care they receive they can easily go elsewhere.

Greeting clients

How a client is greeted can determine the impression they gain of the practice. The greeting is their first point of contact with the practice and it is very important that they feel welcome and confident that the practice is going to help them and their pet. When a client enters the reception area they should be acknowledged immediately by the member of staff on the reception desk – after only three seconds they will begin to feel ignored.

- Smile and establish eye contact with the client and greet them and their pet by name whenever possible.
- Check the time of the appointment and ask them to take a seat.
- Inform clients if the consultation times are running late.
- If dealing with another client or speaking to a client on the telephone, still smile and make eye contact as the client enters, to show that they have been seen.

Difficult clients

Clients can be difficult for a variety of reasons. Sometimes it is because they are anxious or upset, sometimes because they are having a stressful day and sometimes because they just always behave in this way. There are also occasions when clients become aggressive, sometimes because of drink or drugs; this kind of client is not acting in a reasonable manner.

Whatever the outcome of dealing with a difficult client, the encounter should not be taken personally. The client has no personal grudge: they simply took out their feelings or anger on the first person they came across in reception.

Steps to follow when dealing with a difficult client

- **Listen carefully to what they are saying – make sure that their problem or complaint is understood.**
- **Be patient – sometimes they need to get the problem off their chest and the situation is then defused.**
- **Remain calm and use a normal tone of voice with the client.**
- **Never become angry or defensive – this will only worsen the situation, making the client even more difficult to deal with.**
- **Do not pass blame or make excuses – the client will simply not be interested.**
- **Sort the problem out quickly and in a positive manner.**
- **If the client is causing embarrassment, consider asking them to move to a separate room where their problem can be discussed in private (NB: do *not* do this with an aggressive or really angry client).**
- **If unable to sort out the problem easily, seek help from someone in authority and pass the client on to them so that other waiting clients can be dealt with.**

Steps to follow when dealing with an aggressive client

- **Listen carefully.**
- **Stay calm; don't argue or become defensive.**
- **Remain polite at all times.**
- **Avoid any prolonged eye contact, as this can be seen as threatening or challenging.**
- **Seek help from a more senior member of staff if necessary.**
- **Keep your distance (they may be unpredictable) and never make any physical contact.**
- **If the client is likely to be a danger to staff or to other clients, call the police.**

Non-verbal communication

A large proportion of communication is non-verbal. People do not need to speak to show how they feel; their body language can do this for them. When dealing with clients face to face, it is important to be aware of the non-verbal signals that clients are sending and being given. Clients need to be given positive non-verbal messages. This shows that practice staff are listening to them and care about them.

Positive and negative body language

Positive body language includes:

- **Smiling**
- **Eye contact (but not staring)**
- **Facing the person**
- **Open and relaxed body position**
- **No fiddling or fidgeting**
- **Nodding in agreement.**

Negative body language includes:

- **Not making eye contact**
- **Turning away**
- **Not smiling, but frowning or looking glum**
- **Arms folded**
- **Fiddling or fidgeting**
- **Foot tapping or hand tapping**
- **Clenched fists.**

Recognizing positive and negative body language enables better judgement of how to deal with situations and how likely the clients are to accept suggestions or agree to treatment. For example, a client who continues to exhibit negative body language after having the reasons for flea treatment explained to them is less likely to purchase the flea product than the client who is smiling and showing positive body language.

Security and confidentiality

Client records contain large amounts of personal details that the veterinary practice must keep secure and confidential. Most client records are computerized, but there are still paper records in some practices. Either kind of record will contain information such as that listed in the section 'Record keeping' later in this chapter.

The collection, storage and use of this data is controlled by the Data Protection Act 1998, which requires information about individuals to be accurate and relevant and kept secure from unauthorized access or accidental loss. Clients have the right to see the information in the records and to ask for the removal of any incorrect data.

Computer screens in the reception area should be placed in such a position that clients and other visitors cannot read the information displayed. Client details should never be discussed in front of or with other clients or members of the public.

Making and receiving telephone calls

The telephone is a major communication method in veterinary practice. It rings hundreds of times a day and each time it is answered the person who picks it up must use good communication skills.

Answering the telephone

The number of rings

The telephone should be answered after three to four rings. If it is answered before this, the client may be taken by surprise or may think that the practice is not very busy. Letting the phone ring too many times suggests that the practice is not interested in the call or simply too busy to reply.

The greeting

The greeting will be decided by the practice, but generally it is likely to be something similar to: 'Good morning/afternoon/evening, this is ABC Veterinary Practice, how can I help you?' Some practices also require receptionists to give their name to the client in the greeting.

Speaking clearly

The receptionist should speak clearly and not too fast, should sound welcoming and should never use jargon such as 'OK'. The tone of voice is very important, because the client cannot see the person at the other end of the telephone or any of their body language, which means that what is said can sometimes be less important that how it is said. A grumpy or disinterested voice could easily cause the client to feel unwanted or a nuisance.

Identifying the caller and the problem

- Make sure that the caller gives their name and address and the name of their pet.
- Take details of the pet's illness and the treatment or service required so that the veterinary surgeon can prepare for the consultation.
- Listen carefully to enquiries and provide the necessary information, or pass the caller on to a member of staff who can.

Priorities

The phone is always the most important priority. A phone call can mean an emergency and so even if another client is already being dealt with the phone must be answered. Apologies should be made to the client, explaining that the phone call could be a life or death situation. Most clients will be understanding – after all, it might be them making the call one day.

Putting someone on hold

If it is necessary to put a caller on hold:

- Always check that it is all right to do so and wait for their answer. Remember that the call could be an emergency, in which case being put on hold would not be acceptable
- Return to the client at regular intervals and ask if they are still happy to remain on hold. Do not leave them on hold for intervals of more than 30 seconds
- If they are not happy to continue holding, or if it is clear that they will have to wait a long time, offer to phone them back.

Busy times

The receptionist should try not to sound harassed at busy times: the client will hear the stress in their voice and this is not a good advertisement for the practice, as it suggests bad organization. At busy times it may be appropriate to offer to phone back a client who has a particularly complicated query that cannot be dealt with easily and quickly.

Taking messages

It will often be necessary to take detailed messages from clients or other veterinary practices or organizations.

- Always have a pen and paper available.
- Make careful, clear, detailed notes of any message.
- Always take a contact name and telephone number.
- Always be sure who the message was for.
- If any of the message is unclear, ask for it to be repeated.

Making telephone calls

Individuals and organizations who are telephoned need to be impressed by the efficiency of the practice staff.

- Check the practice's policy on making telephone calls: is there a specific time of day when they are made?
- Choose a time when the practice is less busy to make any calls.
- Estimate how long the call will take and make sure that there is still someone available to answer incoming calls.
- Make sure that all the information needed is at hand (documents, names, addresses, figures, etc.).
- Check the telephone numbers to be called and the names of the people to speak to.
- Plan what needs to be said.
- Listen carefully and make notes during the call so that all the relevant information is recorded.
- At the end of the call, write up any other relevant details.
- If the person required is not available, leave a clear simple message, a contact name and number and a time when it would be convenient to be called back.
- If asked to call back, find out what time would be best and make sure that the call is made at the time suggested.

Other electronic communication

Veterinary practices increasingly use other kinds of electronic communication than the telephone. As with the telephone, it is necessary to be familiar with the practice's policy on their use.

Mobile phones

- Remember that the full area code must be dialled on mobile phones before the personal number.
- Become familiar with the use of the practice's mobile phones, how to store and retrieve numbers, messages and texts and how to recharge the phone.

Fax machines

Faxing is an excellent way to communicate larger quantities of information, such as records and reports.

- Always check the telephone number to which the fax is being sent (faxes sent to the wrong address can be embarrassing).
- Many fax machines produce a fax report, which is a useful record of time of sending and destination.
- When receiving faxes, check that the paper roll or tray is not empty.
- Know how to change fax rolls and add more paper and how to deal with paper jams.

Email

Most practices now use external email and many have internal emailing systems. Clients are increasingly using email to contact their practice and sometimes to make appointments. Some practices, with their clients' agreement, send booster reminders, newsletters and so on by email.

Care must be taken not to send unsolicited or confidential information to the wrong email address.

Written forms of communication

Veterinary practices communicate with their clients using a variety of written forms of communication (Figure 9.5).

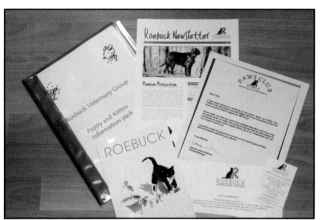

9.5 A range of printed material produced by a practice.

Newsletters

Newsletters are usually produced quarterly and sent to clients or distributed in the reception area. They contain news about the practice, animal health information and often promotional material about products and the practice's services.

Leaflets

Leaflets on various healthcare topics are given to clients for information or to those whose pets may benefit from particular treatments. Leaflets help to distribute extra information and advice to clients and are often used in conjunction with poster displays.

Practice brochures

Many practices produce a practice brochure, which they normally give to all new clients and make available in reception. The brochure gives information about the practice, its staff, its services and specialities, consultation times, payment policy, contact details, emergency numbers and other useful client information.

Booster reminders

Most practices post vaccination reminders to clients to encourage them to bring their pet for its annual booster. Usually the booster reminder takes the form of a card with the client's address on one side and the booster details on the other. The cards are often posted to the pet by name.

Bills

Bills should be paid at the time of treatment. Inevitably this is not always 100% successful and bills have to be sent to clients who owe money at the end of each month. In equine and large animal practice, posting monthly bills is the general practice.

Posting information

Veterinary practices use the postal system to communicate with clients, and to send reports and some laboratory samples. There are various postal options and the choice depends on the need for speed and security of the item to be sent.

- First-class post – normally delivered the next day.
- Second-class post – delivered by the third working day.
- Special delivery – guaranteed by 12 noon the next day.
- Recorded delivery – allows confirmation of delivery of important items.
- Parcel post – for heavier items.

Basic reception work

The receptionist plays an important role in the practice. The job is very much more than answering the telephone and booking appointments; it is varied and demanding and covers both practical and administrative tasks.

Record keeping

Records such as client details, animal treatment and diagnostic results are kept so that a pet's ongoing healthcare is carefully monitored and maintained, and so that previous treatments and complaints can be checked.

Client records

Many practices have computerized client records, while some still maintain client record cards. Whatever format records take, they must be accurate and kept up to date. Whatever system is used, a client's record will have three major parts: general, clinical and financial.

General details of client and pet

The general details kept are:

- Client's name
- Client's address
- Telephone numbers (home, mobile, work)
- Email address
- Pet's name
- Pet's date of birth
- Breed
- Colour
- Sex
- Weight
- Vaccination details
- Flea control details
- Microchip details
- Insurance details.

Clinical details

Clinical details are recorded by the veterinary surgeon, and in some cases the veterinary nurse.

Financial details

All financial details (money owed and paid) must be recorded. This ensures that bills are accurate and queries can be answered easily.

Recording messages

Dozens of messages and pieces of information are received by receptionists every day. They must all be accurately recorded, stored or passed on in the appropriate way.

Client records, X-rays, laboratory reports, equipment details, maintenance records, etc. also need to be filed and stored carefully. These may be filed in a number of ways.

- Alphabetically (e.g. laboratory reports) – by client surname, then initial.
- Chronologically (e.g. X-rays) – by date, year, month, day of month.
- Numerically (e.g. standard operating procedures or protocols) – by sequential numbers, which are cross-referenced to other information.

Recording accidents

All accidents (i.e. incidents involving injury to or illness of a member of staff in the workplace) must by law be recorded in the practice's accident book. The information to be recorded includes:

- Date of accident
- Time of accident
- Place of accident
- Name of injured person
- Job of injured person
- Details of injury
- First aid given
- Consequences (e.g. continued work, went home, went to hospital)
- Name and signature of person who dealt with the accident.

Drugs and batch numbers

Responsibility for recording the movement of drugs to and from the practice (including records for disposal of out-of-date drugs) may fall to a receptionist. Under new EU regulations, practices are required to carry out a detailed annual audit of all the transactions with incoming and outgoing medicines. These records may be inspected. The information that must be recorded includes:

- Drugs dispensed:
  - Date
  - Product name
  - Manufacturer's batch number
  - Quantity supplied
  - Name and address of client
  - Name and address of practice.
- Drugs purchased:
  - Date of purchase
  - Product name
  - Manufacturer's batch number
  - Quantity received
  - Name and address of supplier.

If records are accurately maintained, at the end of the year the amount of each drug purchased should equal the amount dispensed plus any disposed of as clinical waste.

Making appointments

Most practices operate an appointments system but some have what is called an open surgery, where clients can simply turn up and wait their turn to see the veterinary surgeon. Appointments are made either in an appointments book or on a computerized diary, which should indicate appointments available and who the consulting vets are and should be made up for at least four weeks ahead so that advance bookings can be made. Some requests for appointments are more urgent than others (for example, a booster is not urgent while an animal that has been vomiting for 24 hours is).

- Organize appointments efficiently to suit both client and veterinary surgeon.
- Offer clients an appointment that suits the consulting pattern of the practice, thereby staying in control of the appointments.

There is a basic checklist of information needed from the client which helps the veterinary surgeon and aids the smooth running of the appointments system:

- Name of owner
- Whether they are an existing or a new client
- Owner's address
- Name of pet
- What the appointment is for
- Problem or clinical signs
- How long the pet has been ill
- Any other relevant details
- Whether they are bringing one pet or more than one.

This information should be used to decide whether the client requires a single or a double appointment (for example, more than one pet or possibly a first vaccination may mean a double appointment) and how urgent the case may be. The relevant information should be noted on the client's appointment record so that the consulting veterinary surgeon is prepared for the consultation. A sick animal must always be seen on the same day, even if the client has to be asked to come to the surgery and wait because the diary is full.

Taking payments

All small animal veterinary practices expect clients to pay at the time their pet is treated and every client should be presented with an itemized bill at this time. Because so much large animal and equine work is carried out away from the practice, these clients are usually sent monthly accounts. When clients have paid their bills, their account must be credited with the payment.

There are a number of different payment methods.

Cash

- Ensure that the money is valid currency. Banks often provide information on how to check paper money for the following:
  - Watermarks
  - Metal strips
  - Paper quality
  - Printed shapes at the bottom of each note.
- Always check the amount of cash handed over and the change given.

Cheques

- Always watch as the cheque is being signed.
- Check that the signature matches the guarantee card and that the written amount matches the numbered amount.
- Record the cheque card number, expiry date and type of card (e.g. Mastercard, Visa) on the back of the cheque.
- Never accept a postdated cheque.
- If the client makes an error when writing the cheque, the mistake can be crossed out and rectified but the correction must be initialled by the client.
- A cheque will take three working days to clear.

Debit cards and credit cards

All new debit and credit cards are chip-and-pin.

- The chip is a small microchip embedded into the card which holds the cardholder's unique details.
- The pin is the four-digit personal identification number assigned to the cardholder.

When the card is placed in the practice's electronic card terminal the cardholder keys in their pin number, online authorization is given and a receipt is printed.

Standing orders

A standing order is a fixed-amount payment from a client's account into the veterinary practice's bank account on a fixed date. A standing order can be altered by the client. A small number of clients use this method of payment to keep their account in credit.

Direct debits

A direct debit differs from a standing order in that the amount paid into the practice's bank account from the client's account is flexible and can be altered by the practice, depending upon how much the client owes. As with the standing order, a few clients use this method to pay their veterinary bills.

Retailing, marketing and promotion

Veterinary practices depend on good marketing and retailing to boost their business. Practices promote their services and products to clients in a variety of ways.

Product displays

Product displays should be eye-catching and attractive and placed so that they can be seen easily (Figure 9.6). Clients should be able to touch and look at the products, all of which should be priced. There should be neither too few nor too many items on display. Those that do not sell readily or are damaged or gather dust should be removed. Easy-to-sell items should be placed at ground level and the products that the practice wants to sell the most should be at eye level. It is always worth having a small selection of 'impulse buys' near the reception desk. Those who promote and sell the products should be familiar with them and able to talk about the benefits they have for clients and their pets.

Although a good source of revenue, product displays can be tempting for the potential thief. To minimize theft a number of measures can be taken:

- Position displays in the direct view of the staff
- Have dummy boxes of products
- Ensure that clients have to walk past the reception desk to leave the practice.

Promotions

Monthly

These regular promotions are often tied in with the practice's website and newsletter. Posters and wall displays can be used to promote services and leaflets can be made available in reception if the client asks for more information. It is important to talk to the client about these promotions and be able to answer any queries.

Seasonal

Special promotions are often carried out at different times of the year, such as Christmas (Christmas toys), summer (vaccinations) and spring (flea control).

General veterinary

There are an increasing number of annual countrywide veterinary promotions such as Pet Smile Week (for dental care) and National Pet Month (promoting good pet care).

Wall displays

Whatever a wall display is promoting, it should be eye-catching and provide a simple clear message (Figure 9.7). All material should be computer generated and preferably laminated. All the material should be within a frame and should be about 80% pictures and 20% text. Leaflets should be made available to provide extra information.

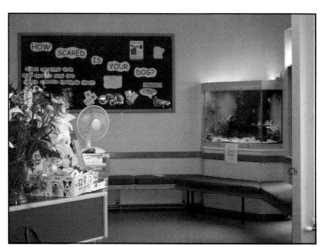

9.7 An information display board in a well ordered reception area.

Practice brochure

The practice brochure contains information about the practice's location, opening times and services to clients. It can be an excellent promotional tool, normally given to all new clients and always available in reception. Many practices use the practice brochure to emphasize to clients the ways in which they provide excellent treatment for sick animals as well as preventive healthcare.

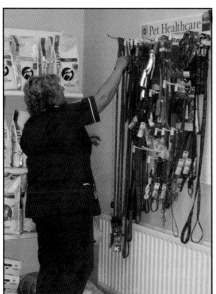

9.6 An eye-catching waiting room display.

Client newsletter

This is often produced on a quarterly basis and gives news about the practice and its staff and information about new services, products and treatments. Some practices send newsletters to all their clients while others send it with booster reminders and have it available both in the reception area and on their website.

Maintaining front-of-house areas

Public areas such as reception are the first parts of the practice that the client sees. The client must have a good first impression of these areas, because the impression they form will be carried through to every other service and facility. If a client has a good first impression they will assume that everything else in the practice meets the same standard – and the converse is also true.

Cleanliness and tidiness

The reception area should always be clean. Regular cleaning times help to achieve this.

- Floors should be mopped a number of times each day, especially in bad weather.
- Surfaces should be wiped and dust free.
- Any animal urine or faeces must be cleaned up and the area disinfected immediately (gloves should always be used when doing this and hands washed afterwards).

Everywhere, including the reception desk, should look tidy and be clutter free (untidiness suggests poor organization and clutter in the wrong place can be a health and safety hazard). Magazine racks, leaflet displays, tabletops and toy boxes should be kept tidy.

The reception area should not smell. Regular cleaning and disinfecting can help to avoid this problem, as can room fragrance products.

Equipment

Reception areas contain equipment such as printers, photocopiers, computers, fax machines and bank card machines. All equipment should be used in accordance with the training given and be maintained in good order. When not in use, it should be switched off according to instructions.

Maintenance

While using equipment, any damage or usage problems should be recorded and reported to the person responsible for health and safety in the practice. Poor maintenance (e.g. cracked glass, broken catches, sharp edges or damaged equipment) creates potential hazards for both staff and the public. It is part of an employee's legal obligation under health and safety legislation to report anything that they feel may be unsafe or cause a health risk.

Waste disposal

Most waste in the reception area will be paper and office waste. This should be disposed of according to the practice's waste disposal procedures. Waste bins should be emptied at least once a day and the waste stored safely to avoid any risk of fire. Waste printer cartridges and toners should be disposed of according to the practice's waste disposal rules. Any animal urine or faeces should be disposed of as clinical waste in the special clinical waste bins or bags provided by the practice.

Displays

As mentioned earlier, information leaflets and products for sale are an important part of practice merchandising. They should always be kept tidy and look attractive. Clients will not look at untidy leaflets or displays, resulting in lost sales opportunities. Old or out-of-date leaflets should be discarded, as should damaged or out-of-date products.

Noticeboards and posters must look attractive, be tidy and be up to date. Nothing should be stuck on reception room walls with adhesive tape, blue-tack or drawing pins. All posters should be at least laminated and preferably framed. Everything on the noticeboard should be current and kept within the frame. Tired-looking or dog-eared notices should be removed. If too much information is put on the noticeboard, clients will not read it all.

Providing information to clients

Clients need all kinds of information about the practice if they are to use it for their pet in the best way possible.

Practice services

Clients need to know about all the services the practice provides to keep their pet healthy. Staff providing this information must be able to explain all these services to the client in detail and answer any questions they may be asked. There are many types of services, including:

- Consultations
- Neutering
- Puppy parties
- Dental clinics
- Vaccination reminders
- Practice nurse consultations
- Annual health checks
- Nutrition clinics
- Older pet clinics
- Behavioural consultations
- Specialist referral consultations.

Practice availability

New clients need to know about:

- Practice contact details (telephone, website, address)
- Opening times
- Booking of appointments
- 24-hour emergency service
- Parking.

Existing clients need to be informed of any changes made to these details.

Practice policies and procedures

Some of the practice's policies and procedures need to be explained to clients, including:

- Bill payment – when and how they pay
- Animal restraint in the reception area – dogs on leads, cats in baskets
- Missed appointment procedure
- Making insurance claims
- Being given estimates for operations
- The euthanasia process and dealing with pet remains
- Hospitalization and pet visiting.

General veterinary advice

The degree of veterinary advice that can be given to clients by nursing and reception staff will depend on the practice, but as a general rule basic pet healthcare and product advice can be given to clients by trained, knowledgeable staff. Examples might include:

- Flea control
- Worm control
- Feeding
- Pet insurance
- Basic dental care
- Microchipping
- Neutering
- Vaccination
- Puppy and kitten care
- Rabbit care.

More detailed clinical information is likely to be given by qualified veterinary nurses and the veterinary surgeons.

Stock control

Good stock control requires an efficient ordering system, adequate stock levels, appropriate storage and careful stock rotation.

Ordering stock

Stock control is based on the principle of maximum and minimum stock levels for each product. This ensures that the practice does not run out of a product but at the same time does not have excess product sitting on the shelf taking up space and tying up money.

Wholesalers deliver stock daily or several times each week. Most manual stock-ordering systems have now been replaced by computerized systems involving handheld equipment that can be programmed with stock levels. Many systems also use bar codes to speed up the ordering system. If stock control is computerized, the ordering can be linked directly to the wholesaler's system; alternatively orders can be faxed or telephoned through to the wholesaler.

Receiving stock deliveries

All stock received must be checked against the original order and the wholesaler's delivery note that accompanies the delivery. The product name, quantity, pack size and sell-by date should be checked against the delivery note. If the delivery note details match the stock received and there are no damaged products, the stock can be shelved and the paperwork filed.

Sometimes not all of the products on the original order will be sent, because some are not available. The wholesaler should always inform the practice of products 'to follow' (to come at a later date) or on 'back order' (on order by the wholesaler).

Storage

Some stock requires special storage conditions and the product label should always be checked for these. For example, some products (e.g. vaccines) must be refrigerated, usually between 2 and 8°C, and placed in the fridge as soon as the delivery has been checked. Other products may require storage away from light.

- All products must be stored in dry vermin-free conditions in a secure building.
- It must be easy to identify the stored products (a typical storage system would be alphabetically on shelves in the practice dispensary).
- Large volume packs of product (e.g. food) may need to be stored elsewhere in the practice.
- Controlled drugs must be entered in the drug record book and stored in a permanently locked drugs cupboard to which only veterinary surgeons have keys.

Stock rotation

All stock is labelled with a sell-by or use-by date. Once this date has passed the manufacturer cannot guarantee the quality of the product and it cannot be used by the practice or sold to clients. Each stock item should be stored in such a way that the package with the shortest sell-by date is used first. Any stock that has an expired sell-by date must be removed and disposed of in accordance with the practice's waste disposal procedures.

Pet insurance

Pet insurance is in the best interests of the pet, the owner and the practice, and clients should always be encouraged to insure their pets. Since January 2005 veterinary practices have had to be authorized by the Financial Services Authority (FSA) before appointed representatives in the practice are allowed to recommend individual pet insurance companies, explain policy details, help clients to complete proposal forms and assist in the completion of claim forms. If a practice is not authorized it can only provide very general information on the advantages of pet insurance.

There are a large number of companies offering pet insurance and it can be very confusing for clients to know which is the best policy for them. The general advice which should be given to clients to help this choice is:

- Make sure that the cover is adequate: check exactly what cover the policy provides (e.g. injury to pet, death, loss of pet, third party insurance, optional extras such as hospitalization or costs to recover the pet)
- Check that the policy does not stipulate time limits for the length of time a condition is covered
- Check the maximum benefit payable per year and per condition
- Check that the insurance continues for the life of the animal and not just until they reach a certain age
- Check for hidden costs
- Check the small print.

Nurses and clients

Generally the nurse will be more involved with the practical side of pet healthcare than the receptionist. Veterinary nurses are often the link between the client and the veterinary surgeon and they will play an important part in communicating with clients in the following areas.

Patient information

Receiving information

Clear and concise information needs to be gathered from the client about their animal's condition if the correct treatment is to be given. The right questions must be asked.

- What is the problem?
- When did it start?
- What signs is the animal showing?
- What is the history of the problem, if any?
- What is the current situation?
- What has been done so far?
- Who saw the animal last?

The nurse should listen very carefully to the client, make notes if necessary, and make sure that all the information has been given and that it has been fully understood. If unsure, it is useful to repeat the problem back to the client just to check that there has been no misunderstanding.

Reporting information

Clients are always anxious about their pet, whether it has been in for an operation or is hospitalized. Animals that have been in for general operations are usually discharged the same day and clients need to know how to take care of their pet while it recovers, what medication it needs to be given and how to administer it. Reports on hospitalized animals may involve giving an update on the pet's condition and sometimes an idea of how much longer it will remain at the practice.

Many clients will be anxious and worried about their pet and so communicating sometimes quite complex information must be done carefully. The animal's progress should be discussed in a supportive way and the nurse should consult a veterinary surgeon if in any doubt. It is important to ensure that the client has understood what has been explained to them.

- Provide the information in clear simple terms. Do not complicate matters unnecessarily.
- If talking to the client face to face, find a quiet place where there are no distractions.
- If reporting on the telephone, take extra care that the client has understood the information.
- Repeat the information if the client appears to be confused.
- At the end of the conversation, always summarize what has been said.

Admitting patients

When admitting animals for operations or hospitalization, the nurse should:

- Make sure that there is a full record of the client's details and the pet's details on the consent form
- Check that there has been no change of address or telephone number
- Make sure that the animal's records are available at the time of admission
- Confirm the procedure for which the animal is being admitted from the records and with the owner
- Make absolutely sure that the owner understands what is going to be done and why
- Complete the consent form in accordance with practice procedure and ask and check that the owner reads, understands and signs the form
- Explain to the owner how and when they can find out how their animal is progressing after the operation
- Take the animal from the owner to admit it, making sure that it is adequately restrained.

Discharging patients

When the owner arrives to collect their animal:

- Check that the animal is ready for collection
- Identify any notes or medication to be sent home with the animal
- Explain to the owner any aftercare that the animal will need and make sure that they understand and are able to carry this out. If there are any questions you cannot answer, refer them to a veterinary surgeon
- Return the animal to the owner together with any medication, healthcare instructions and other belongings such as leads or blankets, making sure that the animal is adequately restrained so that there is no danger of escape.

Euthanasia

Clients are at their most sensitive and vulnerable at this time and need appropriate understanding and sympathy. They should not be judged by their behaviour at this time as it may not be normal. The euthanasia appointment should be made away from normal appointment times, so that the client comes into contact with as few other clients as possible. Some clients will wish to pay for the euthanasia consultation at the time or beforehand, but do not insist upon this unless the practice policy is otherwise.

If the client is very upset by the death of their pet they should be given time to grieve, preferably in a private part of the practice, and careful consideration should be given as to whether they are safe to drive themselves home if they have come by car. Some practices offer pet bereavement counselling and clients can be directed to this service if they ask or can be given contact details of other pet bereavement counsellors.

Nurse clinics

There are many different kinds of nurse clinics. Examples include:

- Nutrition clinics
- Weight clinics
- Dental clinics
- Senior pet clinics
- Adolescent clinics
- Well pet clinics
- Puppy parties
- Dressing changes
- Nail clipping
- Second vaccination.

Nurse clinics provide an excellent service for clients who wish to keep their pets healthy. They are an ideal opportunity to discuss the health of the pet and often highlight problems that would otherwise have gone unnoticed.

- As with any other consultation, explain what the problems or potential problems are, how they can be treated or prevented, what this involves, and how long it is likely to take.
- Make sure that the client has understood any explanations.
- Provide back up leaflets and literature where appropriate.

For more information on nurse clinics see *BSAVA Manual of Advanced Veterinary Nursing*.

Advising clients

Clients can often be nervous or embarrassed about asking for advice, especially from the veterinary surgeon. The nurse can play an important role in reassuring clients and providing advice.

- Always encourage clients to ask questions – ask them if they have any questions or if they need any help, as this opens the door for them to enquire.
- All advice must be given in accordance with the practice's policies and procedures.
- Provide clients with leaflets and literature produced or approved by the practice to help to explain the advice.
- Give clear precise advice – do not leave the client confused or wondering which option to take.
- Explain the benefits of following the advice and the consequences of not following it.
- If the advice required is of a too technical, clinical or specialist nature, pass the client on to the person who can give the most expert advice.
- Always appear confident and professional; this gives the client confidence in the advice and will make them much more likely to follow it.
- Be aware that clients differ in their ability to understand the information they are given – provide the advice and information in the best way and form for the client.

References and further reading

Corsan J and Mackay AR (2001) *The Veterinary Receptionist: Essential Skills for Client Care*. Butterworth-Heinemann, Oxford

Masters J and Bowden C (2001) *Pre-Veterinary Nursing Textbook*. Butterworth-Heinemann, Oxford (in association with BVNA)

Nicholls L and Shilcock M (in press) Client communication and advise. In: *BSAVA Manual of Practical Veterinary Nursing*, ed. E Mullineaux and M Jones. BSAVA Publications, Gloucester

Pease A (1993) *Body Language, 19th edn*. Sheldon Press, London

Shilcock M (2001) *The Veterinary Support Team*. Threshold Press, Newbury

Shilcock M (in press) Professional responsibilities of the veterinary nurse. In: *BSAVA Manual of Practical Veterinary Nursing*, ed. E Mullineaux and M Jones. BSAVA Publications, Gloucester

Shilcock M and Stutchfield G (2003) *Veterinary Practice Management – a Practical Guide*. Saunders, Edinburgh

10

Veterinary terminology

Paula Hotston Moore

> *This chapter is designed to give information on:*
>
> ■ Word roots
> ■ Prefixes and suffixes
> ■ How to understand and recognize common veterinary words
> ■ Common abbreviations

Introduction

Veterinary terminology is a completely new language. This chapter explores how medical terms are constructed. Once an understanding of some basic body parts and their terms are learned, words can begin to be built up. A long, confusing medical term can be broken down into sections to obtain its meaning.

The main section of the word is the *word root* and it is this which gives the word its meaning. A prefix or suffix is added to the word root at the beginning or end to change its meaning.

■ A *prefix* is added in front of the main word root to form the first part of the word. Many words used in everyday language are formed as a word root with a prefix in front (e.g. *tri*cycle; *anti*social; *dis*advantage; *un*acceptable).
■ A *suffix* is added to the end of the word root to form the last part of the word (e.g. mov*able*; charm*ing*; happi*ness*; baro*meter*).

Example

Word root:	MORTEM ('death')
Prefix:	POST ('after')
New word:	POSTMORTEM ('after death')

Some words have both a prefix and a suffix, which combine to alter the meaning of the word root.

Example

Word root:	STRESS
Prefix:	UN ('not')
Suffix:	FUL ('complete')
New word:	UNSTRESSFUL

Many word roots change their spelling slightly to accommodate the addition of a prefix or suffix, to allow ease of pronunciation. This is called the *combining form*.

Example

Word root:	NATURE
Combining form:	NATUR
New word:	NATURALLY (not 'natureally')

The following sections relating to terminology for body systems give:

■ The word root
■ The Greek or Latin origins
■ The meaning.

This is followed by examples of words that combine the root with various prefixes and suffixes to form new words. The prefix (e.g. 'peri~') or suffix (e.g. '~itis') and its meaning are given in the first two columns; the combined word and its meaning are given in the last two columns.

The heart

Word root: **cardia**   From: **Greek *kardiakos***   Meaning: **heart**

~genic	produced by	CARDIOGENIC	arising from the heart
brady~	slow	BRADYCARDIA	slow heart rate
tachy~	fast	TACHYCARDIA	fast/increased heart rate
myo~	pertaining to muscle	MYOCARDIUM	heart muscle
~logy	study of	CARDIOLOGY	study of the heart
~pathy	disease of	CARDIOPATHY	disease of the heart
~megaly	enlargement of	CARDIOMEGALY	enlargement of the heart
~graph	instrument that records	CARDIOGRAPH	instrument that records the heart
~gram	record of	CARDIOGRAM	record or radiograph of the heart
~al	belonging to	CARDIAL	belonging to the heart
endo~/~itis	inner, within/ inflammation of	ENDOCARDITIS	inflammation of the inner lining of heart wall
peri~/~al	near, around/ belonging to	PERICARDIAL	around the heart
myo~/~itis	pertaining to muscle/ inflammation of	MYOCARDITIS	inflammation of the heart muscle
electro~/~graph	having electricity/ instrument that records	ELECTROCARDIOGRAPH	instrument that records electrical activity of the heart
electro~/~gram	having electricity/ record of	ELECTROCARDIOGRAM	a recording of the electrical activity of the heart

Word root: **angio**   From: **Greek *angeion***   Meaning: **vessel**

~oma	tumour	ANGIOMA	tumour of a blood vessel
~gram	record of	ANGIOGRAM	record or radiograph of a blood vessel
~graphy	description of	ANGIOGRAPHY	process of taking a description, recording or radiography of blood vessels
~plasty	reconstructive surgery	ANGIOPLASTY	reconstructive surgery of blood vessels

Word root: **vascul**   From: **Latin *vasculum***   Meaning: **blood vessel**

		VASCULAR	relating to blood vessels
cardio~	pertaining to the heart	CARDIOVASCULAR	pertaining to the heart and blood vessels
~itis	inflammation of	VASCULITIS	inflammation of a blood vessel

Word root: **ven**   From: **Latin *vena***   Meaning: **vein**

intra~	into	INTRAVENOUS	into a vein

Word root: **phleb**   From: **Greek *phleps***   Meaning: **vein**

~itis	inflammation of	PHLEBITIS	inflammation of a vein
~otomy	incision into	PHLEBOTOMY	incision into a vein (to collect blood)

Word root: **haem**   From: **Greek** *haima*   Meaning: **blood**

~logy	study of	HAEMATOLOGY	study of blood
~thorax	chest, pleural cavity	HAEMOTHORAX	blood in the chest
~rrhage	excessive flow	HAEMORRHAGE	excessive flow of blood, process of bleeding
~uria	pertaining to urine	HAEMATURIA	presence of blood in urine
~oma	tumour, growth	HAEMATOMA	accumulation of blood in tissues, forming solid swelling
~lysis	breakdown of	HAEMOLYSIS	breakdown of blood

The respiratory system

Word root: **pneumo**   From: **Greek** *pneumon*   Meaning: **lung**

		PNEUMONIA	inflammation of the lungs
~thorax	chest, pleural cavity	PNEUMOTHORAX	presence of air or gas in the pleural cavity

Word root: **pnoea**   From: **Greek** *pnoe*   Meaning: **breathing**

a~	without	APNOEA	absence of breathing
dys~	difficulty	DYSPNOEA	difficulty in breathing
tachy~	fast	TACHYPNOEA	fast breathing rate
brady~	slow	BRADYPNOEA	slow breathing rate

Word root: **thorac**   From: **Greek** *thorax*   Meaning: **chest**

~otomy	surgical incision into	THORACOTOMY	surgical incision into thorax
~centesis	to withdraw fluid	THORACOCENTESIS	to withdraw fluid from the thoracic cavity

Word root: **rhin**   From: **Greek** *rhis*   Meaning: **nose**

~scope	instrument for examining	RHINOSCOPE	instrument used for internal examination of nose
~itis	inflammation of	RHINITIS	inflammation of the nose

Word root: **laryng**   From: **Greek** *laryngos*   Meaning: **larynx**

~itis	inflammation of	LARYNGITIS	inflammation of the larynx
~scope	instrument for examining	LARYNGOSCOPE	instrument used for internal examination of larynx
~spasm	involuntary movement of muscle	LARYNGOSPASM	involuntary tightening of larynx area

Word root: **trache**   From: **Greek** *tracheia*   Meaning: **trachea**

~otomy	surgical incision into	TRACHEOTOMY	surgical incision into trachea
~itis	inflammation of	TRACHEITIS	inflammation of the trachea
laryngo~/itis	pertaining to the larynx/ inflammation of	LARYNGOTRACHEITIS	inflammation of the larynx and trachea
endo~	inside	ENDOTRACHEAL	inside the trachea

Word root: **bronch**   From: **Greek *bronchos***   Meaning: **bronchi**

~itis	inflammation of	BRONCHITIS	inflammation of the bronchi
~scope	instrument for examining	BRONCHOSCOPE	instrument used for internal examination of bronchi

The digestive system

Word root: **oesophag**   From: **Greek *oisophagos***   Meaning: **oesophagus**

~itis	inflammation of	OESOPHAGITIS	inflammation of the oesophagus
~otomy	surgical incision into	OESOPHAGOTOMY	surgical incision into oesophagus

Word root: **gastr**   From: **Greek *gaster***   Meaning: **stomach**

		GASTRIC	relating to the stomach
~itis	inflammation of	GASTRITIS	inflammation of the stomach
~pathy	disease of	GASTROPATHY	disease of the stomach
~scope	instrument for examining	GASTROSCOPE	instrument used for internal examination of the stomach
~ostomy	surgical creation of opening into part of body	GASTROSTOMY	surgical creation of an opening into the stomach
~pexy	surgical fixation of	GASTROPEXY	surgical fixation of the stomach

Word root: **enter**   From: **Greek *enteron***   Meaning: **intestine**

		ENTERIC	relating to the intestines
~itis	inflammation of	ENTERITIS	inflammation of the intestine
~tomy	surgical incision into	ENTEROTOMY	surgical incision into intestine
~ectomy	removal of	ENTERECTOMY	removal of part of intestine
gastr~/~itis	pertaining to the stomach/ inflammation of	GASTROENTERITIS	inflammation of the stomach and intestines
gastr~/~logy	pertaining to the stomach/ study of	GASTROENTEROLOGY	study of the stomach and intestines
gastr~/~pathy	pertaining to the stomach/ disease of	GASTROENTEROPATHY	disease of the stomach and intestine

Word root: **hepat**   From: **Greek *hepar***   Meaning: **liver**

		HEPATIC	relating to the liver
~itis	inflammation of	HEPATITIS	inflammation of the liver
~cyte	cell	HEPATOCYTE	liver cell
~pathy	disease of	HEPATOPATHY	disease of the liver

Word root: **pancrea**   From: **Greek *pankreas* ('all flesh')**   Meaning: **pancreas**

		PANCREATIC	relating to the pancreas
~itis	inflammation of	PANCREATITIS	inflammation of the pancreas

Word root: **lapar**   From: **Greek** *lapara*   Meaning: **flank**

~otomy	surgical incision into	LAPAROTOMY	surgical incision into the abdomen
~scope	instrument for examining	LAPAROSCOPE	instrument used for internal examination of the abdomen

Word root: **periton**   From: **Greek** *peritonaion* ('stretched around')   Meaning: **peritoneum**

~itis	inflammation of	PERITONITIS	inflammation of the peritoneum
intra~	inside	INTRAPERITONEAL	inside the peritoneum
retro~	behind	RETROPERITONEAL	behind the peritoneum

The urinary system

Word root: **nephr**   From: **Greek** *nephros*   Meaning: **kidney**

~itis	inflammation of	NEPHRITIS	inflammation of the kidney
~logy	study of	NEPHROLOGY	study of the kidney
~ectomy	removal of	NEPHRECTOMY	removal of the kidney
~lithiasis	formation of calculus (urolith, stone)	NEPHROLITHIASIS	formation of a calculus in the kidney

Word root: **ur**   From: **Greek** *ouron*   Meaning: **urine**

poly~	many, much	POLYURIA	passing abnormally large amount of urine
dys~	difficulty	DYSURIA	difficulty in passing urine
an~	without	ANURIA	passing no urine
olig~	few, less	OLIGURIA	passing an abnormally small amount of urine
~logy	study of	UROLOGY	study of urine
~logist	person who studies	UROLOGIST	person who studies urine
~lith	stone, calculus	UROLITH	urinary stone
~aemia	specified condition of the blood	URAEMIA	presence of urea in the blood

Word root: **urethra**   From: **Greek** *ourethra*   Meaning: **urethra**

~gram	record of	URETHROGRAM	record or radiograph of the urethra
~itis	inflammation of	URETHRITIS	inflammation of the urethra

Word root: **cyst**   From: **Greek *kystis***   Meaning: **bladder**

~itis	inflammation of	CYSTITIS	inflammation of the bladder
~otomy	surgical incision into	CYSTOTOMY	surgical incision into the bladder
~lithiasis	stone, calculus	CYSTOLITHIASIS	bladder stone, calculus
~gram	record of	CYSTOGRAM	record or radiograph of the bladder
~graphy	description of	CYSTOGRAPHY	process of taking a recording or radiography of the bladder
~scopy	visual examination of	CYSTOSCOPY	visual examination inside of urinary bladder using an endoscope
pneumo~/~gram	presence of air or gas/ record of	PNEUMOCYSTOGRAM	radiograph of the presence of air in the bladder
chole~/~itis	gall bladder/ inflammation of	CHOLECYSTITIS	inflammation of the gall bladder
chole~/~ectomy	gall bladder/ removal of	CHOLECYSTECTOMY	removal of the gall bladder

The reproductive system

Word root: **testicul**   From: **Latin *testiculus***   Meaning: **testis (plural testes)**

		TESTICULAR	relating to the testes

Word root: **prostat**   From: **Greek *prostates* ('standing in front')**   Meaning: **prostate gland**

~itis	inflammation of	PROSTATITIS	inflammation of the prostate gland
~ectomy	surgical removal of	PROSTATECTOMY	surgical removal of the prostate gland

Word root: **ovar**   From: **Latin *ovum* ('egg')**   Meaning: **ovary**

		OVARIAN	relating to the ovary
~ectomy	surgical removal of	OVARIECTOMY	surgical removal of ovary

Word root: **oo**   From: **Greek *oion***   Meaning: **egg**

~genesis	development of	OOGENESIS	development process of eggs in ovary
~cyte	cell	OOCYTE	egg cell

Word root: **uter**   From: **Latin *uterus***   Meaning: **womb**

intra~	within	INTRAUTERINE	within the uterus

Word root: **hyster**   From: **Greek *hystera***   Meaning: **uterus**

~ectomy	surgical removal of	HYSTERECTOMY	surgical removal of the uterus
ovario~/~ectomy	relating to the ovary/ surgical removal of	OVARIOHYSTERECTOMY	surgical removal of ovaries and uterus

Word root: **metr** From: **Greek *metra*** Meaning: **uterus**

py~	denoting pus	PYOMETRA	accumulation of pus in the uterus
~itis	inflammation of	METRITIS	inflammation of the uterus
endo~/~itis	inner, within/ inflammation of	ENDOMETRITIS	inflammation of inner lining of the uterus

Word root: **oestrus** From: **Latin *oestrus*, Greek *oistros*** Meaning: **female sexual impulse**

		OESTRUS	stage of oestrous cycle when female is receptive to male ('on heat')
poly~	many	POLYOESTROUS	having several consecutive oestrous cycles per annum
mono~	one, single	MONOESTROUS	having a single oestrous cycle occurring two or three times per annum
an~	without	ANOESTRUS	absence of oestrus, reduced ovarian activity
pro~	before	PRO-OESTRUS	stage of oestrous cycle when development of ovarian follicles begins, prior to oestrus

Word root: **vagina** From: **Latin *vagina*** Meaning: **sheath**

per	through	PER VAGINA	through the vagina
~itis	inflammation of	VAGINITIS	inflammation of the vagina

Word root: **mamma** From: **Latin *mamma*** Meaning: **milk gland**

~graphy	description of	MAMMOGRAPHY	process of taking a recording of the mammary gland

Word root: **mastos** From: **Greek *mastos*** Meaning: **breast**

~itis	inflammation of	MASTITIS	inflammation of the mammary gland
~ectomy	surgical removal of	MASTECTOMY	surgical removal of a mammary gland

Word root: **natal** From: **Latin *natalis*** Meaning: **birth**

ante~	before	ANTENATAL	before birth
pre~	before	PRENATAL	before birth
neo~	new, recent	NEONATAL	newborn
peri~	around	PERINATAL	around the time of birth
post~	after	POSTNATAL	after birth

The skeletal system

Word root: **oste**   From: **Greek** *osteon*   Meaning: **bone**

peri~	around	PERIOSTEUM	layer of connective tissue covering bone
~malacia	softening of	OSTEOMALACIA	softening of bone
~cyte	cell	OSTEOCYTE	bone cell
~blast	formative cell	OSTEOBLAST	cell responsible for formation of bone
~lysis	breakdown of	OSTEOLYSIS	breakdown of bone
dys~/~trophy	difficulty/ development	OSTEODYSTROPHY	abnormal bone development
~sarcoma	malignant tumour of	OSTEOSARCOMA	malignant tumour of bone connective tissue

Word root: **myel**   From: **Greek** *myelos*   Meaning: **marrow**

~malacia	softening of	MYELOMALACIA	abnormal softening of bone marrow
osteo~/~itis	relating to bone/ inflammation of	OSTEOMYELITIS	inflammation of bone marrow

Word root: **chondr**   From: **Greek** *chondros*   Meaning: **cartilage**

~cyte	cell	CHONDROCYTE	cartilage cell
~genesis	formation of	CHONDROGENESIS	formation of cartilage
~itis	inflammation of	CHONDRITIS	inflammation of cartilage
osteo~/~itis	relating to bone/ inflammation of	OSTEOCHONDRITIS (OCD)	inflammation of cartilage and bone around a joint

Word root: **spondyl**   From: **Greek** *sp(h)ondylos*   Meaning: **vertebra**

~itis	inflammation of	SPONDYLITIS	inflammation of the synovial joints in the vertebral column
~lysis	breakdown of	SPONDYLOSIS	degeneration of intervertebral discs

Word root: **arthr**   From: **Greek** *arthron*   Meaning: **joint**

~itis	inflammation of	ARTHRITIS	inflammation of a joint
~desis	surgical fusion of bones	ARTHRODESIS	surgical fusion of bones across a joint space
~pathy	disease of	ARTHROPATHY	disease of a joint
~plasty	plastic surgery	ARTHROPLASTY	surgical construction of new joint; remodelling of diseased joint
~otomy	surgical incision into	ARTHROTOMY	surgical incision into a joint
~oscopy	internal visualization of	ARTHROSCOPY	internal visualization of a joint

The endocrine system

Word root: **thyroid**   From: **Greek *thyreoeides***   Meaning: **shield-shaped**

hyper~	excessive, abnormally high	HYPERTHYROID	with excessive amounts of thyroid hormone in the bloodstream
hypo~	abnormally low	HYPOTHYROID	with abnormally low amounts of thyroid hormone in the bloodstream
para~	adjacent to	PARATHYROID	next to thyroid glands
~ectomy	surgical removal of	THYROIDECTOMY	surgical removal of thyroid gland

Word root: **pituita**   From: **Latin *pituita***   Meaning: **phlegm**

hypo~	abnormally low	HYPOPITUITARISM	condition caused by subnormal activity of the pituitary gland
hyper~	excessive, abnormally high	HYPERPITUITARISM	condition caused by overactive pituitary gland

The nervous system

Word root: **neur**   From: **Greek *neuron***   Meaning: **nerve**

		NEURON(E)	nerve cell
~algia	pain	NEURALGIA	nerve pain
~logy	study of	NEUROLOGY	study of nerves
~oma	tumour	NEUROMA	benign tumour of nerves
~osis	denoting a condition	NEUROSIS	functional disorder of the nervous system
~itis	inflammation of	NEURITIS	inflammation of a nerve
~pathy	disease of	NEUROPATHY	disease of the nervous system

Word root: **cephal**   From: **Greek *kephale***   Meaning: **head**

hydro~	denoting water or watery fluid	HYDROCEPHALUS	abnormal increase in the cerebrospinal fluid present in the brain
brachy~	short	BRACHYCEPHALIC	with short wide skull or head (e.g. Pekinese)
dolicho~	long	DOLICHOCEPHALIC	with long narrow skull (e.g. Irish Wolfhound)
meso~	middle	MESOCEPHALIC	with skull intermediate between brachy- and dolichocephalic (e.g. Beagle)

Word root: **encephal**   From: **Greek *enkephalon* ('in the head')**   Meaning: **brain**

~itis	inflammation of	ENCEPHALITIS	inflammation of the brain
~malacia	softening of	ENCEPHALOMALACIA	degeneration or softening of the brain
~pathy	disease of	ENCEPHALOPATHY	disease of the brain

Word root: **mening**   From: **Greek *meninx***   Meaning: **membrane**

~oma	tumour	MENINGIOMA	benign tumour of the meninges
~encephal/~itis	pertaining to the brain/ inflammation of	MENINGOENCEPHALITIS	inflammation of the meninges and brain

Word root: **plegia**   From: **Greek** *plege* ('a blow')   Meaning: **paralysis/weakness**

para~	beside, near	PARAPLEGIA	paralysis of both hindlimbs
tetra~	four	TETRAPLEGIA	paralysis of all four limbs
hemi~	half	HEMIPLEGIA	paralysis of one side of the body (left or right)

The ear

Word root: **aur**   From: **Latin** *auris*   Meaning: **ear**

		AURAL	relating to the ear
~icle	diminutive	AURICLE	visible part of external ear
~scope	instrument for examining	AURISCOPE	instrument used for internal examination of the ear

Word root: **oto**   From: **Greek** *ous*   Meaning: **ear**

| ~scope | instrument for examining | OTOSCOPE | instrument used for internal examination of the ear |
| ~itis | inflammation of | OTITIS | inflammation of the ear |

The eye

Word root: **ophthalm**   From: **Greek** *ophthalmos*   Meaning: **eye**

~logy	study of	OPHTHALMOLOGY	study of the eye
~scope	instrument for examining	OPHTHALMOSCOPE	instrument used for internal examination of the eye
~itis	inflammation of	OPHTHALMITIS	inflammation of the eye

Word root: **ocul**   From: **Latin** *oculus*   Meaning: **eye**

| | | OCULAR | relating to the eye |
| ~motor | movement | OCULOMOTOR NERVE | nerve concerned with movement of the eye muscles |

Word root: **blephar**   From: **Greek** *blepharon*   Meaning: **eyelid**

| ~itis | inflammation of | BLEPHARITIS | inflammation of the eyelid |
| ~spasm | involuntary movement | BLEPHAROSPASM | involuntary spasm or twitching of the eye muscle around the eyelid |

Word root: **conjunctiv**   From: **Latin** *conjunctum* ('joined')   Meaning: **conjunctiva**

| ~itis | inflammation of | CONJUNCTIVITIS | inflammation of the conjunctiva |
| sub~ | under | SUBCONJUNCTIVAL | under the conjunctiva |

The mouth

Word root: **gloss**   From: **Greek** *glossa*   Meaning: **tongue**

~itis	inflammation of	GLOSSITIS	inflammation of the tongue
~pharyngeal	of the pharynx	GLOSSOPHARYNGEAL	relating to the tongue and pharynx

Word root: **gingiv**   From: **Latin** *gingiva*   Meaning: **gum**

~itis	inflammation of	GINGIVITIS	inflammation of the gums

The skin

Word root: **derm**   From: **Greek** *derma*   Meaning: **skin**

epi~	above	EPIDERMIS	outer layer of skin
~itis	inflammation of	DERMATITIS	inflammation of the skin
~logy	study of	DERMATOLOGY	study of the skin
~mycosis	fungal infection of	DERMATOMYCOSIS	fungal infection of the skin

Word root: **kerat**   From: **Greek** *keras*   Meaning: **horn**

hyper~	excessive	HYPERKERATOSIS	overproduction of the horny layer of the skin

Word root: **seb**   From: **Latin** *sebum* ('suet')   Meaning: **sebum**

		SEBACEOUS	containing or secreting fatty or oily matter
~rrhoea	excessive flow	SEBORRHOEA	excessive secretion of sebum

Tumours

A tumour is any abnormal swelling on or in the body.
Tumours are classed as malignant or benign.

Definitions

Malignant tumour	A tumour that invades and destroys tissue in which it originates and then spreads to other sites in the body
Benign tumour	A tumour that does not destroy tissue or produce harmful effects
Metastasis	The spread of malignant tissue to other areas of the body

Classification of tumours

Adenocarcinoma	Malignant tumour of glandular tissue
Adenoma	Benign tumour of glandular tissue
Carcinoma	Malignant tumour of epithelial tissues
Fibroma	Benign tumour of fibrous tissue
Fibrosarcoma	Malignant tumour of fibrous tissue
Lipoma	Benign tumour of adipose cells
Lymphosarcoma	Malignant tumour of lymphatic tissue
Malignant melanoma	Malignant skin tumour of melanocytes
Melanoma	Benign skin tumour of melanocytes
Osteosarcoma	Malignant tumour of osteoblasts
Papilloma	Benign tumour of epithelial cells, often wart-like in appearance
Sarcoma	Malignant tumour arising from connective tissue
Squamous cell carcinoma	Malignant tumour of squamous epithelium commonly affecting skin, mouth and conjunctiva

Abbreviations

a.c.	before food
ACD	acid citrate dextrose (an anticoagulant)
ad lib	*ad libitum* – freely as wanted
b.d.s.	to be taken twice daily
bid	twice daily
BIOP	been in owner's possession
BSAVA	British Small Animal Veterinary Association
BVA	British Veterinary Association
BVNA	British Veterinary Nursing Association
CD	controlled drugs
CNS	central nervous system
COSHH	Control of Substances Hazardous to Health
CPD	continual professional development
CPDA	citrate phosphate dextrose adenine (an anticoagulant)
CPR	cardiopulmonary resuscitation
CVP	central venous pressure
EDTA	ethylenediamine tetraacetic acid (an anticoagulant)
e.o.d.	every other day
FeLV	feline leukaemia virus
FIA	feline infectious anaemia
FIP	feline infectious peritonitis
FIV	feline immunodeficiency virus
FLUTD	feline lower urinary tract disease
FURTD	feline upper respiratory tract disease
g	gram
GDV	gastric dilatation and volvulus
GI	gastrointestinal
h	hour
Hb	haemoglobin
HSE	Health and Safety Executive
IC, i.c., i/c	intracardiac
ICU	intensive care unit
IM, i.m., i/m	intramuscular
IP, i.p., i/p	intraperitoneal
IPPV	intermittent positive pressure ventilation
IU	international units
IV, i.v., i/v	intravenous
KC	Kennel Club
kg	kilogram
kV	kilovolt
mA	milliampere
mAs	milliampere second
mcg	microgram
MCV	mean cell volume
m.d.u.	use as directed
mg	milligram
ml	millilitre
mm	millimetre
mm	mucous membrane
NAD	no abnormalities detected
NPO	nil per os (nil by mouth)
NSAID	non-steroidal anti-inflammatory drug
NYD	not yet diagnosed
o.d.	every other day
p.c.	after food

PCV	packed cell volume
pd	polydipsic
pu	polyuric
q.d.s.	to be taken four times daily
q4h	every 4 hours
qid	four times a day
rbc	red blood cell
RCVS	Royal College of Veterinary Surgeons
RPA	radiation protection adviser
RPS	radiation protection superviser
RTA	road traffic accident
SC, s.c., s/c	subcutaneous
sid	once a day
sol.	solution
t.d.s.	to be taken three times daily
tid	three times a day
TPR	temperature, pulse and respiration
uid	once daily
v	volume
wbc	white blood cell
w/v	weight/volume (percentage of weight of drug per volume of solution)

Terms of description, position and direction

Figure 10.1 shows the common anatomy directions.

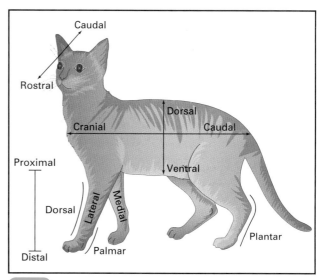

10.1   Anatomical directions and planes.

Abduct	Move a part of the body away from the midline
Acquired	Condition that develops due to external factors
Acute	Condition of sudden onset
Adduct	Move a part of the body towards the midline
Anterior	Relating to the front part of a limb or organ (not in common use)
Axis	Imaginary line through a part of the body about which the part moves
Bilateral	Relating to both sides of the body
Caudal	Relating to the tail end of the body

Chronic	Condition present for some time and with a slow onset
Congenital	Present at birth
Cranial	Relating to the head or front end of the body
Distal	Situated away from the midline of the body
Dorsal	Relating to, being near, or on the back
Inherited	Condition that arises from the genetic makeup of the individual
Lateral	Relating to a part of the body furthest from the midline
Medial	Relating to parts of the body nearest the median plane
Median	Situated in the plane that divides the body into a left and right half
Oral	Relating to the mouth
Palmar	Relating to the back of the front foot
Plantar	Relating to the back of the hind foot
Posterior	Situated at the rear of the body or organ

Primary	Condition that happens first, or that arises from changes within the body part affected and not elsewhere
Prognosis	An assessment of the outcome of a disease
Proximal	Situated close to the midline of the body
Rostral	Relating to the nose or front end of the head
Sternal	Relating to the sternum (the bone lying in the ventral midline of the thorax)
Superficial	On or near the surface
Unilateral	Affecting one side only
Ventral	Relating to the undersurface of the body

References and further reading

Lane D, Cooper B and Turner L (2007) *BSAVA Textbook of Veterinary Nursing, 4th edn.* BSAVA Publications, Gloucester

Lane D and Guthrie S (2004) *Dictionary of Veterinary Nursing.* Butterworth-Heincmann, Oxford

Index

Numbers in *italics* indicate figures; numbers in **bold** indicate boxes.

Index

Index

Index

Index

Skin
disease
in dogs 24, 25
signs of disease *111*
terminology 186
Sleep requirements in dogs 27
Snake bite 162
Snakes
anatomy and physiology 76
breeding 77
handling 77
feeding 76, 77
assisted *80*
sexing 77
Sneeze barriers **89**
Social Security (Claims and Payments) Regulations 1979
102
Socialization of puppies 19
Sodium (dietary) *131*
Soiled patients, bedding 93
Spaying
of bitches 22–3
of queens 43–4
Sprains 161
Standard sanitary operating procedures (SSOPs) 98–9
Standing order payments 171
Staphylococcus aureus, methicillin-resistant (MRSA)
101–2
Sterilization 96
Stings 162
Stock control 173
drugs 149–50
Storage 173
of drugs 149
Strains 161
Subcutaneous injection 143
Suffocation 156

Taenia 22
Tapeworms
in cats 43
in dogs 22
Taurine and cats 47, **128,** 130
Teamwork 11, 164
Techniques
artificial respiration *155*
bathing a dog 126
capillary refill time *110, 155*
CPR *155, 156*
cutting claws *128*
dealing with aggressive dog *118*
giving a tablet *141*
giving ear ointment *146*
giving eye drops/ointment *145*
handling a budgerigar *71*
handling a ferret *67*
handling a gerbil *65*
handling a guinea pig *60*
handling a lizard *78*
handling a mouse *63*
handling a rabbit *57*
handling a rat *62*
handling a snake *77*
handling a tortoise/turtle *79*
health check *109*
intramuscular injection *143*

intravenous injection *143, 144*
introducing dental hygiene *128*
lifting a cat *122*
lifting a dog *120, 153, 154*
physical examination *109*
recovery position *154*
respiration rate *110*
restraining a cat *122*
restraining a dog *120–1*
subcutaneous injection *143*
taking a pulse *110*
taking a temperature *110*
using electric clippers *126*
Teeth
brushing in dogs *26, 128*
in chinchillas 61
in ferrets 67
in guinea pigs 59
in rabbits 55
in rats 62
routine check in kittens *35*
Telephone calls
answering 167–8
making 168
Temperature *see* Body temperature
Tenesmus *116*
Terminology 176–88
Terrier Group *17*
Thirst, describing *116*
Thoracic wounds 159
Ticks on dogs 22
Toilet training for puppies 20
Topical drug administration 145
Tortoises *see* Chelonians
Toxocara canis 22
Toxoplasma 40
Training
classes for dogs 19, 20
dogs for handling 117–18
puppies 19, 20
Training Practices 9
Transdermal drug administration 145
Transporting injured animals 152–4
Triage 151–2, 154
Triclosan 101
Tourniquets 157
Toy Group *18*
Toys
for cats 40, 96
cleaning 98
for dogs 19
Tumours
in dogs 25
terminology 186

Ultraviolet light requirement for reptiles 76
Unconsciousness 158
Urinary system 180–1
Urination
describing *116*
increase/decrease *113*
rate in cats *110*
rate in dogs 24, *110*
Urine in rabbits 55
Utility Group *18*

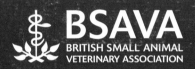

BSAVA

BRITISH SMALL ANIMAL VETERINARY ASSOCIATION

Veterinary Nursing: new edition
the best just got better

BSAVA Textbook of
Veterinary Nursing
4th edition
(formerly Jones's Animal Nursing)

Edited by Dick Lane,
Barbara Cooper and Lynn Turner

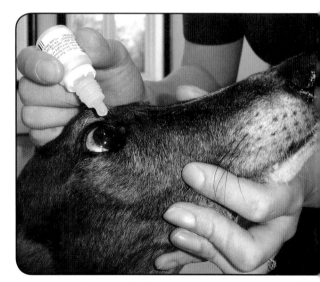

- Updated to reflect changes in RCVS syllabus
- Includes process and models of veterinary nursing
- Tinted tables and boxes highlight key areas
- Full colour photos and illustrations

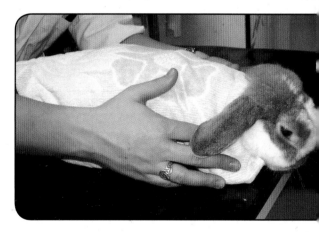

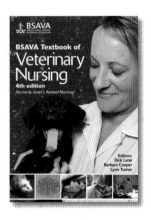

Price: £49

736 pages
ISBN-10 0 905214 89 7
ISBN-13 978 0 905214 89 4

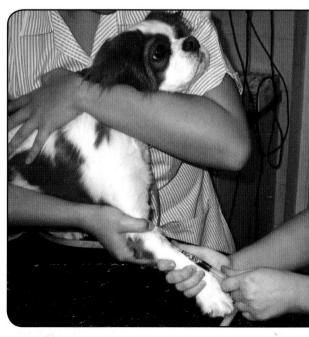

British Small Animal Veterinary Association
Woodrow House, 1 Telford Way, Waterwells Business Park,
Quedgeley, Gloucester GL2 2AB

Tel: 01452 726700
Fax: 01452 726701
Email: customerservices@bsava.com
Web: www.bsava.com